feel
fabulous
forever

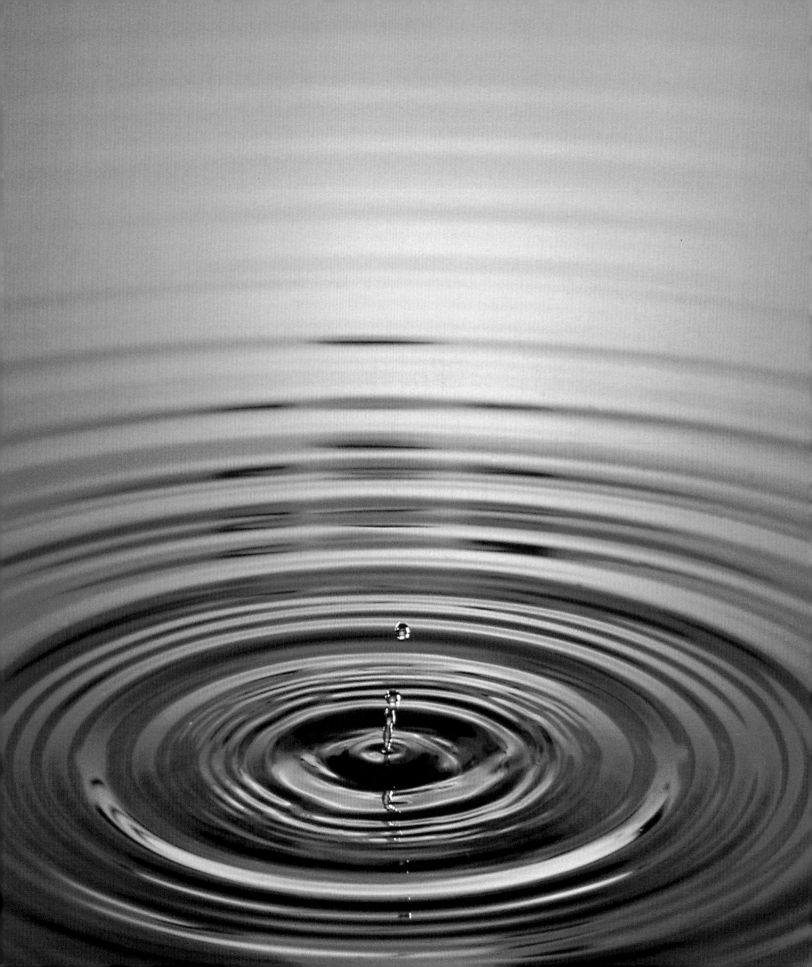

feel
fabulous
forever

THE ANTI-AGEING
HEALTH & BEAUTY BIBLE

JOSEPHINE FAIRLEY AND SARAH STACEY

KYLE CATHIE LIMITED

contents

part two: how to feel fabulous 154

part three: how to be fabulous 226

To forever fabulous (Great-Aunt) Doris Fairley and
(Great-Aunt) Florrie Rowe

Sarah dedicates her part of the book to her
beloved friend Steffie (Stephanie Tepper Cran)

First published in Great Britain in 1998 by Kyle Cathie Limited,
20 Vauxhall Bridge Road, London SW1V 2SA

ISBN 1 85626 285 5

A Cataloguing in Publication record for this title is available from the British Library

Book design by Button Design Co.
Edited by Susan Fleming
Picture research by Nadine Bazar
Proof reading by Beverley Cousins
Index by Alex Corrin
In-house Editorial by Kirsten Abbott
Production by Lorraine Baird
Colour reproduction by ChromaGraphics, Singapore
Printed and bound in UK by Butler & Tanner

a note to readers

The following symbols are used throughout this book:
£ denotes under £10, ££ denotes under £20 etc, * means this item features in the directory
and ** signifies that the experts' credentials are listed in the acknowledgements.

introduction

As health and beauty writers, there is one question we are asked constantly: 'How can I hold back the hands of time?' After writing *The Beauty Bible*, we were able to share some of our insights with friends, family and readers, and it became obvious that there was another book to be written.

As those of you who have read *The Beauty Bible* know, we are clear that beauty requires a two-way approach: what goes into your body and your mind matters just as much as – and, in the long term, more than – what goes on your skin, eyes, hair and nails. Like most women, we love make-up, skincare, fragrance, love the excitement of unwrapping a new product – but we're not always so thrilled with the effect – or lack of it… Our mad idea for *The Beauty Bible* was to test products – 9,000 in all – on panellists. It was the stuff of nightmares (we lived with packing cases for months) but for the first time, we were able to put our hands on our hearts and say 'we think these are the best products and here are our testers' reports'.

When we started researching this book – and had the crazy idea of repeating the Tried & Testeds – one thing kept coming back to us about a category which most women hurtling towards 'middle youth' really want to know about – anti-ageing miracle creams. Yes, the hype – and the hope – is a triumph of the marketing guys' ingenuity and imagination but the truth is that many of the miracle creams tested in *The Beauty Bible*, have notched up amazing scores and rave reviews, even from confirmed beauty cynics.

So we decided to take our research one stage further: to embark upon the biggest survey of anti-ageing products ever carried out, recruiting a panel of over 1,000 women to test state-of-the-art skincare in eight different categories. Our testers, who vary in age from late twenties to eighties, have just one thing in common: they care about their looks. Some were sceptics. Some true beauty-hounds. We divided them into groups of ten, with a spread of ages in each team. In the case of 'miracle' face creams, most of the products were blind-tested: nobody knew if theirs was the latest 'cult' cream – or a bargain brand. We asked them to try the creams on one side of their face, with their usual product on the other. (A challenge that most of them accepted – until the improvements became so obvious that they felt they had to start 'matching up' the other side…) Between them, our teams tested hundreds of different products across the categories – a monumental exercise compared to most magazine Tried & Testeds. (In which, usually, one product is given to one woman, another to someone else – just possibly the beauty department junior, whose only wrinkles are in her t-shirt…) We think you'll be amazed – as we were – by our intrepid panellists' reports…

But looking fabulous is about much, much more than slapping on a face cream. If you don't feel gorgeous inside, you won't look it outside. So we also set about talking to the experts in every field – from make-up to medicine, cosmetic surgery to sleep, haircolouring to hormones, nutrition to fitness, sexuality, and that intangible, but vital quality – peace of mind – to bring you their wisdom on ways to feel, look and be better than ever. And because we all need role models, we interviewed a series of 'inspiring women' – real-life examples of women who embody everything we have come to believe in. They aren't fresh-faced twentysomethings, but women in their forties, fifties, sixties – and way up; shining examples of glowing health, graceful looks and *joie de vivre* – who will, we hope, inspire you as much as they do us…

And by the way, just in case you're thinking 'well, it's all right for them (i.e. us) but what do they know about difficulties?', we just want to say that we do know a bit. Between us, we notch up over 90 years during which we, like most women, have been up and down on the emotional roller-coaster: come through the usual gamut of broken hearts, depression, redundancies, addiction and eating disorders, infertility and childlessness, the deaths of parents, friends, babies. What's more, we have produced two books together and we are still friends today – closer than ever.

We've given you all the health and beauty secrets we know in this book, but the ultimate secret is learning to love the real You: face, body – and soul. Then you will truly **feel fabulous forever**…

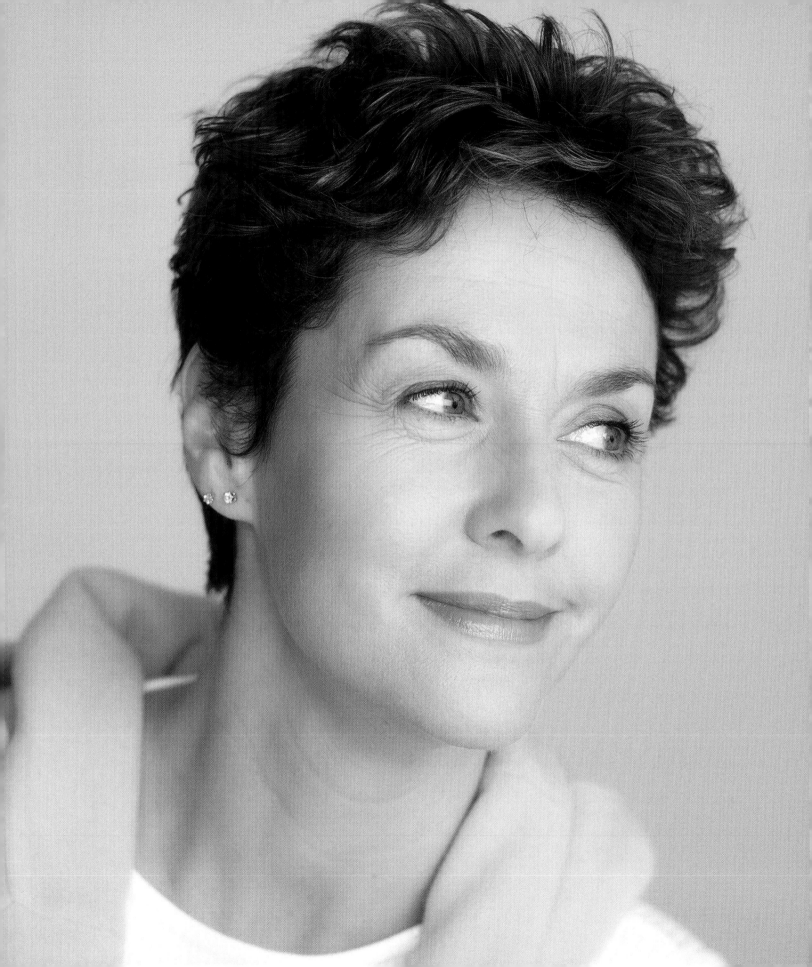

We can thank our lucky stars to have been born in the 20th century.

Once upon a time, wrinkles were an inevitable fact of life. Don't get us wrong:

some lines we love. The only way not to get laugh lines is never to laugh... But

today, we can all beam about the fact that skincare and make-up is up there

how to **look** fabulous

with rocket science, searching for ways to keep time at bay and even turn back

the clock. And – as our 1,000 women testers have discovered – some of it really

works. The dream of younger, fresher, smoother-looking skin has become reality.

So for the truth about ageing from the world's leading skin experts and make-up

artists – and the low-down on the 'miracle' products that make a difference

(whether you're into high-tech or ultra-natural) – **just turn the page...**

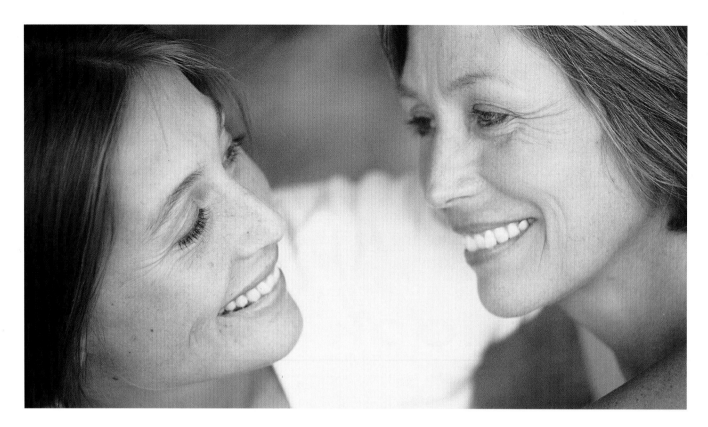

what happens to our skin as we age...

20s Skin is settling down after the hormonal upheaval of teenage years, although oil production may still be relatively high. Towards the end of their twenties, many women experience a gradual shift towards dryness – and notice the very first fan of fine lines around the eyes and mouth.

30s More fine lines develop as collagen and elastin start to break down in the skin and the delicate skin under the eyes begins to thin. The complexion tends to become drier, quicker. Broken veins may start to show up, as tiny red dots – and towards the end of this decade, age spots and brown pigmentation marks may start to appear. Pore size may increase and skin may become noticeably rougher and coarser due to sun damage. Under-eye puffiness can start to become a problem – taking increasingly longer to subside…

40s Deeper lines begin to etch around the mouth and eyes, as well as furrows on the forehead; skin loses more of its 'bounce-back' factor (due to a loss of elastin). Circles under the eyes may grow into pouches. Most women's skins become noticeably drier – although around menopause some women experience teenage-style complexion rebellion in the form of increased oiliness and breakouts. As the start of menopause sets in, skin may become more sensitive – and that may endure till menopause is completed.

50s, 60s and beyond... By now, skin starts to acquire true character: fine wrinkles and lines may deepen into folds in your fifties and sixties as, post-menopausally, there is much less oestrogen being produced. As well as wrinkling, skin can begin to sag and droop – and some women may notice a jowly appearance. In the fifties, skintone is likely to become increasingly uneven, with an increasing number of age- or 'sun-spots'.

how do we age?

According to experts, there are two kinds of skin ageing...

Intrinsic ageing This is the natural, biological ageing that occurs in the skin *without* sun damage – and we have little control over it. (Although a healthy diet, regular exercise, plenty of sleep and fresh air and tackling stress will certainly help.) All of the organs in our body – including skin – become intrinsically aged as the years tick by. Intrinsic ageing causes major changes in our complexions: at 80, for instance, our skin is 30 per cent less thick than at 18. In addition to the structural changes in the dermis and the epidermis, there are other changes that take place as we age: we sweat less as we get older, and there is decreased pigmentation – so older skin can be paler. There is also a loss of muscle tone and a relocation of the fat under the skin's surface, which accounts for the cheeks sinking in as they lose their padding, while little pockets of fat settle in the jowls.

Extrinsic ageing Extrinsic ageing, or photo-ageing, was until quite recently believed to be a fast-forwarding of intrinsic ageing. But differences between the two are now emerging. 'Without the damaging effects of the sun, intrinsic ageing only really starts to show from the age of 60 onwards,' says Dr Daniel Maes, Vice-President of Research and Development for Estée Lauder. But exposure to UV light and pollution speed up ageing, due to the production of free radicals on the surface of exposed skin, damaging the cells. Their attack on the collagen and elastin fibres results in a rough, dry skin texture, deep wrinkles, uneven pigmentation and broken veins. At the same time, new skin cells may be damaged as they form. By the time they get to the outside world, they're already weakened – leaving skin even more vulnerable to future external damage. A vicious circle that speeds up the wrinkling and crêpiness we *think* of as natural ageing – but which is mainly linked with our exposure to the sun, pollution and smoking...

don't fast-forward ageing...

How we age is dependent on two factors: lifestyle – and genes. If your parents aged well, then you will probably go on looking good for your age, too. But how we live – even where we live – can also have a major impact on how we age. Here's how some lifestyle factors can add years – decades, even – to our faces...

Sunbaking – add 20 years. (What more do we have to say?)

Regular solarium use – add 20 years. (According to an increasing body of dermatologists, sunbeds are even more damaging to skin than direct sunlight, because they give out pure UVA rays – which penetrate deep into the skin, causing damage.)

Stress – add 3 years. (A major skin savager, especially as the associated behavioural symptoms – excessive alcohol and caffeine consumption, missed sleep and skipped meals – have detrimental side-effects. Try to reduce stress by finding new ways to relax and slow down.)

Big city living – add 5 years. (Don't think the only solution is to move to the country – try a skin cream rich in antioxidants, instead, to mop up the damage.)

Crash dieting – add 10 years. (Yoyo dieting deprives skin of vital nutrients. If you lose weight quickly, your skin will stretch and sag.)

I've only ever had one wrinkle – and I'm sitting on it.

JEANNE CALMENT
(the world's oldest woman, before she died at the age of 122)

skin enemies – and how to fight them

Much of the damage these do is the result of free radical attack *(see opposite)*...

THE PROBLEMS

Alcohol Drinking alcohol dehydrates the skin and interferes with circulation, robbing skin of moisture and vital nutrients. It can contribute to broken veins *(see p.142)*, particularly over the nose and cheeks. Alcohol also depletes the body of vitamins and minerals essential for a healthy complexion.
The solution: cut down to a maximum of one or two glasses of *good* wine daily and ensure adequate intake of Essential Fatty Acids *(see p.195)*.

Pollution Smog, dirt and the sun's rays bombard skin every day. And according to Toby Mathias, MD, former Head of Occupational Dermatology at the US National Institute of Occupational Safety and Health, 'while there are strict regulations regarding the chemicals we breathe or ingest, little is done to restrict the toxins we touch and handle, or that skin comes into direct contact with.' Our skins are regularly assaulted by free radicals, triggered by everything from burning coal to household cleaning products.
The solution: creams featuring antioxidant ingredients can help neutralise the free radical damage triggered by smoking and chemicals.

Smoking Facialist Eve Lom – among many others – insists she can spot a smoker at fifty paces. 'Their skins are pallid, grey and lined,' she explains. 'Smokers in their forties have wrinkling and sagging in their faces comparable to non-smokers who are in their sixties.' In fact, the *Journal of the American Medical Association* refers to this condition as 'smoker's face'; it's characterised by deep lines around the corners of the mouth and vertical lines in the upper lip – from the repeated action of drawing on a cigarette – and deep lines around the eyes, from squinting through a fug of smoke. *(See p.66 – How to Win the War Against the Big Wrinkler.)*

The skin also has an obvious greyish cast and tired appearance – due to a lack of oxygen supply. This oxygen starvation leads to dehydration, dryness, pallor – and, of course, to wrinkles. As a person smokes, the toxic chemicals enter the body and stick to the skin – and around 4,000 chemical compounds are produced when tobacco burns. Other visible problems resulting from this can include staining, irritation, blackheads and even skin cancer.

The damage that smoking can do to the skin was clearly revealed in a recent study of identical twins where one smoked and the other didn't. Of the 25 twin sets studied at St. Thomas's Hospital in London, the smoking twin consistently had thinner skin than the non-smoking sibling – by as much as 40 per cent. Tobacco may wreak its havoc by constricting blood vessels, damaging gene repair or stimulating the release of enzymes that dissolve the skin's elastic components. Dr Tim Spector, Director of the Twin Research Unit at St. Thomas's, asserts that the chemicals in cigarettes put pressure on the body's metabolism, increasing production of damaging free radicals. 'With time, these speed up the ageing of the cells, breaking down collagen and elastin tissue in the skin. Blood supply to the top layer of the skin may also be restricted.'
The solution: as for other forms of pollution, creams featuring antioxidant ingredients can help neutralise the free radical damage triggered by smoking.

Sun The number one cause of skin damage is the sun. No wonder the face and hands are the first places to show signs of ageing; they are always exposed. Peter Pugliese, MD, a biomedical researcher who has been studying the skin's response to sunlight, believes that 90 per cent of the skin problems associated with ageing are the result of too much sun exposure. These include premature wrinkling, dry leathery skin, distended blood vessels, blotchy pigmentation, and skin cancer. Holiday sunbathing is not the only menace, however. It is constant *daily* exposure to UVA that ultimately leads to long-term damage. 'Research has shown that even as little as 30 minutes UV exposure twice a week during a typical London winter will result in long-lasting damage,' says Nicholas Lowe, Clinical Professor of Dermatology at UCLA.
The solution: daily application of a moisturiser featuring an SPF15, together with antioxidant ingredients that fight the free radical damage.

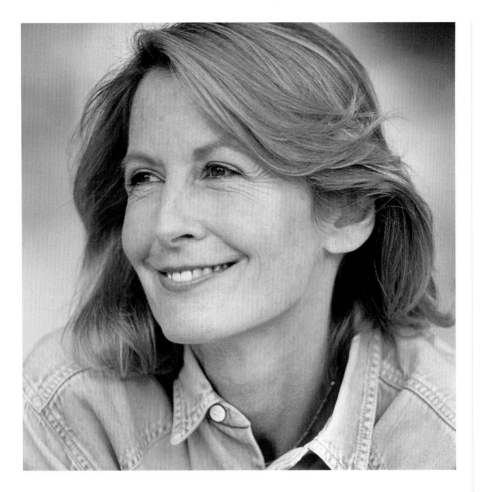

why antioxidants are your best friend

THE SOLUTIONS

There are a couple of words that you will encounter time and again throughout **feel fabulous forever**: free radicals. As far as ageing is concerned, they are Public Enemy No. 1. Our bodies create them naturally – particularly when exposed to sunlight or when we're stressed. Excessive exercise also sets off an avalanche of free radical production, due to an increased intake of oxygen. (Although we're talking running a marathon or mountain-biking up a fairly impressive peak, rather than a brisk daily walk.)

But in the course of modern life, we encounter many more free radicals – in smoke, toxins, chemicals and other pollutants in the air and in our food. What they do is trigger peroxidation – in less than the blink of an eye. (The skin generates free radicals in a millionth of a second if it's exposed to, say, cigarette smoke.) That peroxidation leads to oxidation – which in turn leads to cell breakdown. Cells, organs and tissues break down or decay, resulting in skin ageing and internal disease.

Like 'cellular terrorists', free radicals are highly unstable molecules which are deficient of a negative charge called an electron – so they rush around inside cells seeking that missing electron 'mate' in order to make them stable. During this process, however, they cause other molecules to become unstable – triggering a chain reaction that produces thousands more free radicals.

In the skin, free radicals attack the repair mechanisms, together with the DNA itself (the genetic material responsible for cell reproduction). Free radicals react with protein in the cell's collagen and lipid membrane, resulting in loss of elasticity, slackness, discoloration and wrinkles. The rate at which this damage shows up depends partly on how well skin can defend itself against these destructive free radicals. Young skin generally has sufficient enzymes and vitamins to enable it to neutralise free radicals. From as early as the mid-twenties, however, our natural defence mechanisms become depleted – particularly under emotional or physical stress, so the skin becomes unable to defend itself from attack, resulting in the visible signs of ageing.

The antidote? While the body manufactures some free radical neutralisers, science is still looking at ways of increasing that supply – and the best candidates so far are the antioxidant vitamins. For now, skin creams featuring antioxidants, eating a diet rich in vitamins A, C, E and also taking antioxidant supplements seems to be the wisest insurance policy, working to prevent (and even reverse) damage to the face and body. Which is why you'll be hearing a lot more about antioxidants throughout **feel fabulous forever…**

miracle creams

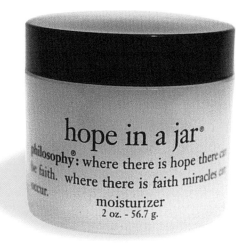

'The wrinkle is a serious disease. Do you know anyone who gets up every morning and worries about illness? But everybody worries regularly about wrinkles...'

LEADING US DERMATOLOGIST, DR ALBERT KLIGMAN

• **Statistic: American women between 30 and 50 spend over $1 billion a year on anti-wrinkle creams.**

As Dr Kligman observes above, millions of women all over the world are obsessed with their wrinkles. Eavesdrop on just about any group of fortysomething women at a glamorous party, or in the hairdresser, and you'll overhear gossip about *this* miracle cream or *that* magic line eraser. There's nothing wrong with that: psychologists have established that when we look better (or just think we do…), we feel better. So wrinkle patrol is about self-preservation in more ways than the obvious. But – crucially – women want to know what really works.

As we age, there are plenty of emotional and spiritual compensations for encroaching lines and wrinkles – wisdom, a more relaxed outlook on life, enrichment of our souls – but the simple truth is that most of us would like to delay the physical and *visible* signs of ageing for as long as possible. And we are prepared to spend billions in that quest.

In the search to satisfy us, the cosmetic companies have raised skincare research to the levels of rocket science – literally; one of the top-selling 'cult' creams in the US was developed by a former NASA scientist. But just consider this: if you're sending a rocket to Mars, you don't know what's out there, don't know whether you'll land successfully, what will happen when you arrive or whether you'll get back safely. Buying anti-ageing skincare is a similar journey into

the unknown – though few cosmetic companies would ever admit the uncertainties or limitations of their products. More practically for the consumers – i.e. all of us – the time and expense involved in finding the creams or lotions, serums or ampoules that really do improve our skins can be incredibly frustrating.

That's one reason we wrote this book – to share with you the secrets your best friend would tell you – if she knew… We cut through the hype, the myth, the blurb and the mystique – and also, for the first time, bring you first-hand experiences of the creams that really work: the results of the Tried & Tested surveys carried out especially for this book by 1,000 women, working in panels of ten, who tested literally hundreds of creams.

BIG BEAUTY, BIG BUSINESS

The beauty industry is mega-business. Every year, it spends billions on research. And to recoup that outlay, it has to earn back billions from the sales of the skin creams that emerge from its high-tech labs. Skincare companies are literally at war to ensure that their product sells the most. And dazzling the consumer (and the journalist) with science is currently their favourite marketing approach.

Before deciding to green-light a launch, many of the leading skincare companies, who already run vast labs of their own, also have prototype products tested independently. This results in stacks of scientific papers, complete with statistically significant figures purporting to show how effective the product is. Those glowing figures are destined for the press and are also widely used in marketing and ad campaigns. Time was when beauty journalists would pretty well reproduce the press release; now they are starting to ask tough(er) questions. So the companies wheel out not only scientific papers but real live scientists to talk about the products. (Although delve a little deeper and you'll often find they or their labs or their research projects have been enriched in some way by the cosmetic companies.)

There's nothing intrinsically wrong in all this. The scientists aren't making up their figures and the companies aren't inventing their claims – although we have discovered some what you might call 'imaginative' research methodology and definitely some embellished interpretations of the results. But the real point is that these results may have very little impact where it counts – on our skins.

Every year, we wade through literally reams of weighty results given to us by skincare companies claiming that their hot anti-ager-of-the-moment delivers a benefit such as '50 per cent reduction in wrinkle depth'. Taken at face value, you'd imagine that the cream made your wrinkles half as deep. But as leading cosmetic dermatologist and researcher Prof Nicholas Lowe explained to us, that's just not the case: 'Very often, the units for the measurement are so small that those changes may not even be visible to the naked eye.'

Furthermore, what the ads almost certainly *won't* tell you is what the women were – or weren't – using on their skin before they started applying the product in question. In some studies we've looked at, the answer is: nothing at all. (Skincare companies frequently ask women to cease using any moisturiser for two weeks or so leading up to the tests.) Now, if you put anything on the skin at that point – even verruca cream – you would instantly get a measurable improvement simply because of the emollient effect of the ointment.

But would you ever guess that from the 'oh-wow-hold-the-front-page!' way those results are presented? Uh-uh…

is it a face cream – or is it a drug?

That's not to say that space-age skincare doesn't work. The great paradox – as we know from our own and our 1,000 testers' experience – is that, as well as the results which are overstated, there are some extremely impressive products out there which actually undersell what they can achieve. Some of the effective high-tech skin creams may be more similar to drugs than cosmetics, penetrating the skin to bring about really noticeable changes.

According to the official definition of the Food and Drug Act of 1936, a drug is a substance that alters the structure or function of any part of the body. In the old days, the skin was seen very much as a one-way street. Today, scientists understand that a cream applied to the skin – or even the ingredients from a patch stuck on the surface – can penetrate deep inside. (This technology is being exploited by drug companies in the shape of skin patches or gels which deliver, for instance, HRT or nicotine.)

If a manufacturer claims that its product will give you a healthy glow, that product is regarded as a cosmetic. But if the packaging or the advertising were to state that the glow is achieved through, say, improved blood flow to the skin, the governments of both the UK and the US would require it to be tested – and then classified – as a drug.

'The game involves not what a product does, but what a company *says* it does,' according to Dr Albert Kligman. (He's the 'grand old man' of anti-ageing skincare, who coined the term 'cosmeceutical'.) If they made more extravagant claims, the products would have to be licensed as pharmaceutical drugs, not cosmetics – which would be prohibitively expensive and time-consuming. (It takes about a decade – and well over £10 million – to get a drug to market.) 'So companies are careful *not* to make any claims that would be considered drug claims,' says Dr Kligman. As a result, there are plenty of anti-ageing products out there that do more than they actually claim to…

now cut through the hype – and find out what really works...

It's because of all the confusion that we've taken a revolutionary approach to writing about anti-ageing creams. Yes, we've spoken to the world's leading experts in skincare. Yes, we've distilled several decades of personal experience to bring you what we consider to be common sense, bottom line advice on ageing. But more importantly than telling you that this or that particular skin cream is going to work wonders on your wrinkles because of its SOD-inhibitor or its mega-dose of phosophosphingolipids (yes, really), we recruited a group of 1,000 age-conscious women to try these anti-ageing products on your behalf. Here are the results...

TRIED & TESTED

BLIND-TESTED MIRACLE CREAMS

These were the skin creams (night and day), the serums, lotions and potions which scored highest of all in our toughest category: 'miracle' skincare. Expensive and cheap, natural and high-tech, well-known brands or lesser names: we called in products of all types and in all price-ranges – more than 100 in all – the most ambitious and wide-ranging survey of anti-ageing creams ever carried out. (We're sure nobody else would be crazy enough to start this!)

Each product was sent to ten women and tested until it was finished – a period of several weeks, usually months. We asked our panellists to use the products on one side of their face only, so they could see the difference. (Or not.) Fascinatingly, the results were sometimes so obvious after a few weeks that the testers felt they had to start 'matching' their complexion by using the cream on the other side, as well. 'I was worried I'd look odd,' said one tester.

Few reported overnight miracles; results were generally seen in anywhere from two weeks to two months. The results often out-performed our (educated) expectations - though it's worth noting that the lowest-scoring product in this category got just 4.12 marks.

We set out to blind-test every product – most products were packaged in anonymous, unmarked jars and bottles – with just a code to tell us who got what. However, in some instances, manufacturers told us that they were unable to supply us with unmarked packaging. So the testers of these products *did* know what they were using. We feel we had to create a separate category for these, as testers could have been influenced by packaging/brand and/or reputation.

So now – what 1,000 women really think about anti-ageing products...

Estée Lauder Advanced Night Repair
8.4 MARKS OUT OF 10 (£££)
This serum is designed to repair at night and to protect by day, with a very high dose of antioxidant ingredients. Used in the daytime – with or without a moisturiser over the top – several testers commented that it made an excellent base for foundation. Advanced Night Repair also features a calming cola nut extract and other anti-inflammatory ingredients 'to help reduce environmentally caused irritation and longer-term damage'. Several testers commented on improvements to the neck and all said they would buy it.
UPSIDE: 'a joy to use this product as I could see improvements after a couple of weeks; a little amount was needed so it went a long way' ◆ 'loved the way my face glowed and looked fresher; did not seem to make a difference to deeper lines, but smaller ones were improved' ◆ 'I think my skin looks more radiant, smoother and younger' ◆ 'I feel really I do look better: I'm more "ironed" on face and throat; after two months I started using it all over my face because the difference was too visible'.
DOWNSIDE: 'the smell could be enhanced a little' ◆ 'doesn't look or appear luxurious'.

Nina Ricci Time Defense Extract
8.4 MARKS OUT OF 10 (££££)
Nine out of ten testers said that they would buy this serum-style product. It is designed to have a 'firming', toning and oxygenating action, making skin smoother and more luminous – so it's targeted at skins that are dry, greyish, wrinkled or have lost tone; however you may need to follow with a moisturiser.
UPSIDE: 'fine lines over my top lip have gone and I would use it again for this reason alone' ◆ 'I know we were asked to use on one side only but when, after five weeks, my pores were closing and fine lines vanishing, I just had to use it all over' ◆ 'my partner thought my skin was glowing' ◆ 'people have commented that I look well, refreshed, brighter, rested' ◆ 'skin was soft and peachy and plumped up'.
DOWNSIDE: 'strange texture – sticky, almost like honey' ◆ 'it was very runny and didn't last as long as I would have expected or liked' ◆ 'I enjoyed using it but feel there have been no real, long-term benefits'.

Neal's Yard Frankincense Nourishing Cream
8.25 MARKS OUT OF 10 (£)
This natural, essential-oil based cream by one of the world's leading aromatherapy beauty companies contains nourishing oils of wheatgerm, jojoba. almond and apricot kernel, together with frankincense and myrrh – renowned for their regenerating and moisturising properties. A rich cream, it can be used at night or as a day make-up base. And although this natural product was one of the highest-scoring products we tested, it was also one of the most accessibly priced.
UPSIDE: 'the original feeling of plumpness has been replaced by a smooth uplift and youthful tightness to my features, yet skin still feels comfortable, has no dry patches or discomfort. Amazing; what happens when I stop using it?' ◆ 'Always felt my skin looked colourless and grey until I tested this product' ◆ 'after two weeks I felt able to go out without foundation – something I've never been able to do before' ◆ 'no adverse reactions – a pleasant surprise because my skin can be sensitive' ◆ 'very noticeable improvement in brightness and translucency – not as sluggish looking' ◆ 'I cannot over-emphasise the healthy and "strong" feeling of my skin afterwards'.
DOWNSIDE: 'took quite a lot of massaging into the skin before it was absorbed'.

Several testers were put off by the slightly medicinal smell of frankincense; others, however, liked it.

Guerlain Anti-Age 12M Time Responsive Care SPF8 (For Dry Skin and Very Dry Skin)
8.07 MARKS OUT OF 10 (£££)
Specifically designed to be used from the age of twentysomething plus, to retard signs of ageing before they even start – so we made a point of sending it to some of our younger panellists. It features caffeine(!), ceramides, vitamin A palmitate and a skin-brightening fruit enzyme complex.
UPSIDE: 'definite reduction in crêpiness around eyes' ◆ 'after 24 hours, skin looked luminous; after two weeks, it had evened out my skintone' ◆ 'fine lines were less noticeable because overall glow had improved' ◆ 'smelt divine, with a luxurious texture' ◆ 'everyone remarked how well I looked – even with the 'flu. I'm addicted' ◆ 'despite being sceptical I was totally converted; I've had loads of comments – is it a coincidence I've got three men interested in me?'
DOWNSIDE: 'nose did become a little red

and flaky' ◆ 'very greasy and it made my normal-to-dry skin look shiny'.

Vichy Lumiactiv
8 MARKS OUT OF 10 (££)
Created to protect the skin from damage – with UVA/UVB filters and antioxidants – and to rejuvenate with fruit extracts. Nearly all testers said they would buy this cream.
UPSIDE: 'skin definitely felt softer and plumper after 24 hours' ◆ 'immediate improvement in texture and brightness; skin definitely looks younger' ◆ 'good quality, light and fluffy, easy to apply and absorbs immediately. Totally hooked and would like to use it all over my body!' ◆ 'used it quite liberally on face, throat and upper chest but it still lasted a long time' ◆ 'fine lines on forehead and around mouth have reduced' ◆ 'my skin is quite sensitive but this cream is fine; left my skin looking radiant'.
DOWNSIDE: 'slightly drying; felt I needed extra moisturiser'.

Decleor Concentré Stimulant
8 MARKS OUT OF 10 (££££)
This aromatherapy-based facial oil features

cinnamon, clove, geranium and thyme essential oils in a jojoba/wheatgerm base, to improve firmness and elasticity. It is designed to be used morning and evening on devitalised or mature skin. Almost all of the testers were impressed enough to want to buy it in future.
UPSIDE: 'found the warmed oil very soothing and gentle to skin; easily absorbed and pleasanter than ordinary creams' ◆ 'lines much smoother and much less noticeable; I think ageing has been halted and rejuvenation begun. I received more compliments than I have in years, especially from the opposite sex!' ◆ 'after two weeks, skin was much brighter and younger-looking; after using the bottle, my skin looks brighter, with an amazing difference to the softness' ◆ 'crêpiness is improved; slight but definite reduction in fine lines and the grooves in my neck were definitely reduced. Tell me what it is – I want more!'
DOWNSIDE: 'getting the prescribed three drops of oil out of the bottle was difficult' ◆ 'the smell – and the fact it was an oil – was offputting' ◆ 'great for very dry skin but my beautician commented on blocked pores'.

For 'logistical' reasons (so the manufacturers told us), the following products were only supplied in the original branded packaging, so we couldn't include them in our strict blind-testing only survey. However, the comments were, as you can see, extremely positive – and, in fact, the highest scoring product of all fell into this category.

Clarins Extra Firming Night Cream
8.57 MARKS OUT OF 10 (££££)
Top-scoring cream of all those sent out but as Clarins were unable to supply product in unmarked jars, we felt testers could have been influenced by Clarins' excellent reputation – and, in fact, all of them said they would buy it. Available in versions for all skintypes or specifically dry skin; the recipe includes essential oils of ylang-ylang and cedarwood, micro-algae and wheat protein. It is hypo-allergenic. Several testers noticed obvious improvements in neck skin.
UPSIDE: 'skin was velvety to the touch when I woke each morning' ◆ 'I have an uneven skintone, scarred from adult chicken pox; people commented for the first time in ten years "your skin's better, isn't it?"' ◆ 'very effective tightener of sagging skin – might make me delay surgery!' ◆ 'skin certainly looks younger – my self-esteem is now much better. Thanks!' ◆ 'the smell is sensuous; I would not have believed that in two weeks I could see a difference or dare to venture out without foundation' ◆ 'my skin certainly felt soft and smooth and it's helped prevent those early-morning "face creases" when

your head's been in a fixed position on the pillow' ◆ 'my husband commented on how young I'm looking'.
DOWNSIDE: no negative comments at all.

Crème de la Mer Moisturising Lotion
8.1 MARKS OUT OF 10 (£££££+)
A lightweight version of the extremely costly cult cream which has caused a sensation in the US, with women joining waiting lists to get their hands on a jar. Is this a triumph of hype over performance? When we analysed results, this product scored deceptively well because of the appealing texture, lovely smell and the fact it makes a great make-up base – but the bottom line was: very little long-term improvement. Several testers did, however, report immediate brightness and softness.
UPSIDE: 'a lovely cream and really perfect for combination or sensitive skins; seemed to calm my skin down. I used the product on one side only and the difference was quite strong – smoother and healthier on the tested side' ◆ 'absorbs beautifully, ready for make-up' ◆ 'excellent; feels wonderful just after application but saw no long-term

changes' ◆ 'this cream was amazingly smooth and light; it had excellent moisturising results and absorbed well. My skin felt really soft and silky, and had slightly more glow – without redness'.
DOWNSIDE: 'no change in the long run, just on application' ◆ 'moisturising effect doesn't last a whole day in the particularly drying conditions of an office'.

Aveda Bio-Molecular Recovery Treatment
8 MARKS OUT OF 10 (£££)
This botanical, gel-like serum contains AHAs and BHAs plus antioxidants and essential oils. Two thirds would buy it.
UPSIDE: 'used on one side of my face, the results were so obvious I had to bring the other side in line; lines from mouth to chin have reduced in depth and my face and neck both look younger, softer' ◆ 'skin under eyes felt firmer' ◆ 'people have commented: "your skin's lovely – you can't be 60!"' ◆ 'crêpiness has improved, especially on the cheeks – slight improvement in bigger lines/grooves'.
DOWNSIDE: caused some tingling and redness; some panellists felt that gave a healthy glow; others saw it as a negative.

what is a serum? (and do they work?)

Today, serums – pumps or vials of potent but lightweight anti-ageing ingredients, often a cocktail of antioxidants or alpha-hydroxy acids – have joined the clutter on our bathroom shelves. Some are designed to be used every day, others when skin is in the doldrums, generating everything from fresh new skin cells to a burst of brightness. But should they be used instead of a moisturiser – or as well as? 'Serums are mostly designed to be used underneath a moisturiser,' John Gustafson of Dickins & Jones explains. 'They may not have enough moisturising ingredients to be used on their own.' Many of the top 'miracle' products that our testers tried were serums – and there is no question that they (and we) are impressed…

TRIED & TESTED

SERUMS

The best of the serum-type products our testers tried.

• **Estée Lauder Advanced Night Repair Protect Recovery Complex**
8.4 marks out of 10 (££££)
• **Nina Ricci Time Defense Extract**
8.4 marks out of 10 (££££)
• **Aveda Bio-Molecular Recovery Treatment**
8 marks out of 10 (£££)
• **Jurlique Herbal Extract Recovery Gel** (see p.48)
7.62 marks out of 10 (££££)

CULT CREAMS

Can any skin cream justify the price of a jacket? Is any mere moisturiser really worth adding your name to a list of 1,600 desperate women – the number at one time waitlisted at Saks Fifth Avenue (where Crème de la Mer is kept under lock and key) for a $155 2oz pot of this cult cream. (Its celebrity following includes **Cher** and **Sharon Stone** – although you can bet *they* didn't have to wait that long…)

The whisperings about favourite 'secret' fountains of youth have swelled into a transatlantic topic of animated conversation. New users flock to these obscure creams by word of mouth – because devotees swear that the product's performance is the cause of all the hype and the *real* reason for their devotion. It makes them hard to find – and frequently sold out. (Which is just the way the people who make them like it. They have no intention of mass marketing their creams or reducing lofty prices; half the appeal of these coveted creams is the thrill of the chase.) Creams with a 'cult' following include Karin Herzog's Vit-a-Kombi range (which one Manhattanite snaps up thirty jars at a time), La Prairie (from Switzerland), Estée Lauder Re-Nutriv Instant Firming Cream, Cellex-C (a vitamin C-based range from America), Kanebo Sensai EX La Crème – as well as Crème de la Mer.

Of course, all moisturisers are basically a mix of oil and water. So how *can* manufacturers justify the price tag – and/or making us wait? According to Lancôme's UK Managing Director Peter Bloxham, 'The quality of the ingredients is a major factor in differentiating between prestige and mass market brands. There are cheap liposomes and

expensive liposomes, cheap vitamins and expensive vitamins.' Estée Lauder's Dr Daniel Maes, who was given carte blanche to create Intensive Lifting Crème (Lauder's 'alternative to the scalpel') agrees. 'Usually, when I'm asked to create a new product, there's a strict budget. This time, I was told: "Do whatever you want." It meant I was able to use ingredients which are normally prohibitively expensive. In reality, the first product I created was a disaster – it was too active, so it was very irritating. So it had to be reworked…'

Adds Peter Bloxham, 'With a prestige brand, you're getting the level of investment in research and development which mass market brands don't match.' Vit-A-Kombi, for instance, was the creation of Nobel Institute epidemiologist Paul Herzog. Crème de la Mer, a rich, sea-kelp-based moisturiser, was developed by a brilliant aerospace physicist, Max Huber, as a treatment for his own face, which was severely burned while he was conducting chemical tests for NASA in the early 1960s. After the cream healed his scars, Huber began selling it on a very limited basis – and after he died, in 1991, Crème de la Mer was sold to Estée Lauder. Impressive stuff.

But before you make long-distance calls, wait months for your name to come to the top of a list or dip into your pension pan to pay for a cult cream, we thought we'd let you in on the secrets of what our testers thought of some of the world's most expensive – and elusive – creams. (NB We felt it was important to include *all* the results in the 'cult' category, even though some of them didn't score particularly high marks. You will see, too, that many had mixed reviews, with some women loving them, others not so keen.)

TRIED & TESTED
BLIND-TESTED CULT CREAMS

Crème de la Mer Moisturising Lotion
8.1 MARKS OUT OF 10 (£££££+)
For the testers' verdict on this, *see p.17.*

Kanebo EX La Crème
7.71 MARKS OUT OF 10 (£££££+)
Only a third of the testers said they would buy this, the most expensive skin cream in the world. (NB Perhaps tha's not surprising since Kanebo were a touch stingy with the amount they gave testers – only a teaspoonful according to one, which lasted a maximum of four days.) However, almost half saw an improvement within 24 hours.
UPSIDE: 'I loved this; it left my tired skin feeling softer and smoother' ◆ 'I would be very happy to use this always, especially as a night cream, but I wouldn't pay a miracle price for it' ◆ 'after three applications my skin looked more uniform in texture, as if I had foundation on – when I didn't'.
DOWNSIDE: 'tingling sensation when I first used the product' ◆ 'very thick and difficult to apply' ◆ 'triggered redness soon after application' ◆ 'very slight stinging that lasts a few seconds after application'.

Cellex-C Serum
7.12 MARKS OUT OF 10 (£££££+)
Very mixed reviews for this serum, which delivers an intense burst of vitamin C to the skin: some of the testers found it irritated their sensitive skins. Less than half the testers said they would buy this in future.
UPSIDE: 'at the end of the treatment period, the side of the face I'd used it on was a lot softer and the skin felt a lot firmer; fine lines were noticeably reduced and there was some reduction in bigger grooves' ◆ 'definitely makes skin look younger; many people have said how well I look. On application it leaves the skin taut and tacky but this disappears if I apply moisturiser; the results are excellent – my skin is smoother and brighter; crêpiness on my neck particularly reduced' ◆ 'my sensitive skin had no problems with this cream, which I think makes skin appear younger'.
DOWNSIDE: 'testing this made my skin prone to redness and produced no visible improvement on my face' ◆ 'it's astringent rather than nourishing and rather drastic for my sensitive, mature skin'.

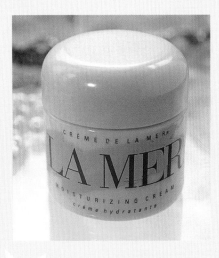

Estée Lauder Re-Nutriv Intensive Lifting Crème
7.1 MARKS OUT OF 10 (£££££+)
This is the top-of-the-line 'star' of Estée Lauder's Re-Nutriv range for mature skins, with AHAs (fruit acids) to improve skin texture, plus extracts of heather, lady thistle, vitamins C and E, milk peptides and grapeseed oil. Almost half the testers said they would buy this cream. And although it scored maximum points with several testers, the average was dramatically reduced by a tester who gave it just one mark, as she found it very drying.
UPSIDE: 'the morning after I first applied it, I looked like I'd had a really good night's sleep' ◆ 'this product really wins, for me, on reduction of crêpiness on the neck – usually a real problem zone' ◆ 'grooves above lips are less pronounced and blotchiness has evened out' ◆ 'it's probably very expensive but definitely did make my complexion younger-looking' ◆ 'skin softness much improved; I can leave make-up off when at home and not feel uncomfortable about my skin' ◆ 'I used this on my hands, too; after two months age spots had faded'.
DOWNSIDE: 'slight flakiness on forehead' ◆ 'a little rich to use under make-up' ◆ 'smell reminded me of some ointment I've used…'

Karin Herzog Vit-A-Kombi 1
6.4 MARKS OUT OF 10 (££££)
The low score for this 'skin oxygenating

cream' – created by the inventor of the iron lung – reflects the fact that while some testers gave it a rave ten, others only awarded it two points – because on its own, it was not sufficiently moisturising for very dry skin. However, it is claimed to balance both dry and oily skins, and so to be suitable for all skintypes.
UPSIDE: 'I feel my skin looks younger, and with prolonged use, the ageing process would be slowed' ◆ 'gives an immediate lifting effect' ◆ 'considerable reduction in fine lines' ◆ 'the glow has come back to my skin and it feels moist' ◆ 'skin looks younger, brighter and firmer, with an even skintone; sun spots faded slightly' ◆ 'within 24 hours I felt the side of my face I had used the cream on was plumper, but it was not really noticeable in the mirror' ◆ 'less obvious crêpiness on the side of my neck I used the cream on'.
DOWNSIDE: 'slight tingling but no irritation' ◆ 'smell reminds me of medicine' ◆ 'no good for my very dry skin, which needs a much richer moisturiser'.

Crème de la Mer
6.1 MARKS OUT OF 10 (£££££+)
Several testers scored this cult cream down, complaining it was complicated to apply: it is designed to be warmed in the palm, then patted into the skin, rather than smoothed on. This is a time-consuming challenge (although the cream does become more runny in hot weather and therefore easier to apply). Other testers felt the results justified the fuss, but less than half said they'd buy it – and two thought it was Nivea…
UPSIDE: 'a great reduction in the depth of frown lines' ◆ 'a definite reduction in bigger wrinkles and softening of fine lines' ◆ 'a big plus: I've used this cream on my cleavage and can't wait to wear low-cut necklines – it has really made a difference' ◆ 'skin looked healthy and glowing after four weeks; a brown mark on my forehead seems a lot lighter; crêpiness on my cheeks has almost gone' ◆ 'must I steal for this?'
DOWNSIDE: 'if the texture of this cream could be improved it would be the perfect anti-ageing product' ◆ 'I had a reaction – swelling and itchiness and it seemed to results in a lot of redness'.

you and your skin – what's really going on?

On a good day, it may look like the calm velvety surface of a bowl of cream, but the skin is a living, breathing, constantly changing organ. The largest we have, composed of billions of cells floating in a salty, watery liquid; half the water in our bodies – over 30 per cent – is found in our skin. Just like the rest of the body, bones and all, skin continuously renews itself. (Every day, we lose about 4 per cent of our total number of skin cells; about 30 lbs of skin in a lifetime.) The big question for older women is *why* skin ages. There are two main reasons: firstly, it simply doesn't renew itself as fast, and secondly, the support structure of collagen and elastin degenerates. Scientists are working on ways of overcoming the problems – but they're not quite there yet...

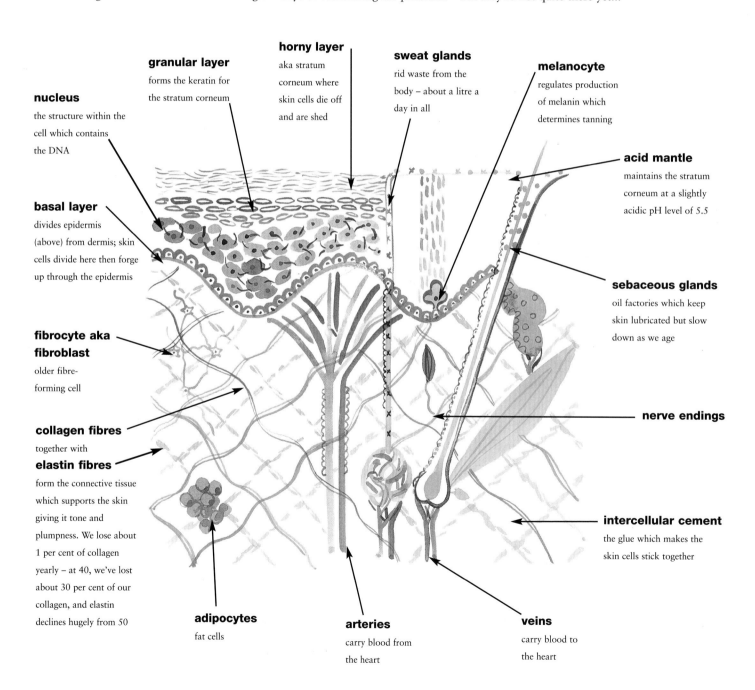

horny layer
aka stratum corneum where skin cells die off and are shed

granular layer
forms the keratin for the stratum corneum

sweat glands
rid waste from the body – about a litre a day in all

melanocyte
regulates production of melanin which determines tanning

nucleus
the structure within the cell which contains the DNA

acid mantle
maintains the stratum corneum at a slightly acidic pH level of 5.5

basal layer
divides epidermis (above) from dermis; skin cells divide here then forge up through the epidermis

sebaceous glands
oil factories which keep skin lubricated but slow down as we age

fibrocyte aka fibroblast
older fibre-forming cell

collagen fibres
together with
elastin fibres
form the connective tissue which supports the skin giving it tone and plumpness. We lose about 1 per cent of collagen yearly – at 40, we've lost about 30 per cent of our collagen, and elastin declines hugely from 50

nerve endings

intercellular cement
the glue which makes the skin cells stick together

adipocytes
fat cells

arteries
carry blood from the heart

veins
carry blood to the heart

SKINCARE – WHO USES WHAT...

Marie Helvin is a fan of Clarins skincare – as is actress and real estate magnate **Fiona Fullerton** whose favourite products are Multi-Active Day Cream, Extra-Firming Night Cream, Gentle Foaming Cleanser and Gentle Eye Make-up Remover. **Donatella Flick** uses cleansers by Estée Lauder, while model-and-rock-star-wife **Patti Hansen** likes Lancaster's anti-ageing Suractif range. **Debbie Harry** – 'Blondie' – is an Aveda addict, and **Donatella Versace** had to buy a whole new range of Aveda skincare because she'd given hers to **Madonna**. Rumour is that **Sally Field**, **Ann-Margret** and **Diahann Carroll** have all used Clinique's Turnaround Cream – and **Jane Asher** likes their bestselling Dramatically Different Moisturiser. Lovers of Decleor's aromatherapy-based skincare include **Shirley Bassey**, **Elaine Paige** and **Lady Lloyd Webber**. Bestselling novelist **Jackie Collins'** favourite is Shiseido Bio-Performance Advanced Super Revitalizer – 'it instantly vanishes on the skin'. **Princess Caroline of Monaco** and **Catherine Deneuve** love cosmetics from 'cult' Parisian beauty house Nuxe*; another 'cult' range attracting celebrity fans is Karin Herzog*: actress **Kate Capshaw** – aka Mrs Steven Spielberg and **Demi Moore** are said to love her oxygenating creams. **Oprah Winfrey** ordered Cellex-C* (a high vitamin C skin serum) from the 1-800 number in the States – as did **Shirley Maclaine**. (**Teri Garr** picked hers up in person at the Joseph Martin Salon in Beverly Hills.) And how does **Isabella Rossellini** get that glow? With a natural-bristled Japanese face brush that makes for ultra-gentle exfoliation...

skincare we love...

We get to try everything. For free. It's one of the perks of this job. (But not always great news for our touchy skins.) Here are the products that we can't live without...

Jo: 'The one skincare product I couldn't live without is Eve Lom's Cleansing Cream, which melts away make-up – an essential step for maintaining luminosity and clarity; two minutes spent cleansing and massaging my skin at night is a better investment than the most expensive cream in the world. Aside from that, I have an entire armoury of skin creams on the go at any one time: in summer, I swear by Estée Lauder's DayWear, a light-but-effective moisturiser with an SPF15, over Jurlique's Herbal Extract Recovery Gel – an antioxidant-rich serum. For winter I like Osmotics Blue Copper cream*, which is excellent under make-up and really improves translucency. I'm a fan of facial oils for my dry skin and use Aesop's Amazing Facial Oil* two or three nights a week; in the city I might use Jurlique Herbal Extract Recovery Gel underneath, as I think my skin needs all the antioxidants it can get. On other nights I slap on a truly blissful, rich (but very inexpensive) Orange Blossom and Rose cream by Verde*, a tiny aromatherapy company I'm very impressed by. I occasionally have bursts of using 'cult creams' Crème de la Mer and Estée Lauder Instant Lifting Cream. It sounds complicated to keep so many pots on the go at one time, but I truly believe in keeping my skin 'on its toes', not stuck in a skincare rut. My other big thing is that – with the exception of my eye zone – I really massage and move the skin around. I personally believe it's good for the circulation, and really doesn't contribute to wrinkling.'

Sarah: 'I'm fairly promiscuous with skincare – a bit of this and a bit of that, with the proviso that, because I have supersensitive skin and eyes that either sting or puff up at the slightest irritant, I dump the product immediately if I feel any tingling. Simpler formulations suit me best. Bioforce's Viola range of cleanser, toner, day and night creams* are a constant standby. I also like Aveda's All Sensitive Cleanser which I remove with a hot flannel. I do try to be scrupulous about cleansing – partly because it feels good. My moisturiser changes but I do like Clarins Extra-Firming Day Lotion, with a vital SPF15. I also use Lauder's DayWear. In summer, I often mix in a dollop of facial self-tanner with the moisturiser, which for me gives more even coverage than self-tanner alone or tinted moisturiser. At night, Osmotics Blue Copper seems to give a noticeable bloom and sinks in like a dream. Biochemist Dr Jurgen Klein, head of natural range Jurlique, advised me that women should use a serum rather than a cream at night to let the skin breathe. So I've been using Clarins Double Serum 38 with good results. Because your skin changes all the time, it's important to match products to what you need that day or night, climate or season. I put extra cream on my cheeks and forehead when they feel dry to the fingertips. Because I'm allergic I often get puffy eyes – ice cubes and the Green People's Eye Gel* are pretty effective. And I slather cream – of practically any sort – on my neck down my bosom.'

simple skincare shifts

Skin changes as we age. But many of us hang onto outdated beauty regimes because of habit, inertia or simply the lovely smell of a particular moisturiser. But our skin's needs change with the years – and we need to adapt with them.

The twin skin shifts linked with ageing are reduced sebum production (for all but a few very oily-skinned women) – so skin is no longer as well-lubricated – and thinning of the skin, which means moisture escapes more easily. Some women actually experience a surge in oiliness around menopause as hormonal changes kick in – but for the *majority* skin becomes progressively drier with the years. Changes to watch for are tightness, itching, dry patches, redness, flakiness, fine lines – or the fact that your make-up seems to be 'evaporating' after you've put it on.

It's vitally important not to get stuck in a skincare rut, believes John Gustafson** of Dickins & Jones. What worked for you at 20 almost certainly won't do the trick at 50. 'Every single time you go to replace a product, talk through your skincare routine and see if it needs an update. And personally,' he says, 'It's vital to change products when you get to the end of a jar or a tube, rather than simply sticking with what works. Otherwise, skin gets "lazy".'

Cleansing As oil production is slowed, an ultra-efficient cleanser may start to do its job *too* well, stripping away too much moisture. Most experts believe that around fortysomething, most women should leave soap – and even foaming cleansers – behind. 'Nobody over the age of 12 should be using soap on her face,' decrees Marcia Kilgore, of Manhattan's Bliss Spa. The age-appropriate choice is a richer lotion or cream formulation. Many of these can be rinsed away with water, so you needn't forgo that fresh feeling. (Avoid extremes of too-hot and icy cold water, however, as these can make skin more prone to spider veins.)

Cotton wool often leaves traces of cleanser behind so top facialist Eve Lom's prescription is a muslin washcloth dipped in hot water and used to remove cleanser; repeat the action three times. 'When skin is warmed, use the cloth to rub gently away at patches of flaky skin, especially in the folds of the nose and chin.' Eve believes this is also the only daily exfoliation your skin needs. *(See Exfoliation, right.)*

Toning Alcohol-based toners are a definite no-no. (You might as well use paint stripper on a mature skin.) For freshness, try rosewater or orange flower water, look for the words 'gentle' or 'alcohol-free' on skin fresheners or ask for a product which is alcohol-free and/or suitable for mature/ dry skins. Susan Harmsworth, of aromatherapy-based skincare line E'SPA, suggests facial spritzers in place of toner – but look for mists with essential oils or hydrating ingredients as well as water. (These are also terrific instant cool downs for hot flushes. Try keeping yours in the fridge.)

Exfoliation The idea behind exfoliation is to slough away the dead surface layers which make skin appear dull, revealing brighter, newer, 'younger' skin underneath. This is achieved in several ways: manually – using an exfoliant scrub or a washcloth – or chemically, with an enzyme-based or fruit-acid-based product, or a vitamin-A product like Retin-A or Retinova *(see pp.30–31)*.

But – a *big* but – exfoliation should be carried out very gently on mature skins. Our sensitive skins do not respond well to the *regular* use of AHA/fruit-acid based products.

cleansers – who uses what

Former Estée Lauder 'face' **Willow Bay** and early-rising US anchorwoman **Joan Lunden** swear by Lancôme's Efacils Gentle Eye Make-up Remover. According to her favourite make-up artist, Tricia Sawyer, **Sharon Stone** is totally hooked on Shiseido's Pure Cleansing Water. **Leslie Kenton** *(see pp.202–203)* has been using Eve Lom's Cleanser for more than fifteen years. 'It's totally different from other cleansers. It's more like an emulsified oil – it's amazing…' **Shirley Conran's** somewhat unusual alternative? Cooking oil. 'You don't need to spend money on products,' she insists. 'The secret is to be lavish with tissues.' (But because dressing-table aesthetics are still important, she decants her oil into Chanel bottles…)

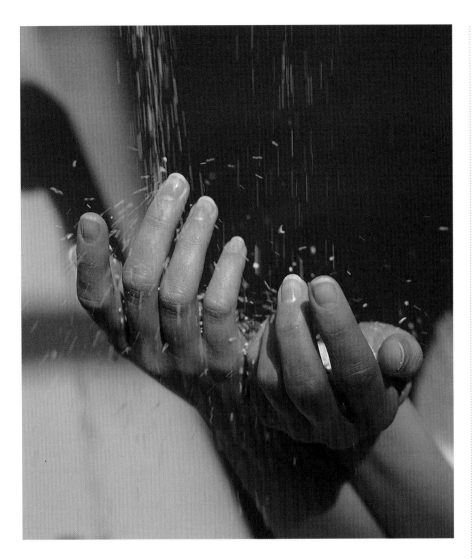

Although some of our testers (*see p.35*) were impressed, we strongly feel that those extra skin layers were put there for a very good reason – protection. As the skin becomes less able to retain moisture and keep out irritants, it makes no sense to turbo-charge the 'thinning' process, exposing skin to chemical and environmental assault.

We believe in Eve Lom's approach (*left*) but if you do use a manual exfoliant scrub, make absolutely sure that it has no sharp exfoliant particles – such as crushed nut kernels – which may literally scratch the skin.

Protection Undoubtedly your greatest ally in the war against wrinkles is strict daily use of a reflective sunscreen with SPF15 or more – often now found in moisturisers – to protect your skin and possibly reverse existing damage. (*More on sun p.26.*)

Antioxidants have also been found to offer protection against free radical damage and a moisturiser with an SPF15 *plus* antioxidant ingredients is now widely accepted as your skin's best insurance policy. (*Discover more about antioxidants on p.13.*)

Everyday treatments All moisturisers combine water with oil, using ingredients that mimic the skin's natural sebum. Many women are happy simply to use a moisturiser that tops up the skin's water level and creates an almost imperceptible barrier trapping moisture in, where it can plump up fine lines and prevent a papery, dry look. We prefer to combine moisture with protection (*as left*). Whatever you choose, the rule of thumb is that mature skins need frequent application of moisturiser, morning and night. Don't neglect your neck and your décolletage, use a special eye product for the eye zone, and *avoid* moisturising the folds of the nose, where an excess of moisturiser can contribute to the development of open pores. But when it comes to moisturiser, contrary to almost all our other advice: *more* is more, used sensibly. (*See p.159 for advice on night creams, and turn to p.49 for details of skin replenishing facial oils – of which we are both big fans.*)

Masks and special treats If your skin isn't too sensitive and you like the occasional skin-brightening, mood-soothing effect of pampering yourself with a face mask, go right ahead. The one *caveat:* choose moisturising masks, which don't set on the skin, rather than clay-based masks which dry out – and dry your skin out, too. Weekly or fortnightly is usually enough for most mature skins.

International socialite **Mouna Al-Ayoub** loves this Middle Eastern face mask recipe. 'Lemon and sugar are cooked at a high temperature, then cooled. Applied to the face and peeled off, it takes away all the dead skin cells and leaves your skin feeling soft.'

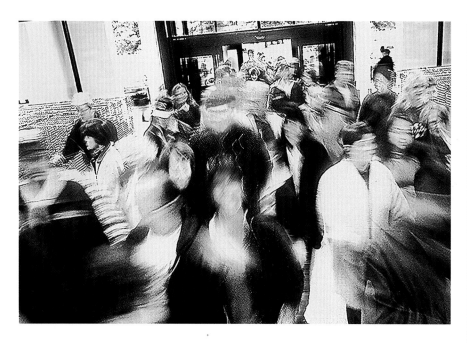

SHOPPING FOR SKINCARE

Our advice would be: don't buy a skin cream purely on the basis of a fancy graph. More important is to rely on your senses. Try the product before you buy it – on your hand, and preferably your face – to establish, firstly, how it feels on your skin and, secondly, whether it has the effect of making it feel and/or look smoother/softer/more hydrated. Trust your nose: do you like the fragrance? If possible, persuade the sales assistant to give you a sample so that you can try the product at home.

John Gustafson, of Dickins & Jones – who has completed the training programme of over 40 skincare companies – gave us this insight. 'Different companies have different policies on sampling anti-ageing products. When asked for samples, some companies have a strict policy: "Tell them that because it's a long-term product, a mere sample won't give them enough time to see a result." Certainly, I'd agree with that – but a sample is at least going to let them know if they like the texture, if they like the smell, or if they have a reaction to the product. So if a sales assistant says, "Oh, we don't give out samples of this product", say "Would you mind if I brought in a little container and you gave some to me?" Then if they start saying, "I'm sorry but it's not hygienic and the product won't keep well like that," reply that you're willing to take that risk if they are. I think it is significant that the real heavy-hitters in the beauty industry, the more expensive lines (such as La Prairie, Estée Lauder, Kanebo) are usually more than willing to sample their products – because they trust them implicitly. Yes, it is expensive to give out samples. But these companies are confident that if you use their product even for only two days a week for two weeks, you'll see sufficient results to want to come and buy them. And for the most part,' he concludes, 'you *will*...'

take it back!

You wouldn't think twice about taking a dress back if it fell apart after you'd worn it a couple of times. But most women never dream of returning a cosmetic that isn't working for them. Now, there are limits to what you can expect: you probably won't get very far in your quest for a refund if your complaint is that the skin cream which promised to work miracles in ten days hasn't made a blind bit of difference to your face. 'But if a beauty consultant has sold you a moisturiser which she told you would be adequate for your dry skin, for instance, and it's not, ask for a refund,' says John Gustafson. You should *definitely* ask for a refund, adds John, if a product triggered an adverse reaction, even a minor one. Another good reason to take skincare or make-up back is if packaging is difficult to open, or delivers a wastefully large splodge of expensive moisturiser from the nozzle, because it has been badly designed.

Remember, your comments also give valuable feedback to cosmetics companies and help them to meet the consumer's needs in future. Except for items such as safety-sealed fragrances, returned skincare purchases are usually sent back to their individual manufacturers, who reimburse the stores. (One less reason to hesitate). According to Juanita Doran, of Saks Fifth Avenue, 'this is often the only way companies get feedback from customers. A lot of problems, such as inconvenient dispensers or hard-to-open jars are caught this way. After a particular item has been returned a lot, I'll often see changes, like redesigned packaging, being shipped to stores six months down the line.'

can you mix and match products?

At some stage when you're skincare shopping, you can be sure that a beauty consultant may try to sweet-talk you into buying an entire, matching regime – complete with heart-stopping price tag – from the company she represents. Well, don't fall for it. With refreshing honesty, Christina Carlino – founder of the Philosophy cosmetics range – admits: 'I'm not a believer that you have to use everything from the same line. I'd love to say it was true, but it isn't anything we can prove or verify.'

Confirms John Gustafson, 'The reason people try to sell you the entire range is: that's their job. Most skincare lines do *not* work synergistically – that is, you won't get extra benefits from using the whole range together. Probably the best reason for buying products from one line is that you love the packaging.'

However, there are some products which definitely *don't* go together – and that's where the advice of a consultant may be extremely valuable. Advises John: 'You shouldn't buy an exfoliant product *and* an AHA/fruit acid cream, or you'll be stripping off too many layers of skin.' The motto is: when in doubt, ask questions. But be prepared to walk away empty-handed if the sales *spiel* whirrs into overdrive.

'It is very hard for women to get independent information,' acknowledges John. So his advice is this...

▷ 'I always say: if it starts sounding like a chemistry lesson, leave. What I want is someone who'll say, "Look, Mrs. Bloggins, if you take this product away now, by tomorrow you should find your skin is softer and smoother and by next week you'll find the fine lines are starting to soften." Practical, nitty-gritty explanations. What I don't want to hear is that it's an asymmetric carrier system with a time-release novasphere action.' The question you need to ask is: 'What am I going to see if I take your advice and buy the product?'

▷ 'If you're going in for a moisturiser, tell the consultant that – and ask her to help you choose the right one for your skintype. If they start trying to sell you a whole line of other things, be firm and say, "Today I just need a moisturiser, thanks."'

▷ 'Try to take the time to visit two or three counters and ask the same questions.'

▷ 'Another good idea is to ask whether any of the consultants are beauty therapists; many are, and they may sometimes have a deeper understanding of the products. If the answer is "yes", then say to the assistant serving you: "I don't mean to insult you, but would you mind if I spoke with them? I have some questions that may be a bit technical." She shouldn't find that at all offensive – and should trust their products enough to be able to do it.'

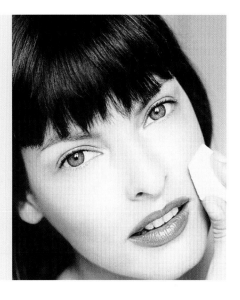

'Yardley face', supermodel **Linda Evangelista**, is in her early 30s – so really too young to qualify for this book. But she gave us a piece of skincare advice we find irresistible. 'I have a "wardrobe" of moisturisers,' Linda told us. 'In the morning, I don't just do things on automatic pilot: I really look at my skin, touch it, analyse what it needs. If I've been travelling or in the sun, I probably use a richer moisturiser. If I'm going to be outdoors working, slather on a high-protection sunscreen. But some days my skin doesn't seem so "needy" – so I'll just use a lighter moisturiser.' Our experience is that skin *does* change – not just with the seasons, but from day to day and week to week, due to diet and hormonal cycles. And it pays to tune into your complexion – and give it what it really needs...

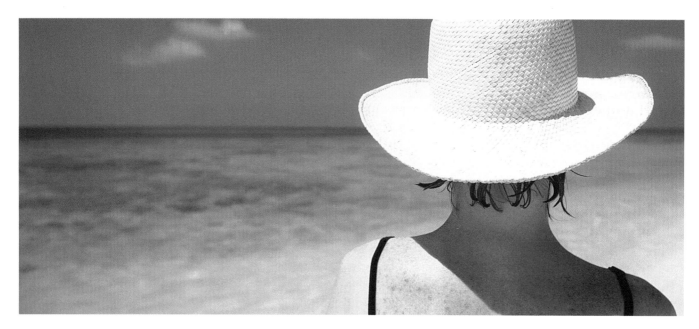

safe sun

When it comes to the links between suncare, skin cancer and ageing, there's so much confusion and misinformation that it's tempting to bury our heads in the sand. (While leaving the rest of the body to fry.) But in the war against skin ageing, sun protection is our greatest ally – and it's never too late to start.

According to Dr Anthony Quinn**, 'There is some evidence that you can actually reverse some of the damage sun does, even in later life. When patients in Australia with what's called actinic keratoses – pre-cancerous skin lesions – started to use effective sun protection, those lesions were reduced, even at a relatively late stage.' And although to date there is little statistical proof backing up the idea that fine lines and wrinkling will also slightly diminish if you religiously slather on Sun Protection Factors, the cosmetic industry is working hard to come up with data that will confirm that belief.

But isn't only Fear Of Wrinkles that should make us slip on a t-shirt, slap on a hat and slop on sun protection. Skin cancer statistics are soaring; over 30,000 people in the UK develop the disease every year; in the US, by the year 2000, according to Professor Elaine Rankin**, one in 90 people will get malignant melanoma – the potentially deadly form of skin cancer. (Which is why it's so important to report absolutely any changes in moles to your doctor.)

Sun protection is our best insurance policy against this. But since there has been a lot of publicity about the fact that malignant melanoma is linked with childhood exposure, many women throw caution to the sea breeze and go on tanning. But as Dr Quinn explains, 'Other non-melanoma forms of skin cancer are linked with cumulative exposure – so that's a very good reason to practise a lifetime of sun avoidance, rather than lie back and say, "Oh, well, the damage is done, I might as well go on spit-roasting." It's *never* too late.'

The minimum daily protection you should be wearing is Sun Protection Factor (SPF) 15 – on face and body. For our experts, this is the 'magic' number. The higher numbers can actually be misleading, they say, because above SPF15, the numbers aren't truly representative; in fact, they are only a *little* more powerful than SPF15.

Get in the habit of wearing an SPF15 on your face, year-round. There are many excellent day creams on the market that now have built-in SPF15. Choose your daily moisturiser from one of these.

Wear an SPF on your lips, too.
The lower lip is ultra-vulnerable to skin cancer, so lip sunscreen is a must.

When shopping for sunscreen, always look for 'broad spectrum UVA/UVB' protection.
Sunshine has different kinds of ultra-violet radiation: UVA and UVB. UVA is linked with the *ageing* effect of the sun and UVB leads to *burning*. It is vitally important to have protection from both kinds of rays. UVB protection is standard; effective UVA protection still isn't.

Look for an SPF based on reflective ingredients, rather than chemical sunscreens.
According to Dr Quinn, 'There are two kinds of sunblock available. One is *reflective* – also known as a *physical* block, with minerals which bounce back UV light before it hits your skin. The other type is a *chemical* sunscreen, which works by absorbing the UV light on the skin's surface. If you have sensitive skin, reflective blocks may be better because the chemical kind can trigger sensitivity when they interact with the sun. A lot of people who think they have heat rash are actually allergic to their sunscreen.'

Apply sunscreen before you go to the beach or sightseeing.
This is particularly important if you are pale or freckled. If you leave putting your sunscreen on until you've set up on the beach, for instance, you may already have been exposed for long enough to get sunburn.

Slap it on.
The key is to apply it liberally – an ounce is needed to cover the whole adult body – and *not* to rub it in too hard, because you lose some of the protection.

If you are on the beach, reapply your sun protection frequently.
If you're wearing sun protection on your face, probably under make-up, and exposing your skin only briefly throughout the day, then you don't need to reapply. But as soon as you are likely to be in the sun for longer periods of time, you *must* reapply sunscreen frequently. This is because the sun itself breaks down the protective ingredients in the cream – reducing its effectiveness.

Practise a lifestyle of sun avoidance.
'A sunscreen is useful – but it's only part of the picture,' advises Professor Rankin. 'Think like the Latin people. Avoid strong sunshine in the middle of the day, use your head – and put a hat on it! Wear an SPF15 – and never just lie in the sun.' Adds Dr Quinn: 'In theory, an SPF15 allows you to stay out in the sun fifteen times longer without burning than you could if you left your skin unprotected. But, says Dr Quinn, 'my advice is to head for the shade *long* before that.' If you do reach your "limit", you have to come out of the sun, or risk a real burn – unless you are naturally very dark-skinned. You *cannot* slap on more sunscreen and get extra protection.

Avoid sunbeds.
According to Dr Quinn, 'We don't yet have concrete evidence that sunbeds cause skin cancer – because we just don't know the long-term effects of large doses of UVA exposure, which is what these beds give you. But there is an impression – from skin cancer patients – that there may be a link.'

A fake tan gives no protection.
Although some fake tanners claim to offer a (low) level of sun protection, this is very short-lived. 'You must still remember to wear SPF15 *whenever* you go outdoors,' says Dr Quinn.

Remember: there is no such thing as a safe tan.

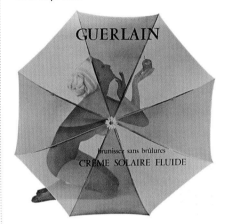

SUNCARE – WHO USES WHAT...

Famous faces know to protect them. So fans of Chanel's glamorously packaged, only-available-in-the-US suncare line include **Sharon Stone** and **Geena Davis**, who target vulnerable areas with Chanel Protection Instant Spot Protector. (For after-sun, Fredric Brandt – a dermatologist who's treated **Cher** and **Madonna** – suggests Clarins After Sun Skin Conditioner to his patients.) **Faye Dunaway** protects her skin with a minimum of SPF30 sunscreen. And **Barbara Daly**, OBE, who gets to see celebrity skins up close (so she sees just what sun exposure can do to them) insists on Lancôme and Clarins sunscreens, with an SPF25. 'From the first day of April to the last day of September, I won't set foot outside without a sunscreen,' Barbara says.

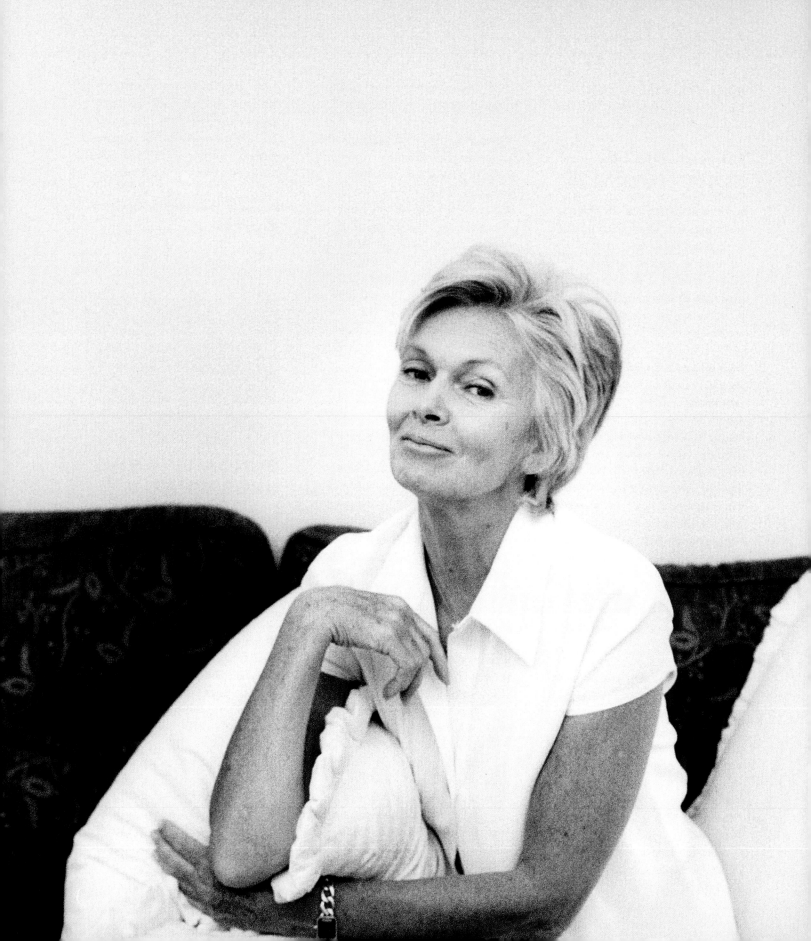

Bernadette Rendall

We are inspired by Bernadette Rendall – the hard-working, fabulous, fiftysomething PR for Chanel – because of her sparkling charm and pure French chic. (Not to mention the fact that she'll happily and unselfconsciously face the world – never mind the postman – without make-up.) Like so many Frenchwomen – in whom beauty and elegance are schooled from an early age – Bernadette learned from her mother the secrets of everlasting beauty and effortless elegance. And now, in turn, she is an inspiration to her three grown-up children...

'I love what Mademoiselle Chanel said about beauty, which is that it must start with the heart and soul, otherwise cosmetics are wasted. My mother taught me about beauty care until it became as natural as brushing my teeth. I would sit and watch her; from a very young age she had me using cleansing milk instead of soap, as I have a fragile skin, and encouraged me to use moisturiser. One of the big lessons she instilled in me was to treat my skin very gently and never to pull. Today I use Chanel Douceur Lactée cleansing milk and Hydra-Sérum moisturiser, but I have two sisters in Paris who are always trying to get me to try things. So for a nourishing cream, I use Pier Augé creams and a German brand called Biodraga; they are very rich and well suited to my dry skin. But I don't mind about laugh lines; I have always laughed and made jokes and I am perfectly happy if my face tells that to the world.

'My neck is my real obsession, and I moisturise it whenever I can. It's the one thing I don't like about getting older; other than that I am very comfortable in my skin. There's not much you can do about necks. I have seen women who've had them "fixed" surgically and it doesn't really work. I haven't had cosmetic surgery because I'm frankly frightened of it. So it's creams, instead. But I don't feel the need to wear make-up. Maybe a little powder and eyeliner and lipstick if I'm having my photo taken. For me, a white shirt is better than any make-up for what it does for my face. I like pearls for the same reason: they literally light the face. And I don't wear black any more because I find it drains my complexion; I think that's true for many women of a certain age. Navy blue is much softer.

'My big regret is spending so much time in the sun. For about ten years I lived in the Far East and as I tan easily, I'd be out there on a boat with nothing to protect my skin but a dab of sun cream on my nose. Today I wear a sunscreen of at least SPF25 and am always telling my daughter to be ultra-careful about going in the sun.

'Frenchwomen are brought up to be quite disciplined. My mother was naturally slim and I've inherited those genes, but I am still very careful with what I eat. My mother was divine, but strict – and it was the best thing that could have happened. As children, my sisters and I were always impeccably dressed; she was hot on manners and the way we sat, spoke – and ate. We had to have cheese for calcium and fruit for vitamin C. And whether or not you like it at the time, it establishes good habits that last a lifetime. I try to remember what Maman said about eating fruit and cheese every day, and I am very careful about fat. I certainly never drink a drop of alcohol if I'm on my own, or eat cake or chocolates unless it's a special occasion.

'My big thing is walking; I get off the bus early or walk to meetings and take the stairs instead of the lift: ten minutes here and there soon adds up. I wear flat Chanel pumps so I don't have an excuse for a taxi – and they mean I can walk *fast*. Because I have started to feel my back lately, I have started to do gentle tummy-strengthening curl-ups, to strengthen the middle area.

'What I love about growing older is that I am so much wiser. I know I don't look thirty any more, but I still feel it inside. I am still enthusiastic and mad, can jump up and down and be crazy, but I am much calmer in my decision-making and the way I judge people – more peaceful altogether. You trade a little elasticity in your face for a lot of calm and wisdom.'

drugs for your face

Women now have another choice in anti-ageing skincare, as dermatologists start to prescribe potent creams to hold back time...

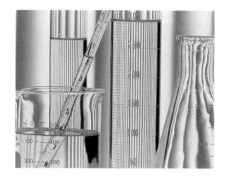

RETIN-A

A decade ago, news broke that a cream designed for treating acne could alleviate the fine lines and rough texture of sun-damaged skin. Derived from vitamin A, Retin-A (aka tretinoin) catapulted us into the age of the cosmeceutical, when changes brought about by skincare are more than short-lived plumping of fine lines with mixtures of oil and water.

Retin-A still only has a licence as an anti-acne cream – but that doesn't stop dermatologists prescribing it for wrinkles if they believe it would be effective, so long as they don't *promote* the drug for this unapproved use. (In other words, you won't get clinics advertising that they prescribe Retin-A for anti-ageing.) Many doctors – and patients – believe the cream makes wrinkles less obvious; it may also reduce the appearance of age spots.

But there's a flipside: irritation. In the most publicised research project on Retin-A to date, at the University of Michigan, in the US, more than nine out of ten patients developed serious enough skin irritation to warrant withholding the cream from them for a few days. In the end, three of the forty patients in the trial found the irritating side-effects so intolerable they withdrew from treatment altogether. (And it's worth noting: some patients using Retin-A for acne stop because

they find breakouts preferable to the side-effects of the drug.)

Irritation is especially high during the first two weeks of treatment, when redness, itching, slight burning and scaling are common. Because skin is thinned, water loss may be speeded up – and it may be easier for irritants to enter the skin, creating reactions to products that the complexion got along just fine with in the past.

Because Retin-A causes a gradual thinning of the top layer of the skin, it allows greater penetration of UV light; some of the vital protective layers are no longer there to do their job. So everyone who is given Retin-A should also be warned to wear a sunscreen *at all times* and never to expose her face to the sun. And the bottom line is that anyone wanting to maintain the benefits will have to go on using the cream for life.

So would *we* put it anywhere near our faces? We would not...

what Retin-A did for me

AGE: 58
PROFESSION: HOUSEWIFE

'I read about Retin-A about eight years ago when it was hailed as a potential new "wonder treatment" for wrinkles. Like most women my age, I grew up

not realising the dangers of lying in the sun, and though people generally think I look good for my age, I do have some wrinkles and crêpiness that are entirely down to sun-worship. So when I read about Retin-A, I was off to my doctor like lightning. He offered to write a private prescription – then sent me off into the wide blue yonder. I certainly didn't get any instructions about how to use it, or any side-effects.

'The cream was to be used at night, with a small quantity patted into the skin; I went home and slapped it on, expecting to wake up looking wonderful. But I soon realised that it was too strong to use every night, since it was making my face look quite red – like I'd been out in the sun; it was also itchy and irritated, so I cut down to every other night instead.

'Within a couple of months, my skin did look a little smoother and slightly "plumped up" – but the effects weren't very dramatic. I persevered for a while and then decided that Retin-A was no better and no worse than other expensive skin creams, and gave up using it on a regular basis. I still occasionally use it for a mini-treatment – if I want my skin to look brighter for a special event – but wasn't convinced enough to go on using it on a regular basis. On balance, my experience is that you have to treat Retin-A with caution.'

RETINOVA/ RENOVA

Although Retin-A has never been officially sanctioned in the war against wrinkles, a younger cousin – Retinova (known as Renova) created headlines as 'The First FDA-Approved Fountain of Youth', when the US Food and Drug Administration sanctioned it for use to reverse the effects of sun damage. Suddenly, even the government was saying there really is hope in a jar. So Retinova is now promoted with glossy literature extolling its anti-ageing virtues. Some of these, to our amusement, feature totally identical pictures of the same women. In one, we could clearly see that her wrinkles had been air-brushed out by photographic techniques, rather than high-tech skincare.

Renova contains the same active ingredient, a derivative of vitamin A, but in a more cosmetic-like, moisturising base. The most recent studies into Renova – funded by the manufacturers, Ortho Pharmaceuticals – have documented an improvement in the appearance of fine wrinkles, mottled pigmentation and roughness in 42–63 per cent of the test subjects who used the cream for six months. After 12 months, two-thirds of the test subjects whose skin responded to Retinova were able to maintain their skin improvements when they switched from daily to weekly applications. But that means weekly *forever*, unless you want to get back all your original lines, mottling and sallow skin.

The irritation level is said to be 'moderate', with potential for mild redness, itching and scaling, as with Retin-A. Retinova also increases the skin's vulnerability to the sun, so those who are using it should become wedded to sunscreen and wear hats on sunny days. Be aware, too, that among women of colour, both Retinova and Retin-A may cause dispigmentation (lightening, mottling or darkening of the skin). It is extremely important to follow the instructions, use only the prescribed dose – and to follow the sensible rules laid out here. And once again, we wouldn't dream of putting this very new drug anywhere near our sensitive skins.

what retinova did for me

AGE: 46
PROFESSION: MANAGER FOR HAIR SALON GROUP

'I suppose, over my lifetime, I've had an average amount of sun exposure and I was beginning to notice lines and wrinkles. So about four years ago, I went on Retinova. I was prescribed it by a doctor in a cosmetic surgery clinic. He was very careful to make

how to use Retin-A

If you do decide to opt for Retin-A or Retinova, it is very, very important that you use it in the correct way to minimise adverse reactions such as excessive redness, flaking and irritation. As Dr Patricia Wexler, leading Manhattan dermatologist, told us: 'Just because a little Retin-A/Retinova may be a good thing, a lot is definitely not better.' However, we have heard many, many instances of women walking out of a doctor's surgery with a Retin-A prescription – and not a word of advice about how it should be used and how to incorporate it into a skincare regime. So here are the rules:

• Ask your doctor where you should apply it: face/arms/neck/eyelids (upper and lower) hands/chest. Apply only where he/she tells you.

• Do not get the cream into the eyes; if you do, rinse with running water and wash hands.

• Always test a small area with the cream first; if it stings excessively or itches, contact your doctor.

• Use a sunscreen every day with an SPF (Sun Protection Factor) of 15. The sunscreen should ideally have a three (***) or four (****) star UVA rating. Every morning after washing or showering, apply the sunscreen to the sun-exposed skin of the face, neck and hands. In the summer, on outdoor days, or snow-skiing in the winter, use a waterproof sunscreen with an SPF25–30. The sunscreen should have a three (***) or four (****) star UVA rating. (Dr Nicholas Lowe suggests sunscreens by Ambre Solaire, Neutrogena, Nivea, Piz Buin, Soltan or Uvistat.)

NB Retin-A is not recommended for pregnant women because of a risk that vitamin A derivatives *may* cause birth defects; it should also be avoided by women who are breast-feeding.

sure that I knew exactly how much to use, and from that moment on I couldn't put my face in the sun except with a high SPF. Now I never venture outside without an SPF30.

'I was told that some people can expect mild side-effects – in my case, what felt like dozens and dozens of horrible tiny little spots under the surface of the skin, over the first few weeks of the treatment. You could hardly see them – but I could feel them. Apart from that, there was no redness or itching. I never really got to the point where I thought, "something's happening" – but I would say now that my skin isn't ageing at the same rate as people around me, and I'm sure that's down to the Retinova.

'I used the prescribed amount of cream – a pea-sized dollop – every other night, building up to every night after about a month; you use it instead of a night cream, because it's quite emollient. I stuck with that regime for about a year and then, when I felt I'd achieved the maximum benefits, cut back to a maintenance programme of two or three times a week. More isn't necessarily better.

'The real difference to my skin was that in the past I'd always felt I needed to wear foundation. After about a year on Retinova, I got to the point where I felt confident enough with my skin to go bare-faced: there was a new clarity and a kind of glow, as well as being smoother. It wasn't a massive, overnight improvement; it was very, very gradual – and nothing to make me go, "Golly, that's amazing". But I'm very happy with my skin and I've recommended Retinova to girlfriends. I don't think it's turned the clock back – but I'm fairly sure it's stopped it ticking forwards...'

(NON-PRESCRIPTION) VITAMIN A...

Recently, the skincare companies have been turning to other vitamin-A-derived ingredients and using them in anti-ageing formulations. These vitamin A derivatives – confusingly and variously called retinol or retinyls (such as retinyl palmitate and retinyl linoleate) – have gained popularity because it's thought they work like Retinova and Retin-A, without the irritation. And we anticipate much more widespread use of retinol and retinyls in future anti-ageing skincare. When asked for their predictions about which were the 'most promising' skincare ingredients that we are likely to see more of, several leading dermatologists pointed to these vitamin A derivatives – 'spot-targeted' at specific problems, such as reversing 'sun spots' or reducing fine lines and wrinkles around the eye zone. (For now, however, retinols and retinyls are the skincare equivalent of using a machine gun to aim at a bullseye.)

VITAMIN C

There are two possible reasons for putting vitamin C on your skin: protection and treatment. As an antioxidant, vitamin C applied to the skin can help protect it, neutralising some of the damage done by free radicals caused by UV exposure and pollution.

But much higher concentrations of vitamin C – up to 10 per cent – are also being squeezed into skincare. Dermatologists now believe that these larger, 'therapeutic' doses of topical vitamin C (L-Ascorbic acid, ascorbyl palmitate or magnesium ascorbyl phosphate) can help repair skin and encourage collagen growth and repair – thereby increasing skin firmness and helping to smooth out fine lines and wrinkles. In addition, vitamin C has been reported to inhibit our bodies' production of melanin – the stuff that products not only a tan, but also freckles and sun spots. In the US, some doctors are also prescribing vitamin C after laser surgery, to quicken recovery.

You will probably never see – with a naked eye – any improvements to your skin from using creams which merely feature small doses of vitamin C as an antioxidant; they're just designed to prevent future damage. (See A-C-E Protection, opposite.) But even as a treatment, in high concentrations, don't expect overnight miracles; Jeffrey Rapaport, MD – a Fort Lee, New Jersey dermatologist – says 'Vitamin C isn't a quick fix. It's a slow process, often taking six to nine months before you see results.' Skincare manufacturers, however, would like to persuade us that two months is the maximum it takes to see benefits.

And vitamin C has a couple of downsides. It can be very unstable and rendered ineffective by exposure to air. The leading cosmetics manufacturers claim, however, to have developed delivery systems which can get the vitamin into our skin intact, for instance with hermetically sealed ampoules or patches (see p.36).

In high doses, vitamin C can also irritate and even burn sensitive skin, particularly when combined with other high-tech ingredients. If you use a prescription vitamin A cream like Retin-A or Retinova, warns Dr Patricia Wexler, use it at the opposite end of the day to your vitamin C cream.

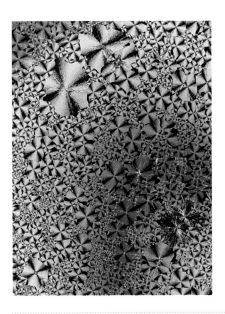

VITAMIN E

Beauties have long sworn that simply breaking open a capsule of vitamin E and massaging it into their skin has a gloriously anti-ageing effect. (On the other hand, experts point out, vitamin E – particularly in the synthetic form – can cause contact sensitivity, so it doesn't suit everyone.) But scientists are still trying to unravel its mysteries and work out why vitamin E may be effective.

Like vitamin C, vitamin E is an antioxidant, helping to fight sun and smog damage when it's formulated into skin creams. (Look for it on the label as d-alpha tocopherol – the natural form – or tocopheryl acetate.) According to dermatologist Dr Nelson Lee Novick, MD, author of *You Can Look Younger At Any Age*, 'What we can say at the present time is that, at least in lab studies, vitamin E can block the sunburn in laboratory animals when applied to the skin – even up to eight hours after exposure. It is also able to decrease skin thickness and sensitivity after sun exposure, and to have direct sunscreening properties when applied before exposure.' So for now, vitamin E is particularly being looked at for its role in sun protection.

A-C-E PROTECTION

When the beauty world was summoned to the Foreign Press Association for a press conference recently, from all the fanfare and fuss you'd have thought World War III was about to be launched. And, in a way, it was: war on wrinkles was being officially declared.

Dermatologists have long believed that topical applications of carefully – balanced doses of vitamins A, C and E – as well as other antioxidants like green tea and pine bark – may have an effect at preventing skin damage, by 'mopping up' the harm done by UV light and pollution. Now, they are coming up with the data that begins to confirm this educated hunch.

At that press conference, we were presented with the results of an ongoing eight-year French study – Su.Vi.Max (The Supplementation, Vitamin and Mineral Antioxidant Trial), run by a non-profit group of independent French scientists and dermatologists. The skins of 160 women in Tours, Toulouse and Grenoble were looked at over 18 months. Half applied an antioxidant cream (formulated by Estée Lauder); the others had a placebo moisturiser (also Lauder-formulated) – and nobody was allowed to wear extra sun protection. Several tests were carried out to measure improvements, including skin 'imaging' (a mask being taken of the skin before and after), and ultrasound.

It was a small sample (but statistically significant) and what the experts saw was a total surprise: not only did the topical antioxidants help protect the skin against ongoing damage from pollution and UV rays (resulting in a 23 per cent reduction in the formation of new lines and wrinkles), but in the group given the real antioxidant cream, the skin began to repair itself – resulting in a very, very small reduction in lines and wrinkles of an average of 8 per cent.

It all sounds impressive, on paper. Certainly, the results grabbed head-lines. But when challenged by us later, Estée Lauder's Dr Daniel Maes conceded that no, this doesn't actually translate to a *visible* improvement. Nevertheless, he told us, what they saw thrilled the scientists. 'We were concerned with prevention of *future* damage; this wasn't designed as a treatment,' he told us. But what happened, the scientists believe, is that shielding the skin with antioxidants enabled it to get on with the task of repairing itself. However, to experience any real benefit, antioxidant protection must be worn every single day. Always. Or you can kiss any benefits goodbye. 'But if women were only going to do one thing for their skin, I would say, absolutely: use an antioxidant,' Dr Maes concludes.

Although it's still early days, we are sufficiently convinced of the benefits of antioxidants to take them internally and slather them on our skins – religiously. Conscious that, for now, antioxidants are probably the best insurance policy we can invest in for our skins and, indeed, our health.

the AHA phenomenon

At the beginning of the nineties, AHAs – alpha-hydroxy acids – began to create a skincare stir, spawning a thriving, multi-million dollar industry. Today, you can find these ingredients – derived from sugar cane, wine, sour milk or fruit (e.g. apples or grapes), or synthetically produced – in virtually every skincare product from face creams to foot scrubs. The names of the acids include lactic, malic and glycolic acid.

These ingredients have made the cosmetic industry rich and many women happy – because AHAs may reduce the visible signs of ageing and sun damage. By dissolving the 'intercellular glue' that binds dead, flaky skin cells, AHAs gently peel away the uppermost layer of skin – revealing a smoother, newer, more youthful-looking complexion underneath. On Asian and black skins, they may also be used to treat ashiness.

However, as these acids achieved widespread usage, concerns began to emerge. Some reports suggest that AHAs may in some instances even be harmful, triggering burning and irritation. There are bigger questions, too: could they slough off too much of the skin's outer layer – leaving it vulnerable to sun damage? Just what are the long-term effects? Nobody knows – because this is new science.

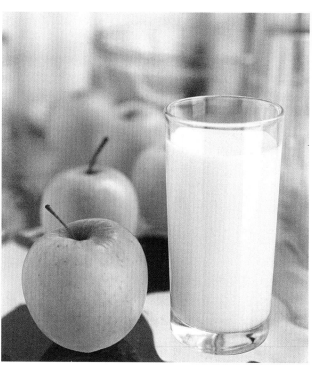

According to the Food and Drink Administration's Stanley Milstein, PhD, 'If these products do even half of what they say they do, it's possible they should be classified as drugs, not cosmetics.' Dr Albert Kligman, the leading dermatologist and skincare researcher, is pushing for more research into the side-effects of AHAs.

In fact, after the first wave of AHAs – and the first wave of AHA-related problems – some of the recent entries into the AHA market trumpet the fact that their formulations feature 'gentler' AHAs, or have added skin-calming ingredients such as green tea. Other manufacturers have begun to use BHAs – beta-hydroxy acids – instead (for instance, salicylic acid), which they herald as being kinder to the skin, although these may also cause sensitivity in vulnerable women.

Some experts believe that the ability of fruit acids to reduce the appearance of wrinkles actually *comes* from this irritation; the skin may thicken to protect itself – and so looks less wrinkled. Others claim this thickening is due to stimulation of collagen production.

Our personal experience with AHA products has not been very happy. Although both of us have seen some skin-brightening, we have experienced redness, scaliness and a kind of 'facial dandruff' – perhaps a sign of the speeded-up exfoliation process the fruit acids famously trigger. We find the only way we can use them on our sensitive skins is as a fortnightly 'face treat', to brighten skin; problems arise when we use them for more than one day/night at a time. But we do know women with more resilient skins who get on very well with AHAs.

Meanwhile, use some common sense. At any sign of redness, itching or irritation, stop using the product immediately. It is always a good idea to do a patch test before using an AHA behind the ear or near the hairline. Allow the product to sit for 24 hours and repeat. If there is any irritation – redness, swelling or itching in the area – you may want to think twice about using it on the rest of your face.

In addition, be cautious in the following areas…

• Increased sun sensitivity

There is growing evidence to suggest that many AHAs make users more vulnerable to sun damage. John Bailey, Director of the Office of Cosmetics and Colors at the US Food and Drug Administration, has cautioned: 'If you're using AHAs, always wear a sunscreen with SPF15 or higher.'

• Non-Caucasian skin

No research has been published about the risk levels for ethnic skin type groups. If you are unsure, test AHA products on your arm for several days and check for any pigmentation changes before applying to your face.

• Other medication

No research has been done on how AHAs interact with some drugs, but their use may be contra-indicated if you are using any drug that increases your skin's sensitivity to sunlight, such as Accutane, or tetracycline.

• AHA overload

More is not necessarily better. Observes Estée Lauder's Dr Daniel Maes, 'We're so used in this business to saying "more is better", but in this case, *less* is actually better.' In formulating products for Estée Lauder, he prefers to use low concentrations of spot-targeted AHAs which actually *stay* in the top two or three layers of skin, where they're less likely to cause problems. If you are using one AHA-based product in your skincare regime, don't be tempted to seek greater results by adding an AHA cleanser, peel or mask into your skincare regime – and stick with reputable companies.

TRIED & TESTED
BLIND-TESTED AHA CREAMS

Because of the high level of interest in AHA creams, we felt it important to test what's out there on the market. So these are the products that our skincare testers were most impressed by – along with their reports. (NB We avoided sending any AHA-based products to members of our testing panel who declared on their initial form that they have sensitive skin.)

Aveda Bio-Molecular Recovery Treatment
8 MARKS OUT OF 10 (£££) – *see p.17*

Vichy LumiActiv
8 MARKS OUT OF 10 (££) – *see p.17*

Gatineau Strategie Jeunesse Intensive Wrinkle Treatment
7.6 MARKS OUT OF 10 (£££££)
A 'dual-phase' treatment: a day serum and a richer night serum. It contains a 'phospho-hydroxy acid' – actually, derived from apple; Gatineau say that it's specifically designed not to irritate. More than three-quarters of the testers said they would buy it.
UPSIDE: 'the results were very good and noticeable to myself and friends' ◆ 'after two weeks, my skin was clearer, brighter and more translucent, though there was no softening in lines' ◆ 'I couldn't believe the difference; my skin is smoother and lines less noticeable on the side I've used it on'.
DOWNSIDE: 'tingles after every application and skin slightly red on each side of nose' ◆ 'I developed a pimply rash beneath the skin after four days – so I discontinued it; I don't normally suffer from sensitive skin'.

Yves Saint Laurent Fruit Jeunesse
7.5 MARKS OUT OF 10 (£££)
This water/silicone emulsion contains 2.5 per cent gluco-hydroxy-acid, a compound AHA offering what they described as 'minimal risk of irritation'. This product received mixed reviews; some thought it was amazing, while others were unimpressed. Nevertheless, three-quarters of the
testers said they would buy this cream.
UPSIDE: 'after two weeks my skin felt much firmer; I liked it very much though found the texture rather runny. I really believe I look younger and the people I work with say so, too' ◆ 'lines are softer-looking and bigger grooves, especially round mouth and chin, are less harsh-looking' ◆ 'want more! Skin looks "dewy" and pinker' ◆ 'vast improvement around mouth and nose' ◆ 'my skin looks a lot brighter, fresher and smooth as a baby's bottom'.
DOWNSIDE: 'it was a bit tacky and greasy and my make-up slid off' ◆ 'texture rather sticky and caused slight redness'.

Estée Lauder Re-Nutriv Intensive Lifting Crème
7.1 MARKS OUT OF 10 (£££££+) – *see p.19*

Estée Lauder Fruition Extra
7 MARKS OUT OF 10 (£££)
An updated version of what was one of the first mass-market AHA products on the counter, offering what Lauder describe as 'impressive results, faster, more precisely and with even less irritation'. (However, a couple of the testers reported a burning sensation immediately after use.) It features a combination of four alpha- and beta-hydroxy acids plus vitamins A, C and E and green tea extract. For use morning and evening under a moisturiser.
UPSIDE: 'my skin looks much better and younger – the fine lines have almost disappeared' ◆ 'friends ask if I'm using new make-up – my skin feels glowing, has improved elasticity and looks brighter; I feel more attractive because I'm sure I look younger than my age' ◆ 'colleagues at work comparing one side of my face with the other say that the side I've been using the cream on is definitely younger and less lined-looking'.
DOWNSIDE: 'didn't like the strong smell of perfume and the texture felt quite astringent' ◆ 'a burning sensation after using this – so I stopped'.

the beauty buzz

We bring you the inside track on some of the beauty breakthroughs that have women rushing to the counters...

PATCHES

One of the newest waves in anti-ageing skincare grew out of the drug industry: the dermal patch. In the old days, skin was regarded as a one-way street: we saw it as letting *out* sweat and toxins while performing the task of protecting our inner organs from the elements. But in the last decade, doctors have woken up to the skin's ability to absorb ingredients with the right size (i.e. not too big) molecule – and the potential uses for transdermal patches, probably best known for their application as HRT and nicotine patches to help smokers quit.

Today, patches are being infused with skincare ingredients for localised application, designed to be worn on the skin for anywhere from ten minutes to overnight. Their manufacturers claim that these patches are a more efficient method of delivering skincare ingredients than traditional lotions or creams. Their assertion is that the creams ensure a localised application of a high concentration of ingredients because they can be applied directly to specific 'problem' areas, i.e. around the eyes or on the forehead. Being able to pinpoint delivery zones can help avoid problems. For instance, Gene Goldberg, Senior Vice President at Doak Dermatologics (who make dermal patches), says: 'When you put a cream near your eyes, it might irritate if you put it too close.' Using a patch, he says, prevents that type of irritation.

'The skin patch takes a medically proven delivery method and applies it to skincare,' says Steven Porter, co-founder of the pioneering cosmetic dermal patch company Osmotics. 'The limiting factor with topical application of vitamins is the delivery system. Some unstable ingredients – for instance, certain forms of vitamin C – immediately react with the oxygen in the air; the ingredients 'decay' and become less effective, so they're not appropriate for use in a cream.'

However because the patches are packaged in air-tight envelopes, the ingredients don't come into contact with oxygen until they are applied to the skin.

But how long will results last? As with just about any cosmetic, you have to keep on using them to maintain any benefits. According to the manufacturers, the side-effects (if any) are minor; they include a risk of irritation for the small percentage of the population allergic either to topical vitamin C, or to the adhesive used in patches.

In the glamour stakes, these are pretty much non-starters; if you thought that going to bed wearing white gloves over hand cream was a passion-killer, try facing your partner for a goodnight kiss with what looks like an elastoplast slapped on your forehead/laugh lines.

But don't just take our word for it. We sent some of the leading patches on the market to our testers. See opposite for what they thought...

OXYGEN CREAMS

Having sold us on acids and vitamins, the cosmetics industry is now peddling oxygen as the ultimate element for skin. Yes, skin needs oxygen. Every breath we take helps to make our skin glow. But in the US, in particular, (where skin 'fads' tend to take a grip before the rest of the world) there has been a surge of interest in skin creams and facials that, supposedly deliver more oxygen to the skin than it is able to take up through the bloodstream, i.e. simply through breathing.

According to a spokesman for Lancaster Cosmetics, who have an entire range of oxygen-based lotions and potions (many of which did very well in the Tried & Testeds in this book) 'As we age, the walls of the capillaries which deliver oxygen to the skin start to thicken.' This also slows down cellular regeneration, so that skin becomes thinner, wrinkles and brown spots start to appear. Marcia Kilgore, founder of Manhattan's Bliss Spa and the Remède skincare range, insists: 'You can measure the level of oxygen in your skin with a pulse oxymeter. And if you measure oxygen levels in your skin before and after applying one of these creams, they're markedly higher after. So there is something to it.' In agreement with Kilgore is New York plastic surgeon Paul Lorenc, MD, who instructs his patients to use Karin Herzog's Vit-A-Kombi cream before and after surgery, 'because they heal faster – especially smokers'. Not everyone is convinced, however. Harold Swartz, MD, PhD, a scientist at Dartmouth, New Hampshire, whose research centres on oxygen, observes: 'There is certainly no data that I know of that suggest the skin starts looking old because the cells aren't getting enough oxygen – and that if you could somehow just return the oxygen to them, everything would be hunky dory.'

Incorporating oxygen into a skin cream has been a real cosmetic challenge, as it is very unstable and actually 'escapes'. The first scientist to succeed was Nobel Prize-winner Dr Paul Herzog, creator of the iron lung for polio patients. His patented formulation means oxygen can be tightly locked into a cream even when exposed to air. For your skin, this is alleged to mean destruction of acne-causing bacteria, increased collagen production – and a more radiant complexion. (His wife, Karin Herzog, now markets creams using this technology under her name.)

Used in facials, meanwhile, oxygen is pumped onto the surface of the skin via a metal tube from a tank, at 180 million particles a second. According to New York dermatologist David Orentreich, MD, 'there's no way taking a little jet of oxygen and blowing it on the skin can make that oxygen penetrate the skin. It just bounces off.' It is, however, a fantastic antiseptic – and that's where its value lies in salon treatments, which can introduce infection (as women who 'break out' after facials know very well). An oxygen facial – a favourite of models like **Cindy Crawford** and **Christy Turlington** and film stars like **Uma Thurman** – leaves a genuine (if short-lived) glow. (Which is why there's an 18-month waiting list at Bliss Spa for oxygen facials.)

We'd certainly go back for one of these heavenly treatments. But we still believe the best way to deliver oxygen to the skin is to take a brisk walk.

TRIED & TESTED
PATCHES

The high cost of these products meant that we were given just a few to test – so each set of patches went to three women. The results were as patchy – sorry! – as the products. Nothing achieved a unanimous success and some scored very low indeed. Our conclusion is that though patches are a promising innovation, the technology has some way to go. Some products could be great if you wanted a short-term boost – but we'd recommend them before a two-hour drinks party rather than a dinner party, as the benefits seem extremely short-lived!

Glico-Lift Full Face Patch
7.6 MARKS OUT OF 10 (£££)
Available for full face, neck, lip or eye zone. Designed to be applied on alternate nights to pre-cleansed skin and left for about half an hour. To maintain, treatments should be repeated several times a year. Patches are impregnated with glycolic acid (an AHA) and collagenic plant protein, which should infuse the skin exfoliating dead cells, plumping out complexion and helping to reduce fine lines.
UPSIDE: 'feels similar to a face mask – but it doesn't crack' ◆ 'a slight improvement and after more treatments they could be even more noticeable' ◆ 'I would definitely recommend this product; it left skin smoother and firm, although it has a drying effect; my mum and sister said how much smoother my skin looked'.
DOWNSIDE: 'tight like sticking plasters' ◆ 'very hot and tingly straight after patches removed – slightly pink skin' ◆ 'quite uncomfortable peeling the patches off – ouch!'

Wrinkle Miracle Eye Pads
7.5 MARKS OUT OF 10 (££)
Gauze pads soaked in healing plant extracts, which were first developed to help skin healing after plastic surgery. Designed to be applied to cleansed skin, left for 30–45 minutes, then removed, with the promise that they rapidly reduce the appearance of fine lines, wrinkles and eye puffiness.
UPSIDE: 'Didn't like the smell or the feel – very greasy, ointment-like substance, with no feel-good factor – but laughter lines were reduced and skin plumpness increased around eyes' ◆ 'couldn't believe the difference in crêpiness after one application, which improved progressively' ◆ 'the puffiness under my eyes was vastly improved'.
DOWNSIDE: 'Quite an unpleasant experience' ◆ 'overall good but messy'.

Eyesential Under Eye Enhancer
7.5 MARKS OUT OF 10 (£££)
A rollerball tube glides over the skin leaving behind a layer of lotion that dries and tautens; said to temporarily erase puffiness. Once applied, you have to avoid any facial movement for one to three minutes. A mix of silica, magnesium and water, manufacturers claim this is a favourite with Madonna, Lauren Hutton and make-up artists.
UPSIDE: 'after two hours, fine lines had disappeared; my eye zone definitely looks younger – and my whole face! I'd never have believed it if I hadn't seen it with my own (gorgeous!) eyes' ◆ 'reduced the puffiness'.
DOWNSIDE: 'felt unpleasantly taut at first; de-puffing lasted for less than four hours' ◆ 'after four hours, the crow's feet and bigger lines had started to reassert themselves'.

The Wrinkle Miracle Lip
6.5 MARKS OUT OF 10 (££)
The lip version of the eye patch mentioned above; it is placed on the top lip – looking very odd indeed – but said to reduce fine lines and wrinkles.
UPSIDE: 'immediately softer and a little plumper – my top lip didn't look quite so pinched' ◆ 'after two weeks the results were so good that I would use them regularly' ◆ 'easy to use; skin looked plumped up and moist – not surprisingly because the patches are so moist and sticky'.
DOWNSIDE: 'the foil patches are hard to open and patches difficult to get out'.

NB The lowest scoring product in this category earned just 5 marks.

FIRMING CREAMS

Anyone can get firmer skin – simply slather egg whites on your face. But 'firming' is one of the new beauty product buzzwords – and an infinitely alluring one to those of us who are losing the 'bounce-back' factor. Technically, tautness of the skin is measured by lab technicians attaching black suction boxes against women's cheeks and dropping small metal balls against their faces. Elasticity is measured by the distance the ball bounces.

Firming creams tend to merge various skincare innovations, with the aim of tightening, toning and smoothing slack skin using one luxurious product. (So firming creams tend to be expensive.) Some that did well in our Tried & Testeds (*see p.16*) include Nina Ricci Time Defense Extract and Guerlain 12M. All are rich in protein – often from plants like soya, wheat or peas (rather than the cow and sheep extracts often used in the past), usually working with oil to seal moisture in the skin. Many also have antioxidant vitamins to gobble up cell-ravaging free radicals. Different from 'Instant Face Wakers' (*see p.161*), firming creams are designed to show benefits after regular use over anything from a fortnight to a month or more.

looking after your eyes

Regardless of what comes out of your mouth, your eyes speak the truth. They smile. They glare. They show stress. They cry. And they give the game away about your age...

The skin surrounding the eyes is the thinnest on the body, as fine as an eggshell and at least four times thinner than the skin on the soles of your feet. This means that the moisture evaporates easily – and precisely because eyes are so expressive, the skin around them forms wrinkles faster than elsewhere on the face. The eyelids themselves have some of the thinnest skin on the body – between a half and a quarter of the thickness of your cheek. Blood vessels are close to the surface. There is less elastin and only a thin band of collagen. What's more, eyelids get an exhausting workout, blinking between twelve and twenty times a minute. They even move while you sleep. And then there's the barrage of abuse that eyes are subjected to: contact lenses, mascara, eyeliner, marathon sessions at the computer, smoke-filled rooms and sunlight. No wonder our eyes start to show up signs of ageing sooner than anywhere else...

Depending on your habits, the first signs of ageing around the eyes can appear as early as your twenties or as late as your forties. Non-smokers who keep to the shade and wear sunglasses are, genes willing, going to have younger-looking eyes than their smoking, sun-worshipping peers. 'But the good news is that you can effect tremendous changes in the eye area,' says Debra Jaliman, MD, a dermatologist and clinical instructor at Mount Sinai School of Medicine in New York City. 'As easily as you can damage the eye skin, you can fix it. Everybody can improve its appearance, to some degree.'

While we are, in general, fans of simple skincare regimes rather than bathroom shelves cluttered with dozens of lotions and potions, there is definitely a case for using a separate eye cream from your regular moisturiser for the eye zone. 'It's important that products used near the eyes be appropriate for this sensitive area, where stinging and burning can happen all too easily,' says New York-based dermatologist Dr Karen Burke MD, PhD. That's why some ingredients regularly used in facial moisturisers – like fragrance, certain emulsifiers and emollients – are eliminated from eye products. (Key words to look for, if you have sensitive eyes and aren't sure whether a product will suit you, are 'hypo-allergenic', 'fragrance-free' and/or 'ophthalmologically tested' – which means that the product has been screened for ingredients that might trigger eye sensitivity.)

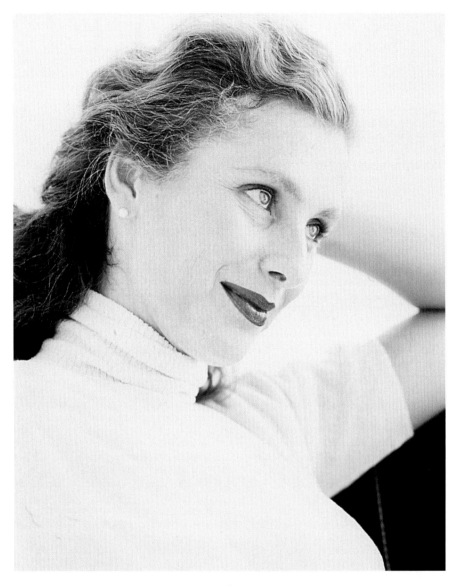

The skin around the eye area presents another problem in that it loses moisture easily but can't tolerate heavy products; this is because the oil glands in the eye area are fewer in number and smaller in size than those on the rest of the face. Use of too-rich cosmetics (or not removing make-up efficiently) can be a contributing cause to the development of milia, small sebaceous cysts which look rather like whiteheads under the eye, and can be unsightly. (*See Getting Rid of Milia p.136.*)

Most importantly, the eye area should be protected from future damage. We are big fans of sunglasses with very wide arms, which are the most effective way of shielding the eye area. An SPF15 sunscreen is also advisable. Here's the conundrum, however: most sunscreens advise you to avoid the eye area, because of the very real potential for stinging. But dermatologist Joseph P. Bark, MD, author of *Your Skin: An Owner's Guide (see Directory)*, believes we

should be using sunscreen around the eyes, regardless. The key is to find a suitable formulation: to minimise the potential for stinging, try different SPF15 moisturisers (on your hand), trying to identify those which go fairly matte after application, as these are less likely to travel into the eye itself. Many lightweight daily moisturisers now incorporate an SPF15 sunscreen (the magic figure); these are more suitable for the eye area than summer 'beach'-type sunscreens, which tend to be greasier. Or look out for specially designed eye products that contain sunscreens, which are starting to turn up within cosmetic ranges as the manufacturers respond to our angst about sun damage to the eye zone. The ideal regime is to use a basic, light moisturiser with sunscreen on the entire face – including the eye zone – during the day, and at night, try a specialised eye product.

Turn-back-the-clock eye treatments, meanwhile, are mostly designed to be worn at night. However, the big challenge is how to find an eye cream that effectively tackles fine lines and wrinkles – yet isn't so rich that it triggers irritation. There is a baffling number of options, featuring ingredients from high-tech liposomes to antioxidants via AHAs – and whether targeting wrinkles, dark circles or puffiness, many eye cream manufacturers now tap into the botanical trend by using ingredients like rosemary, ginseng, green tea and rosewater.

So we asked our panel of 1,000 women testers to try out literally dozens of eye creams for us over a period of several months. Here are their eye-opening conclusions...

TRIED & TESTED

─── EYE CREAMS ───

Shiseido Benefiance Revitalising Eye Cream
8.2 MARKS OUT OF 10 (££££)
A rich moist-feeling cream targeted at mature skins, it's said to reduce the appearance of fine lines and boost resilience, used (in small amounts) morning and night. It contains hyaluronic acid, ginseng extract and what Shiseido term 'revitalisers'. (Double Dutch to us, too.) Almost all the testers said they would buy this product. One tester even sent us a diagram of how the laugh lines on the lower eye now lift upwards instead of drag downwards when she is smiling!
UPSIDE: 'Having tried many eye creams, I feel this one is way up among the top' ◆ 'improved crêpiness around the inner eye' ◆ 'skin around my eyes looked much softer and less puffy within a day' ◆ 'fine lines reduced, skin smoother' ◆ 'the product seems to flatten out lines' ◆ 'just what I need when nearing fifty and attempting to look youthful' ◆ 'excellent: eye area looks much firmer and smoother after 14 days' ◆ 'greatly reduced crow's feet' ◆ 'my eyes are very sensitive and I wear contact lenses, but this didn't sting' ◆ 'hooded eyelids seemed to improve and skin noticeably softer'.
DOWNSIDE: 'fiddly lid' ◆ 'instruction leaflet difficult to follow – no outrageous claims though' ◆ 'made my eyes sting a little – use sparingly' ◆ 'using too much at night means puffy eyes the next morning'.

Gatineau Treatment For Eye Area
8.16 MARKS OUT OF 10 (££££)
This serum can be used morning or evening or once a week as a special booster treatment with accompanying eye compresses. The blurb boasts that dehydrated collagen capsules react with the skin's natural moisture and swell 'rather like popcorn to 15 times their size', thus visibly puffing out wrinkles, deep-set lines and laugh lines. It contains what Gatineau refer to as 'second generation grafted AHAs' (designed, as much as anything, to blind with science, we feel). Nevertheless, every single tester we sent this product to said that they would buy it.
UPSIDE: 'within minutes of first using this cream, my eyes looked and felt younger; after two weeks, I decided I wanted to use it

forever' ◆ 'very easy to use; liked the measured amount from the pump dispenser; lovely smell' ◆ 'it was very economical as only a small blob is required' ◆ 'under-eye area became progressively firmer and less puffy – a definite improvement' ◆ 'the puffiness is distinctly reduced and I look distinctly less tired' ◆ 'significant improvement after a week and steady improvement since' ◆ 'a cool, refreshing gel, good for an instant lift' ◆ 'fine lines were definitely less apparent' ◆ 'my slight crêpiness disappeared and I saw a definite improvement in the skintone'.
DOWNSIDE: none of our testers gave us negative feedback on this product.

Guinot Eye Cream
8 MARKS OUT OF 10 (£££)
Based mainly on plant extracts, this cream includes horse chestnut, chamomile and cornflower to soothe, refresh and help decongest the blood vessels and reduce dark circles under the eyes. According to Guinot, their eye-care products are suitable for use even on sensitive eyes and by contact lens-wearers. Three-quarters of the testers said they'd buy this cream.
UPSIDE: 'didn't improve puffiness – as promised – but really worked wonders on skin above my eyes, making eyes look "lifted" and younger-looking' ◆ 'fine lines very much improved, heavier lines too' ◆ 'the most noticeable difference was in crêpiness – most noticeable when using eyeshadow' ◆ 'packaging, texture and smell of this cream are very appealing; the added bonus of it actually working is wonderful'.
DOWNSIDE: 'not necessarily any better than my usual, cheap cream; had to stop wearing mascara during the day as I looked like a panda' ◆ 'took a long time to absorb into the skin and needed lots of massaging'.

Estée Lauder Uncircle Eye Treatment For Dark Circles
8 MARKS OUT OF 10 (£££)
*This lightweight, refreshing gel-cream for morning and night is specifically designed to tackle the tough problem of dark circles, as well as relieving dry skin and smoothing away fine lines. It uses fish cartilage extract (also now being tried out as a cancer

treatment – and as a skin supplement), plus a litany of natural extracts (including antioxidant green tea). Soft-focus cosmetic technology reflects light away from dark circles. Half the testers said this worked wonders on their dark circles, the other half said it didn't – but three-quarters said they'd buy it.*
UPSIDE: 'dark circles look better after 24 hours and improved progressively' ◆ 'very dramatic effect within 24 hours: eye area looked much younger, under-eye "uplifted"' ◆ 'dark circles diminished – does what it says' ◆ 'on visit to the hairdressers's, could bear to look at my eye area without flinching!' ◆ 'easy to apply, has a very pleasant feel and goes in quickly' ◆ 'might possibly lose my job as Panda for the Worldwide Fund for Nature!' ◆ 'I think it's brilliant: lines much reduced, even when smiling'.
DOWNSIDE: 'I put too much on one night and my eyes puffed up by next morning' ◆ 'very disappointing on dark circles'.

Helena Rubinstein Existence Firmnesse Firming Eye Structurer
7.77 MARKS OUT OF 10 (£££)
This transparent, ultra-light gel claims to be a triple-whammy with an anti-puffiness, anti-shadow and antioxidant action, delivering an immediate benefit. It is suitable for even the most fragile skintypes and is fragrance-free. Two-thirds of the women who tried this cream said they'd buy it.
UPSIDE: 'couldn't believe the difference in just 24 hours; I'm over the moon – that's the truth' ◆ '100 per cent improvement: the slack skin above my eyes has really firmed up, giving my whole face a more youthful look' ◆ 'the cream is a must: I use it morning and night because it makes the skin feel as if it's being "lifted" and reduces puffiness' ◆ 'all-round improvement' ◆ 'pump dispenser gives you the right amount every time' ◆ 'I was impressed that the gel actually did what it said it would in the leaflet – which was written in layman's terms' ◆ 'I feel more confident wearing eye make-up and not drawing attention to age-related wrinkles'.
DOWNSIDE: 'slightly alcoholic/medicinal-type aroma, offputting at first' ◆ 'didn't feel it did anything for wrinkles, bags or dark circles'.

RoC Activ Pur Eye Contour Cream
7.6 MARKS OUT OF 10 (££)

This light gel-cream is dual-action – it's also designed for use on lips. It has been tested by ophthalmologists and, RoC say, can be used safely by women with sensitive eyes and contact lens wearers – even though they admit that it may 'tingle' on first application. Its principal active ingredient is pure vitamin A, vitamin B5 and vitamin E, with glycerine; it's meant to be dabbed on lightly once-daily, morning or evening. Just over half the testers said they would buy this product.

UPSIDE: 'lines underneath my eyes are definitely less visible, even the deeper ones – and it eradicates early morning puffiness' ◆ 'I've just returned from a mission to Bosnia where I met lots of new people, who all thought I'm younger than I am; I could have my pick of toyboys!' ◆ 'I think I can start using sparkly eyeshadow again after using this cream' ◆ 'there was a definite but slight improvement in fine lines and crêpiness' ◆ 'very economical – a little goes a long way' ◆ 'it took many weeks of use but I did notice a reduction in fine lines and puffiness'.

DOWNSIDE: 'packaging is very unattractive, although it's simple and easy to use' ◆ 'I would have liked to see results sooner; if I hadn't been testing it for this book, I wouldn't normally have gone on using it'.

Clarins Eye Contour Balm
7.5 MARKS OUT OF 10 (££)

This light, non-oily formulation, containing rosewater, shea butter and cereal grain extracts, is said to soften signs of ageing around the eyes. It also has light-reflective micro-pigments to give an immediate 'soft-focus' effect to lines, thereby making them less visible. Should be applied every evening. Three-quarters of the testers said they'd buy it.

UPSIDE: 'lines and wrinkles are not going to disappear without surgery, but this cream does everything it claims before you have to go under the knife' ◆ 'absorbed very well into the skin, leaving a velvety surface for foundation' ◆ 'plumps out crêpiness and smooths fine lines immediately but effects only last as long as balm is on the skin' ◆ 'fine lines appear plumped up'.

DOWNSIDE: 'a nice light, soothing cream but certainly no miracle product' ◆ 'had to stop after two days – bloodshot, itchy eyes'.

NB The lowest scoring product in this category rated an average of 1.75 marks.

eye-care how-to

The last thing the delicate eye area tissue needs is any product – or action – that tugs, stretches or irritates. Elsewhere on the face, we have always felt that a bit of massage and stimulation is good for the complexion. But the eye area is so fragile and vulnerable that it needs constant TLC.

• Be gentle. Avoid paper tissues, which actually scratch the eye skin, and seek out soft and natural cotton wool. (We actually prefer organic cotton, when we can find it; since cotton has a huge number of pesticides used on it, we would rather the residues didn't get anywhere near our eyes.) Q-Tips can be very useful for removing make-up from the base of the lashes without rubbing; Chanel teaches its cosmeticians to remove eye make-up with a remover-saturated cotton swab, vertically rolling from eyebrow to lashline until the make-up is removed. For under the eyes, horizontally roll another cotton swab from the outer corner to the bridge of the nose.

• You can also try the 'lash-rolling' trick, to avoid having to swipe cotton wool back and forth across the eye area to cleanse away make-up: apply your specially targeted eye make-up remover (most facial make-up removers just don't do the trick), wait a few seconds while it dissolves your mascara and then roll the residue very gently from your lashes, using your fingers or a cotton pad. In addition, avoid the use of waterproof mascara unless you are likely to get wet or to cry; the fact that it is harder to remove (even with special removers, in our experience) makes it likely that you will tug and pull the eye area more than you would to remove a non-waterproof formulation.

• Make sure you apply creams correctly. You don't need to apply a cream directly to the eyelid or underneath the eye; fine lines act as conduits, like a 'wick' drawing products towards the eye. (Which is why so many women experience irritation with eye products.) Instead, apply creams and gels in minuscule dots on the orbital bone (circling the eye); all in all, you probably don't want to use anything more than the size of a grape seed. Use the bone that surrounds the eye as a guide; the product will gradually work its way to the rim of the eye through the action of blinking.

• Don't rub the cream into the skin, whatever you do, or you're likely to create more of the very wrinkles you're trying to erase. 'Let the product do the work, not your fingers,' suggests Caroline Pieper Vogt, Vice President of Education and Retail Services at Clarins. 'Use a light tapping motion to apply it. You want to stimulate circulation but not drag the skin.'

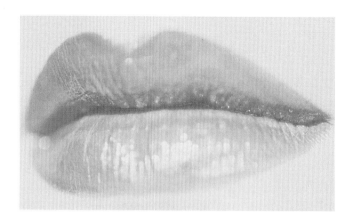

lip service

The skin on your lips (as those of us who look in the mirror and see an ever-deepening network of lines spreading across our pout already understand) is different from the skin elsewhere on the body. In fact, it isn't even skin at all, according to the experts.

Explains Michael S. Kaminer, MD, Director of Cosmetic Surgery at New England Medical Centre, 'It's a mucous membrane and, as such, is missing certain things like sweat glands, sebaceous glands and hair follicles.' Because the skin on lips is thinner and lower in melanin than the skin on the rest of the face, it needs a special protection squad to shield it against wind, sun and cold.

The good news is that your lipstick may help do just that. Men are seven times more likely to develop lip cancer than women – because we wear lipstick, and they don't. A survey by Dr Janice Pogoda and Susan Preston-Martin of the University of South California showed that women who apply opaque lipstick more than once a day cut their risk of lip cancer in half. 'Lipstick pigment is a UV barrier,' says Dr Rino Cerio, a consultant dermatologist at The Royal London NHS Trust Hospital. (And the more richly pigmented the shade, the more effective it is.) If you don't want to wear lipstick, use a lip balm with special UV filters, offering a minimum SPF15; ideally, it should have a sticky, waxy look and feel because this means it will stay on better. (Our personal favourite is Aveda Lip Saver.) Remember to apply both lipstick and lip balms regularly, because eating, drinking, talking and lip-licking all remove lip products fast. (Try to get out of the habit of lip-licking, incidentally, because the repeated wetting and drying actually dehydrates lips.)

As with every zone of the body, protection against future damage is vital. But what can we do to reverse the signs of ageing – those lines and fissures that worsen with the years? All of a sudden, our lips are being targeted with an avalanche of time-defying lip products, designed to smooth, soften or even plump up our pouts and featuring high-tech anti-ageing ingredients like AHAs, vitamin E and vegetable waxes for softening.

But do they work? Dermatologists we spoke to tell us, for instance, that it's impossible to penetrate the lips with moisture, precisely because the 'skin' is different to elsewhere on our faces; all a cream can do is trap the moisture that's naturally there. So we asked our panel of 1,000 women to try anti-ageing lip products. Read their lips: here's the low-down on what worked...

Cher can't leave the house without Aveda Silk Lip Essence – while Michelle Pfeiffer apparently prefers Shiseido Lip Conditioner. Like many celebrities, Anjelica Huston keeps a tube of Kiehl's lip balm in her handbag for on-the-go lip-slicking...

TRIED & TESTED

ANTI-AGEING LIP PRODUCTS

NeoStrata Lip Conditioner
8.12 MARKS OUT OF 10 (£)
This twist-up, clear, lipstick-style balm with SPF8 features gluconolactone, an AHA (fruit acid) said to be suitable for use even on clinically sensitive skins. Half the testers said they would buy this rich formulation, many liking the lack of discernible smell or taste.
UPSIDE: 'fine lines around the mouth are much less visible and lips seem plumper, soother and are no longer dry' ◆ 'the lines seemed to fade because the dryness and cracking went; my lips seemed to stay moist and supple' ◆ 'at the end of the treatment period, my lips do look younger, softer and in better condition; I liked using this product and because it doesn't smear, I could put it on without a mirror' ◆ 'stopped my lips being dry or cracking and gave me smooth, soft lips' ◆ 'almost immediately after application, lips seemed to "plump out"' ◆ 'more comfortable immediately'.
DOWNSIDE: 'this product was fine on its own but lipstick wouldn't "stick" on top' ◆ 'just a lip salve for winter – too thick to wear with lipstick; greasy and heavy, went onto teeth' ◆ 'all lipstick colours looked lighter and some "softer" lipsticks tend to bleed'.

Guerlain Lip Balm
7.7 MARKS OUT OF 10 (££)
This balm – originally formulated as a nipple cream and still with its original marzipan-tasting recipe – is now more popular as an intensive lip treatment, to use at night, or during the day without lipstick. Just under half the testers said they'd buy this product.

UPSIDE: 'magic! Good for two hours, no sign of feathering or discoloration; the best lip balm I've ever used and I even like the unusual smell' ◆ 'lips much softer, less flaky and pleasantly moist' ◆ 'lips are softer and not so dry at the corners' ◆ 'a definite improvement immediately after use; my lips appeared pinker and slightly plumper' ◆ 'I usually suffer from cold sores in winter but haven't while using this product' ◆ 'my lips and surrounding area immediately felt lovely and "alive"; lip texture looked better too' ◆ 'at 53, I have a maddening problem with lipstick bleeding but this helped very much' ◆ 'living outdoors, I used this all the time – especially in the wind' ◆ 'rapidly reduced flakiness'.
DOWNSIDE: 'colour and smell rather offputting' ◆ 'felt heavy and greasy on the lips – four out of ten for comfort' ◆ 'delivered much more than you need for a single treatment' ◆ 'spoiled the look of very matte or pearly lipsticks'.

Caudalie Grape Seed Lip Conditioner
7.6 MARKS OUT OF 10 (£)
This extremely inexpensive twist-up balm contains antioxidants from grape seed – alleged to be 50 times more powerful than vitamin E, 20 times more powerful than vitamin C. Claimed to be a good lipstick base, it can be applied whenever lips feel dehydrated or chapped. Just over half the testers said they'd buy this product.
UPSIDE: 'lips seem plumper – I like the effect' ◆ 'I suffer from dry lips normally and this product was the only one that helped' ◆ 'definite reduction in lines

above lips' ◆ 'lips looked very smooth'.
DOWNSIDE: 'slightly greasy texture which had to be blotted before applying lipstick' ◆ 'no better or worse than any other lip product I've tried' ◆ 'not keen on the strong smell of cocoa butter'.

Lancaster Oxygen Lip Balm
7.37 MARKS OUT OF 10 (££)
This clear, lipstick-style product uses Lancaster's patented oxygen delivery technology, combined with vitamin E. Although not the top-scoring product, it worked brilliantly for some women – more women testing this said they would buy it than any other tested.
UPSIDE: 'the best lip product I have used; long-lasting tube and the velvety texture made lips immediately smoother and softer; also helped my lipstick stay on significantly longer' ◆ 'no taste or fragrance so particularly pleasant; I'm outdoors a lot but no dry lips' ◆ 'lips smoother, plumper and fine lines filled slightly' ◆ 'at the end of the trial period, my lips look a little plumper, more conditioned and less dry; slight difference in fine lines around lips' ◆ 'bleeding of lipstick eliminated; non-greasy consistency greatly liked by my partner' ◆ 'very good light-textured base for lipstick: feeling of smoothness and moisture'.
DOWNSIDE: 'felt – though didn't look – slightly greasy on lips; no difference in appearance' ◆ 'pleasant product to use but didn,t have any long-lasting effects'.

NB The lowest scoring product in this category averaged just 3 marks.

necks

Even a great face can be brought down by a neck that looks a little crêpey, wrinkled or saggy. Cosmetics may help. (And failing that, we have advice on the perfect clothing cover-ups...)

Our neck, like our hands, gives away our age in a flash. The skin of the neck tends to be dry and fine because it has only a small number of fat cells and meagre supplies of sebum (the skin's natural moisturiser) – making for a neck that becomes highly prone to crêpiness and dryness, getting increasingly less Nefertiti-like with the years. What's more, because we move our necks constantly, the collagen and elastin which keep the skin firm are loosened.

'Necks are very often neglected,' observes Christina Carlino, founder of the Philosophy skincare line. What she recommends is incorporating your neck – and your décolletage – in your daily skincare regime, sweeping your cleanser in gravity-defying movements *up* the neck to remove the day's grime. 'Most importantly,' observes Christina, 'the neck can experience insidious sun damage.' Stephen Kurtin, MD, a New York dermatologist, agrees: 'The neck gets a lot of sun and is less able to tolerate it than other areas of the body.' So a broad-spectrum SPF15 moisturiser, applied religiously to neck and décolletage, is a must for shielding the skin – although it won't significantly reverse any accumulated damage.

Another age giveaway can be telltale brown stripes that appear on either side of the neck. These, explains Dr Karen Burke, are linked with

perfume usage: ingredients in some fragrances (specifically psoralens from bergamot oil – a common fragrance ingredient) stimulate the natural tanning ability of the skin, resulting in the stripes. Her advice is *not* to wear fragrance (which is also very drying, because of the alcohol content) on your neck if you are likely to be exposed to UV light. Instead, try lightly spritzing it on your clothes. (Your wrists, however, aren't vulnerable to this streaking.)

For lined faces, cosmetic surgery is a viable option. But in the experience of women we know, neck-lifts are often disappointing. To be truly effective, the procedure would probably leave you with a zip-like scar at the back of the neck; as it is, the 'ringlet' lines on the neck (aka 'lines of Venus') – which are there from birth but worsen as we age – are hard to fix with surgery. Some women have experienced line-softening effects with chemical peels, but these aren't a universal rave with the women who've tried them, either. (As one woman interviewed for this book told us: 'Several of my friends have all had their necks "done" – and all of them have been less than thrilled with the results.')

The good news, then, is that some of our testers were extremely impressed with the line-smoothing power of the neck creams they tested

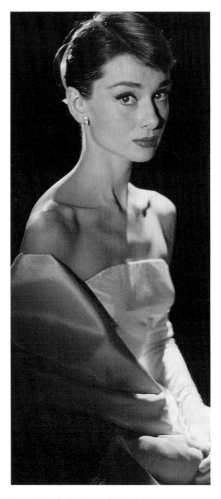

(*see Tried & Tested Neck Creams, opposite*). Facial oils are another great age-defying secret (*see p.49 for Aromatherapy Associates' prescriptions*). However, our advice is that the very best way of defying crêpiness is to use neck lotions and potions not just once, not just twice, but several times daily, to keep the moisture level topped up and maintain the appearance of smoothness. And if you really want to maintain a soft and sinuous neck, try yoga. We have noted that women who regularly do yoga remain more swan-like and have more chiselled chins than women who don't – well into their eighth and ninth decade...

TRIED & TESTED

NECK CREAMS

**Elizabeth Arden Ceramide Lift
For Face & Throat**
8.62 MARKS OUT OF 10 (££££)
*The active ingredient in this firming lotion
is a vitamin A derivative, retinyl linoleate,
in a ceramide formulation designed to
restore resiliency and firmness – both
immediately and over time – and also
reduce the appearance of age spots. In
trying this lotion, our testers concentrated
on the challenging neck zone. All of the
testers said they would buy this product.*
UPSIDE: 'crêpiness is reduced and neck
definitely appears softer – very impressive'
◆ 'it did give an almost immediate
improvement in texture; over time, the skin
on neck (and face) improved greatly, mainly
in softness – skin felt like velvet – plus
reduced dryness' ◆ 'after two weeks, fine
lines and crêpiness disappeared, skin supple
and smooth – I loved it and would highly
recommend it' ◆ 'improvement in tendency
to redness and dry skin and my skin is
smoother and plumper, although it didn't
work for sagginess of neck; I'm not
surprised – plastic surgery might!' ◆ 'every
area of neckline that catches sun easily and
was very crêpey has vastly improved'.
DOWNSIDE: 'slightly greasy – took longer
than expected to sink into skin'.

Clarins Neck Cream
8.5 MARKS OUT OF 10 (£££)
*A very light cream with revitalising marine
algae extracts, moisturising mallow and
ginseng and olive extracts, said to have
a toning effect. (Hence the promised
'firming'.) It can be used morning and/or
night. All but one tester said they would
buy this rich – but rapidly absorbed –
cream. Testers raved about the smell.*
UPSIDE: 'loved this cream: texture superb,
fluffy and rich – and a small amount goes a
long way. My neck looked firmer and the
texture of skin vastly improved' ◆ 'after two
weeks, skin was less dry, fine lines had
disappeared and a very deep line seemed
less deep; after two months, the centre
crêpey part was firmer and more taut' ◆ 'I
love the smell and always looked forward
to using it as it gave me a "lift"; I would
cup my hands over my face and just breathe
in!' ◆ 'I'll definitely buy this product as I
feel as though I can't live without it and

that my neck looks younger than my forty-
nine years' ◆ 'skin less like old chicken; I
now happily wear lower necklines; it hasn't
got rid of wrinkles but that would be
impossible; as a professional violinist I
spend up to six hours a day with violin
clamped under chin. Result: rough, red
mark on neck – but this is looking a lot
less livid now and the skin around it less
damaged' ◆ 'even my partner noticed the
difference – and I'm getting lots of hickeys
on my neck now, because of it!'
DOWNSIDE: 'the product claimed that
blemishes became less apparent but mine
did not. My skin did not look younger and
smoother after two months'.

**Estée Lauder Re-Nutriv Firming
Throat Cream**
8.4 MARKS OUT OF 10 (£££££+)
*This light-textured cream is specially
formulated to tone and firm the dry and
wrinkle-prone neck area, using many of the
same ingredients as the matching eye cream;
it can be worn day and night, unlike some
richer creams. The key active ingredient is
vitamin A palmitate to speed up cell
renewal. All but one of the testers said they
would buy this product.*
UPSIDE: 'sustained improvement in jawline,
which is less saggy, though normal neck
creases unaffected and upper chest no
different' ◆ 'skin definitely firmer and more
elastic, with fewer fine lines and less
crêpiness; jaw-line more distinct' ◆ 'puffs up
crêpey bits to make them look more even,
less lined' ◆ 'my neck is much less bumpy and
crinkly' ◆ 'marvellous!! This has saved me
£4,500 for the facelift I had booked, which I
have cancelled; my favourite dress shop asked
if I had a new man because I looked so alive!'
DOWNSIDE: 'smell!' ◆ 'jar looked full but
had a false bottom' ◆ 'no noticeable
difference in brightness or lessening of
grooves/lines' ◆ 'texture a bit heavy for
daytime' ◆ 'my hair looked a little stringy
where it had touched the treated area'.

Decleor Neck Firming Gel
8.21 MARKS OUT OF 10 (£££)
*This transparent, non-sticky gel promises
immediate and long-term firming results,
achieved by natural extracts including soft
wheat, green algae and soy. It should be

used morning and night after cleansing.
All but one of the testers were impressed
enough to want to buy this product.*
UPSIDE: 'neck skin felt noticeably softer
and looked smoother after using this light,
easily absorbed gel' ◆ 'wonderful smell;
neck feels definitely smoother and less
crêpey after nearly two months' ◆ 'I don't
think my neck looked better but it felt
smoother' ◆ 'I also did a test on my hands
and felt that the gel was excellent for them'
◆ 'I'm a pensioner, but I have definitely lost
my "chicken" scraggy neck; my friends are
most impressed'.
DOWNSIDE: 'if too much gel is used the
neck becomes sticky' ◆ 'would prefer a
cream that sinks in rather than having to
hang around for ten minutes while the gel
is absorbed'.

Prescriptives Uplift Active Firming Cream
8 MARKS OUT OF 10 (££££)
*This is part of Prescriptives problem-solving
Px As Needed range. It's designed to give
both an instant 'uplift' effect and ongoing
improvements. Ingredients include
hydrolysed milk protein (said to work in
much the same way as Cling-Film!), heather
extract and centella asiatica, increasingly
used for its apparent ability to stimulate
collagen and elastin production. It can be
used daily or as a weekly mask. Again, all
but one panellist said they'd buy this.*
UPSIDE: 'absorbed very quickly, nice
texture; after two weeks, skin is much
smoother and softer; fine lines less
noticeable' ◆ 'the discoloration on my neck
has improved; I don't expect miracles but
this cream has some kind of magical
ingredient!!' ◆ 'it improved tone and colour;
made my neck look brighter than its usual
grey; my husband stole some for his face –
and liked it' ◆ 'I love this cream; the smell
alone would sell this product; even my
dentist noticed the difference!' ◆ 'lovely,
fresh, orange blossom smell' ◆ 'overall, one
of the best products I've ever tried'.
DOWNSIDE: 'my daughter and I honestly
can't say there is any noticeable difference,
even though I followed all advice and
instructions; I did so hope for a miracle'.

NB The lowest scoring product in this
category rated 5.5 marks out of ten.

THE BIG COVER-UP

Trompe-l'oeil tricks are a godsend to the woman who feels her neck is looking more turkey-like with every passing season. (That includes us.) So we asked Betty Halbreich, author of the truly brilliant *Secrets of a Fashion Therapist** and Director of Solutions at Bergdorf Goodman (where she works as a fashion consultant to some of Manhattan's best-dressed women) for her suggestions for clever cover-ups. As Betty told us, 'These all work – and help make a woman feel more comfortable in her skin…'

• 'The turtleneck sweater and mock turtleneck remain the No. 1 disguise for a wrinkled neck. However, the mock neckline has a clean, flatter look without creases. These are harder to find than turtlenecks, so I often invert the overlap of the turtleneck, turning it inside. It is much smoother-looking, and lengthens the appearance of the neck. The problem most women have with both kinds of neckline is that they buy a sweater with a too-tight neckline, which causes bulges – and more wrinkles! So beware…'

• 'Jewellery is a wonderful foil. Chokers – whether real or faux – are wonderful, in pearls, diamonds, old or new. (But again, not too tight.) I use pearls – ropes of them – strung round the neck three or more times; the extra-large ones "fill up" the neck and look great. I also work with three or four strands of beads, twisted around the neck. Very feminine – and a good cover.'

• 'Collars can be helpful. The mandarin collar or Nehru stand-up collars are terrific; they should perch just under the jaw-line, where they look very good in profile. Any jacket with a stand-up collar seems to shadow the neck.'

• 'I'm the original scarf-lover. True, they can be hard to get the hang of, but once conquered, they hide a multitude of wrinkles. A simple exercise: take a long oblong scarf or piece of soft fabric and wind it around the neck twice, very loosely. It then becomes a frame around the face. I find chiffon, soft-cut velvet, cashmere and any diaphanous fabric is easiest to manipulate. A scarf used kerchief-style, placed under a regular shirt collar and tied high helps the older neck.'

• 'I often use men's collars – nicely starched shirts – with the collars flipped up. Then slip a string of pearls or a thin gold chain around the neck, resting just above the breast-bone, to "break up" the line.'

• 'For evening, a long maribou scarf, four to six feet long, wound round the neck, is beautiful (think old Hollywood movie-star-style).'

• 'Last – and certainly not least – great make-up and a terrific haircut can work miracles and draw attention away from the neck. Hair can be feathered into the neck or cut below the jaw-bone to distract from neck problems. And most important of all is the way a woman holds herself, neck straight and standing tall, looking directly ahead when she enters a room. That's what people look at: attitude, posture, clothes – then the neck comes way down the list!'

when fatter is more flattering…

Over 40, it's said, a woman must choose between her face and her backside: the thinner you are, the faster your face will appear to age. 'A thinner person will always appear older than someone who is plumper,' says Richard Fleming, MD, a plastic surgeon in Beverly Hills. Fat plumps out wrinkles and may mask other age-related changes, such as loss of bone mass in the jaw and cheek. Super-lean women wrinkle more noticeably and sag sooner because they have so little fat in their faces that every little breakdown is magnified on the skin's surface.

Changes start showing in the early forties, when women begin to notice what surgeons refer to as 'skin redundancy' – those creases and folds that can add years to your looks. This is due to the breakdown of various tissues of the face: everyone gets some muscle shrinkage, so the skin over the top sags. Second, weakened muscle tone causes some of the fat on the cheekbone to slide down, deepening the 'smile line' between nose and lips. Third, bone loss and the breakdown of supportive collagen reduce the underlying frame of the face – and by now, skin is too lax to shrink-to-fit. (Since collagen breakdown is accelerated by sun damage, tanning fans show these changes earlier.)

Worst off, according to experts, are women who abruptly lost large amounts of weight in their thirties or beyond; they will look older than if they had never lost the weight, because the extra skin will just hang. Yo-yo dieting is another culprit that can accelerate the development of jowls and folds.

nature -v- rocket science

Every woman longs to be a natural beauty. On most of us, however, Fate played a cruel trick: looking natural can often mean looking – well, older. Which means we need a little extra help – in the form of lotions, potions and dream creams. The good news for would-be natural beauties, however, is that while high-tech nanospheres and liposomes are enjoying a moment of cosmetic glory, there are some highly effective nature-based cosmetics on the market – if you know where to look for them...

Those in the truly natural beauty industry – outside the big mainstream companies – claim that a lot of the high-tech skincare on the market has been rushed to the marketplace without any research into the long-term effects of using particular ingredients – let alone the cocktail of ingredients that go into a cream. Dr Jurgen Klein, the founder of Jurlique, points out: 'The skin is an absorbent organ. I think everyone should think hard about what they put on their skin. If you wouldn't eat it, it may not be such a good idea to slap it on your face or body.'

It's worth remembering that until just a few years ago, boffins professed themselves baffled as to why aromatherapy was so effective, musing that it was linked to the effect of smell on the brain. 'But now,' explains leading aromatherapist Danièle Ryman, 'there is no longer any question: aromatherapy works on the body and the psyche via the bloodstream, not just because of its pretty smell.'

Homoeopath Lynne Crawford has found that many of her clients are suffering from toxic overload, which she believes can be linked back to beauty products. 'They go straight into the bloodstream and end up clogging the liver and kidneys. Of course it will have an adverse effect on your health,

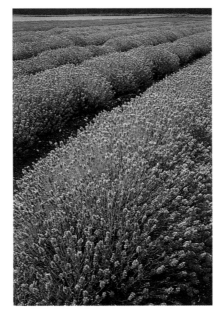

as well as, eventually, your looks.'

And in the long term, worries Dr Klein, the ingredients in some high-tech skincare might – just might – actually turn out to turbo-charge the ageing process. 'When you assault the body with a lot of unfamiliar chemicals that it's not evolved to deal with, this activates the body's defences. We should use this immune system only when it's needed – not challenge it on a daily basis.' In the same way, he feels, if the skin's immune system is being challenged regularly by an avalanche of unfamiliar chemicals, it may ultimately turn out to age more quickly

than if you weren't using that potent anti-ageing cream. It is fair to say that Dr Klein is regarded very much as a radical by the skincare industry. But it's certainly food for thought. Even Estée Lauder's Dr Daniel Maes believes that anything which creates an inflammatory reaction in the skin – such as a flare-up in response to a new skin cream – actually damages skin.

Dr Klein's advice is to concentrate on protection. 'Sun protection and skin creams featuring antioxidants like vitamin C and E – which protect against pollution, radiation and the carcinogens in cigarette smoke – are your best weapon against ageing,' he insists.

There is another reason to consider turning to 'greener' skincare: if you take your empties to the bottle bank, recycle your newspapers and at least *try* not to drive when you can walk, it is a logical step to consider the ecological implications of what you put on your skin.

It reassured us that, while blind-testing 'miracle creams', our 1,060 volunteers discovered that some of the natural ranges of skincare performed as impressively as those which came out of the multi-million-dollar skincare labs. So turn the page to discover some of the top-ranking nature-based creams...

TRIED & TESTED

─BLIND-TESTED NATURAL MIRACLE CREAMS─

Neal's Yard Frankincense Nourishing Cream

8.25 MARKS OUT OF 10 (£) – *see p.16*
Neal's Yard's range is not 100 per cent synthetic-free, but is formulated to use the absolute minimum of preservatives required. This product – featuring anti-ageing frankincense essential oil – scored extremely impressive marks, well above many of the pricey and/or high-tech creams on the market.

Aveda Bio-Molecular Recovery Treatment

8 MARKS OUT OF 10 (£££) – *see p.17*
Aveda have a strong commitment to using non-petrochemical ingredients (petrol-derived ingredients which are in widespread use within the beauty industry), preferring to use botanical products. They also have a policy of supporting environmental charities.

Decleor Concentré Stimulant

8 MARKS OUT OF 10 (££££) – *see p.17*
Although this aromatherapy-based company do use synthetic ingredients and preservatives in some of their products, this particular cream is an all-natural oil.

Jurlique Herbal Extract Recovery Gel

7.62 MARKS OUT OF 10 (££££)
A gel/serum-style product from a leading all-natural Australian beauty company who grow their herbs organically and have a reputation for high-performance ethical products, formulated without petrochemicals, preservatives and solvents. This gel features a high concentration of antioxidants from green tea, grape seeds and turmeric. Just over half the testers said they'd buy this product.
UPSIDE: 'it certainly seemed to plump up the surface of the skin on application; skin also felt smoother and tauter with a shiny look' ◆ 'I am allergic to many skin products but this one made my skin feel fantastic; a friend at work thought I looked ten years younger after using it' ◆ 'after two weeks, texture and brightness had improved; it works like an instant pick-me-up' ◆ 'lines around my eyes visibly reduced. My husband commented my skin looked different' ◆ 'this serum is a dream to use and feels lovely; my foundation went on more smoothly and stayed on better. Even my daughter said how nice my skin was – this is definitely a compliment!'
DOWNSIDE: 'gave too tight a feeling if you used three drops as opposed to two' ◆ 'didn't like the smell or the watery, runny texture'.

is your skincare genetically engineered?

When we asked some of the leading skincare companies what the Next Big Thing in the development of anti-ageing skin creams was going to be, they answered: 'genetic engineering'.

We were shocked. The world of skincare is science at its most high-tech and, for the most part, we wholeheartedly support their research into how our skins age – and what we can do to minimise the signs. But several leading skincare companies are already using genetically engineered ingredients and bio-engineering techniques to create 'new generation' skincare. In many cases, this means using a bacteria or a fungus whose DNA has been 'tweaked', to create molecules (for instance, the moisturising ingredient, hyaluronic acid), rather than obtaining the raw materials from plants or animal ingredients, as they did in the past. The bacteria/fungus is then de-activated – and the resulting ingredient put into a skin cream.

We feel there are real risks involved in the science of genetic engineering – for instance, the creation of bacteria or viruses which could be released into a world that is unready to deal with them. Genetic engineering was developed originally to try to help victims of serious life-threatening inherited diseases, such as Huntingdon's Chorea. Developments in medical laboratories are scrutinised closely and research takes place over decades. We hope cosmetics companies are as scrupulous. But in food – the field of commercial genetic engineering we know best – this is simply not the case, and products are being rushed to the market without any medium- or long-term guarantees of safety. Genetic engineering may prove to be entirely safe and beneficial to humankind, but at the moment we – in common with many scientists and lay people worldwide – do not believe the proof is there.

When the Prince of Wales gave a speech in support of organic farming, he called genetically engineered foods 'Frankenstein foods'. Do we really want 'Frankenstein face creams'? If you are concerned about genetically engineered skincare, make your feelings known to the manufacturers. (In the meantime, you may want to consider switching to one of the natural products that did well in our Tried & Tested Miracle Creams, above.) Our panel of testers considered several to be outstanding.

anti-ageing aromatherapy facial massage

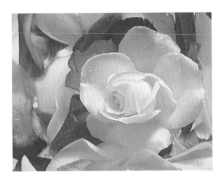

Aromatherapy oils may be Nature's greatest de-ager, restoring suppleness and vitality to even the tiredest skin. We love the effect they have on our weary complexions – and flagging spirits. So we asked leading aromatherapists, Aromatherapy Associates, (who were the late Princess of Wales's aromatherapists-of-choice), to give us this at-home facial massage, using essential oils. It's bliss...

'Aromatherapy massage and essential oils can be extremely beneficial as part of an holistic anti-ageing programme,' explains Aromatherapy Associates' Germaine Rich. 'They can be relaxing, detoxifying, stimulating and supportive to the immune system. They help support and balance the body's metabolic functions. And essential oils help balance the emotions, at the same time.' And depending on the oil – or combination of oils – chosen, they can be tremendously beneficial for the skin. Beat that.

But if you've shied away from facial oils because you're worried they'll leave your face slick-shiny, be reassured. 'The oils are absorbed very rapidly into the skin – leaving it softer, smoother and nourished,' explains Germaine. As an alternative to a night cream, you might want to make up a facial oil using any of the seven anti-ageing essential oils listed, and apply a few drops nightly to the face. But be careful to keep the oils away from the eyes. 'Apply to the skin of the brow-bone and the lower eye socket bone,' advises Germaine. 'The oils will still travel inwards to smooth and nourish the eye skin, but if applied too close to the eye, they may cause sensitivity.'

ANTI-AGEING ESSENTIAL OILS

Frankincense
An excellent skin tonic, particularly valuable for mature, wrinkled skins. Useful for healing wounds. Working on the emotions, frankincense has an uplifting and clearing effect, giving a sense of rising above problems and clearing negativity.

Geranium
Brightens dull skin and balances combination skins; antiseptic and anti-inflammatory. Uplifting, it's one of the best all-round tonics for mind and body.

Lavender
Excellent first aid remedy for cuts, bites, bruises and burns. The most useful and popular of all essential oils, lavender can help counter depression, anxiety, tension, shock and emotional distress.

Neroli
Speeds up cell replacement so is extremely useful for rejuvenation, and in the treatment of scars and stretch marks. Distilled from orange blossom, neroli has a calming, strengthening and euphoric effect – and is an excellent tonic for emotional exhaustion, depression, insomnia, shock and stress.

Patchouli
Helps skin cell renewal so rejuvenating for mature or prematurely aged skins, 'turkey neck' or on scar tissue; an effective antiseptic, it can be used on inflamed or infected conditioners such as weeping eczema, dermatitis, ulcers. Relaxing yet reviving, patchouli is a warming and stimulating oil.

Rose otto *(Damask rose)*
Excellent for all skintypes but particularly beneficial for sensitive, highly coloured or ageing skins; it is also an extremely effective antiseptic. Strengthens fragile capillaries and so is particularly useful for rosacea. A spiritually uplifting and protecting oil.

Sandalwood
A soothing, lubricating oil ideal for sensitive, dry or neglected skins. Nourishes and protects older, papery skin. Good for anxiety/insomnia caused by emotional distress.

THE BASE OILS

Before you apply them to the skin, essential oils should be diluted with 'base' (or 'carrier') oils. (There are a few exceptions to this rule: tea tree, lavender and frankincense are safe to apply neat.) Use any of the following, or a combination of the oils. Experiment to find the blend that you prefer. 'Vegetable oils provide skin with nutrients, essential fatty acids – and have specific therapeutic properties,' explains Germaine. The following oils are widely available and particularly recommended in anti-ageing formulations.

Evening Primrose Oil	Regenerative and good for prematurely aged skins; using the contents of capsules – from health food stores – may be the most practical method
Jojoba liquid wax	*(more commonly known as jojoba oil)* Penetrates well leaving a protective, non-sticky, nourishing film; good for dry, sensitive skins and allergies
Sweet almond oil	Light and nourishing, with vitamin E and high in vitamin A, it helps relieve itching, soreness, dryness and inflammation
Wheatgerm oil	Featuring vitamin A and high in vitamin E; antioxidant. Good for dry, mature and prematurely aged skin and scar tissues

For facial oils, use a 1–3 per cent dilution, being sure to measure carefully. So to each 15ml of base oil, you add 3–9 drops of essential oils. 'Start with a 1 per cent dilution, and then move up to 3 per cent when you are familiar and comfortable with the oils' effect.' Essential oils are potent, explains Germaine, and in too high a concentration may in cause sensitivity. 'But even if you have very sensitive skin, you can use them: the most suitable oils for touchier complexions are sandalwood and rose.' Once you've mixed your facial oil, keep it in a glass bottle and out of direct sunlight, Germaine advises. Choose from any of the oils listed on the previous page – or blend two or three together, always staying within the dilution guidelines.

THE AROMATHERAPY MASSAGE

'To get maximum benefits, try to schedule the session so that it doesn't matter if the hair becomes oily,' says Germaine. 'Otherwise, tie the hair back from the face and remove clothes, so that the shoulders and décolletage can be treated. Cleanse and refresh the skin of the face and neck before you start.' She suggests doing the massage once a week (although facial oils can be used, without the massage, every night).

1 Rub one drop of frankincense essential oil over the palms. Start the massage on the head, to release tension.

2 Deeply massage scalp all over with fingertips to release tension; really get the skin moving over the scalp.

3 Place the pads of your spread-out fingers just on the hairline and make deep 'draining' movements from the hairline to the crown, starting at the forehead and temples and moving backwards through the hair. Do the same from the base of the skull, trailing fingers through to the ends of the hair. 'It gets the circulation going and releases tension,' explains Germaine. 'You can almost feel your scalp buzzing, straight away.' (If you prefer, wash hands before starting the actual massage.)

4 Pour about 5ml of blended oil (see box) into the palm of the hands. Rub the hands together and apply the oil with both hands in long, sweeping movements, across the décolletage, round the shoulders, up the neck, across the cheeks, over the nose and the forehead. Cover the whole area to be treated, circling the eyes lightly with the ring fingers being careful not to get the oil close to the eyes. Repeat the movements until the oil is well spread and the skin is warmed.

5 With the fingers of the right hand, knead the upper left arm, shoulder and up the back of the neck to behind the ear. Repeat on the right side with left hand. 'We all carry a lot of tension in our shoulders – and that can show up on our faces,' explains Germaine, 'so this is a very important part of the massage.'

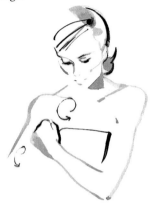

6 With the knuckles make circular, sweeping movements to the neck, shoulders, chest and upper arms. (If you are tense, this can be quite painful. That's normal.) Do one side at a time.

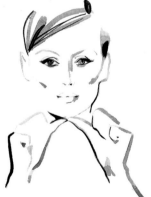

7 With the fatty pads of your thumbs under the chin, apply pressure up against the jaw-bone from the point of chin to the corner of the jaw-bone, moving the thumbs a short distance at a time. 'When you find an area that's sensitive or tender, just keep working on it gently, until it eases up.' Repeat the procedure from chin to jaw-hinge.

8 Place the pads of your fingers just on the jawline, gently touching (with the little fingers meeting). Press, then move the fingers along slightly. Press again. Keep moving the fingers to the edge of the jaw; go back to the beginning and start again. (For this – and the next two steps – be sure you aren't moving your fingers *over* the skin, but actually moving the skin and underlying muscle with the tiny circular movements.)

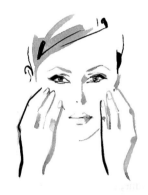

9 Using the pads of the fingers, which are now separated, make tiny, tiny circular pressures on the cheeks, in rows from the jaw-bone up to the top of the cheek-bone. Your little fingers should end up under the middle of each eye.

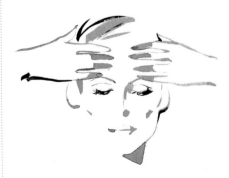

10 Using the pads of the fingers, apply small circular pressures in lines across the forehead, starting at the centre and finishing at the temples.

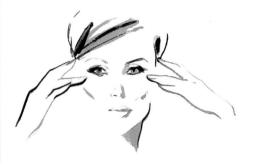

11 With the tips of your ring fingers, circle around the eyes on the socket-bones, inwards under the eyes towards the nose, up onto the eyebrows and outwards, to complete the circle. 'Do this ultra-lightly – absolutely no tugging,' says Germaine.

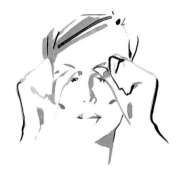

12 Place the thumbs just underneath the inner brow-bone and apply pressures upwards along the ridge of the eye socket, moving the thumbs slightly each time. Keep going till just about the mid-point of the brows. 'This is especially soothing if you suffer from headaches or eyestrain,' Germaine explains.

13 Place the pads of the fingers on the lower ridge of the eye socket-bone, and press. Then move the fingers slightly outwards and press again. Repeat.

14 Rub hands together vigorously and then cup the closed hands over the eyes. Take several deep breaths and sigh out tension.

Lisbeth Damsgaard

Lisbeth Damsgaard inspires us as a true natural beauty: pioneering founder of one of Europe's leading back-to-nature cosmetics and natural food brands – Urtekram. This Danish beauty (b. 1950), mother of Vanessa and Patrick (b. 1975 and 1980), is a shining example of what a truly healthy, organic lifestyle can do to make a woman glow from within...

'In the late sixties, young people were heading to India in droves – but because I wanted to study the system of healthy eating called macrobiotics, I headed for Japan. My imagination had been fired up by a slogan – "Eat Brown Rice and Make Revolution" – and I wanted to learn about the idea that food is your best medicine.

'Everyone gets the wrong idea about macrobiotics, thinking it's terribly strict. I learned that everyone's body needs different fuel, and that after you start to eat pure, clean, natural, fibre-rich food, your body starts to tell you what it needs to balance itself. Today, I eat a lot of seaweed, tofu and miso – "superfoods" – and I believe that my diet is the reason I feel so healthy.

'When I got back to Denmark, I opened a macrobiotic restaurant, juggling it with my social anthropology studies at university. The restaurant was an instant success; so many young people in Copenhagen wanted to eat healthily, at that time, I had queues down the street. Soon after, I met my husband Ronnie McGrail, who'd bought a little grocery store down the road and was introducing natural foods. He asked me to work with him. That was the start of Urtekram, one of Europe's first organic companies. In our cupboards today, you'll find only organic food. You have to clean up your own back yard before spreading the word to the rest of the world...

'I really worry about the number of chemicals that we are exposed to in daily life. And I started to question: if I care about what I'm putting in my body, shouldn't I be equally concerned about what I put on my skin? So Ron and I started playing with recipes and formulations, looking at old books, to develop effective cosmetics made with food quality ingredients – then finding ways to give them shelf-life without using chemical preservatives, using techniques like reducing the water in the recipe and using essential oils like rose.

'The products have won awards for being the most ecologically friendly shampoos, conditioners, body lotions and cleaning products it's possible to create. Now I'm working on skincare, including totally plant-based sunscreens. But at the moment, I'm using Carrot Cream by German natural company Logona*. When it comes to make-up, I'm interested in performance: I think Dr Hauschka* mascara is a good natural choice, but I'll often buy Helena Rubinstein or Christian Dior.

'Ronnie and I always liked to hike in the mountains, but it isn't practical when you're running a business and have small children. So we took up orienteering – following a course with a compass, a map and a stop-watch. It's an activity the whole family can enjoy. What I love is that when I'm trying to get to the next check-point, I am concentrating so hard it takes my mind off everything else. Once a week I also go to a two-hour exercise class with about 30 women of all ages in our village: stretching, weights and gentle aerobics and it's just fun.

'I'm not good at meditating but I try to find windows of time for myself. Sleep is crucial; I try to get seven hours. Friends laugh because in our old house, the bed was on the verandah and we would sleep outdoors on even the coldest night, snuggled under the duvet – but in our new house, we sleep indoors with all the windows and verandah doors open. I'm a slow riser so the older I get, the earlier I rise, to ease myself into the day. That private time with a cup of kukicha tea and a book, listening to birds, is essential to my well-being...

'I believe if you are active and take care of yourself, that's what counts. I am not so concerned about how I look; it's how I feel that's important. I laugh a lot. I love life; even if things are bad I always feel I want to hang on till the last breath – and I try to walk on the sunny side of the street.

'I feel it's important to go forwards and enjoy the adventure of ageing. Not look back with regret...'

skin supplements

Over the last few years, there has been a steady stream of nutritional supplements which claim specifically to improve your skin. Imedeen was the trail-blazer, followed by – among others – Renewal, Seven Seas Collâge, Caudalie, Nourella, NutriSkin Advanced Skin Nutrition, AnDante and Perfectil. Among the benefits of such products are said to be increased smoothness, reduction of coarse wrinkles, redness and fine lines, fading of age spots and increased skin thickness.

The problem with any supplement is that only a small percentage of whatever you take will end up on your skin. The dedicated skin supplement doesn't whizz straight there, bypassing, for instance, your pancreas and gall bladder. (Any more than any other supplement does.)

Much as with miracle creams, the marketing departments and PRs shower beauty editors with stacks of research to back up the claims. If you have the time and expertise to look at these closely, they often show only the most minute improvements – which probably wouldn't be visible to the naked eye. And it's likely that the more significant improvements found in research will be on women who were not already eating a good diet and/or taking other supplements – data that is almost never revealed by manufacturers.

We started out intending to test skin supplements for this book. In the end, we didn't for two reasons. Firstly, when we approached the manufacturers, they were – unlike the skincare companies – reluctant to let us have adequate supplies for a panel of ten women per supplement. Secondly, the manufacturers' own data shows that these supplements almost always take several months for any effect so a reasonable study period would be six to nine months: and, as we said, the manufacturers were not keen on giving us supplies for that amount of time. (Or could it be that they weren't that confident of their product?)

Before we tell you our opinion, here are the views of two authorities on nutrition and skin. Consultant dermatologist Dr Ian White, speaking for the British Dermatological Association, concluded they were basically a waste of time – and money. (Most of the rest was unprintable...) Nutritionist Kathryn Marsden, author of a book on skincare, said that, although you might benefit if you were taking no other supplements and/or you were not eating well and/or were under stress, a better option would be a really good multi-vitamin and mineral supplement. These contain antioxidants, usually a major ingredient in dedicated skin supplements.

Kathryn also recommends a supplement of Essential Fatty Acids (EFAs, also described as the active ingredient GLA, gamma linolenic acid, *see p.195*). Our experience is that these can have a rapid effect in improving skin feel. Kathryn herself takes Femforte and Mega GLA by Biocare, plus Blackmore's Bio-C. She also recommends Solgar's Advanced Antioxidant Complex – 'it's excellent' – and PharmaNord's Bio-Antioxidant.

However, Kathryn did notice a difference to her skin when she took Imedeen for three months. 'I wasn't taking any other supplements at the time and I was very stressed so I may have needed those nutrients but I did think I saw an improvement.' Imedeen, like Nourella, NutriSkin and Renewal, contains marine fish protein, (pulverised dogfish heads in the case of Imedeen) and the suggestion is that compounds in these can effectively improve skin texture. Supporters point to the fact that Japanese women who tend to have thick healthy skins habitually eat fish bones.

We have also had improvements with Imedeen – these showed up differently for all of us: skin firmness for Kathryn, thickness for Sarah, and a 'plumper' look to the skin for Jo. But it took time: three months for Kathryn, four and a half months for Sarah, and three and a half months for Jo.

A woman friend of ours, a health professional now in her fifties, swears by Imedeen because she says it helps her crocky back as well as her skin. An independent scientist admitted that this is entirely possible because, as we point out above, a supplement affects not only the skin but other organs as well.

In summary: dedicated skin supplements are very unlikely to harm anything except your purse but you are probably better off taking a good multivitamin and mineral supplement plus EFAs than buying a skin supplement alone. It goes without saying that your skin will benefit most from good food, fresh air and water – plus our favourite, lots of sleep. But we have all personally had good experiences with using Imedeen.

In the future, however, we may find that there is some hope in a pill – based on plant extracts. Stephen Terrass, Technical Director of Solgar, lists the compounds he believes may help make a difference...

THE NAMES TO WATCH

Stephen Terrass' hot tips

Never exceed recommended dose and if you feel you are experiencing any sensitivity or apparent reaction, consult a nutritionist. (*For more on supplements see p.204.*)

1 Proanthocyanidins
(a class of plant flavonoids) • protect skin collagen and enhance its repair • free radical scavenger • protect capillaries at skin's surface

2 Sulphur-based antioxidants
(e.g. l-cysteine, alpha lipoic acid); sulphur is a major component of skin, hair and nail tissue • protect against free radical damage • have a potent detoxifying effect

3 Carotenoids
(e.g. alpha and beta carotene, lycopene, etc.) • certain carotenoids reduce UV damage to skin tissue • protect against free radical damage • certain carotenoids enhance skin integrity through conversion to vitamin A

4 Essential nutrient antioxidants
(e.g. vitamins A, C and E, selenium, zinc) • protect against free radical damage • enhance collagen repair • generally promote skin healing

5 Detoxifiers remove toxins which may, for example, interfere with skin cell repair or trigger specific skin disorders such as acne, psoriasis, etc. Different compounds work on different parts of the body – liver (milk thistle, l-cysteine); cellular (try barley grass, chlorella, broccoli extract; intestinal (try psyllium seed husks, pectin)

flower power for face, body and soul

The way we feel in mind and body – both short- and long-term – is mirrored in our faces, according to London-based holistic facial therapist Joy Salem. ('No wonder my face looks like a map of the world,' commented 50-ish novelist Elizabeth Buchan.) Joy prescribes an individual regime for each client using facial massage, manual lymphatic drainage plus Dr Bach's flower remedies to restore tone, flexibility and colour and bring both sparkle and calm to the face. Dr Edward Bach's flower remedies were some of the first to be used in the West at the beginning of the twentieth century. He discovered that the extracts of various flowers were particularly effective at helping people deal with negative emotional states. Like **Madonna**, **Twiggy** and a galaxy of other stars we are both devotees of flower remedies so we asked Joy to give us the Dr Bach Flower Remedies which she felt would be most helpful to women at menopause. Take four drops in pure water at least four times daily, especially first and last thing, or as often as you feel the need.

Walnut Very useful at any time of change in our lives; helps us to move forward and to adapt to upheaval.
Mimulus Helpful in allaying day-to-day fears; eases tension until hot flushes subside and equally helpful for shy people who blush easily.
Impatiens Can restore calm and replace irritability with peace. **Larch** Use when you feel unable to cope any longer and also when you feel self-conscious and that all eyes are on you. **Crab Apple** Good when you're feeling hot and sticky during a hot flush, when your bed seems much too warm at night, or at any time when you are negatively obsessed with your looks. **Olive** Use when you feel irritable after losing sleep because of hot flushes. **Gentian** For despondency accompanying bouts of sleeplessness caused by discomfort at night.
Cherry Plum Helps keep extreme hormonal emotions under control.
Hornbeam Good when you feel suddenly overwhelmed by lethargy and fatigue. **Willow** Use against over-reaction and over-sensitivity to insignificant matters which can often turn to self-pity and crying, particularly if you feel past your 'sell-by' date, or opportunities have passed you by, or that you are of no more use since your children have grown up and left. **Sweet Chestnut** Helps deal with the deep sorrow that can arise from the feeling that life from now on will be full of emptiness and that you have missed opportunities. **Star of Bethlehem** For grief over lost youth and the feeling that part of you has died. **Schleranthus** For mood swings, indecision and volatility; helps restore emotional stability. **Rescue Remedy Cream** To counteract vaginal dryness and soreness during intercourse due to reduced levels of oestrogen.
NB Joy points out that if you are going through a really difficult time there is no substitute for consulting an experienced qualified practitioner in Dr Bach Flower Remedies.

facial fitness

Most doctors work themselves into a sweat explaining why facial exercises can't work. But many women swear by the gravity-defying powers of facial aerobics, even using them as an alternative to going under the surgeon's knife. So we asked Eva Fraser, the bestselling queen of facial workouts, to share some of her easy-to-follow facial exercises to get you glowing and fix specific facial flaws. (Find them also in her new book, video and audio cassette package, *Eva Fraser's Facial Fitness**)...

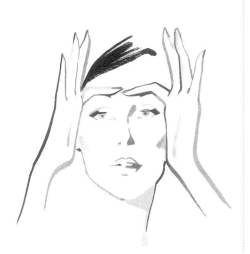

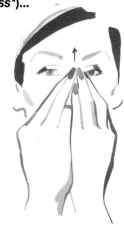

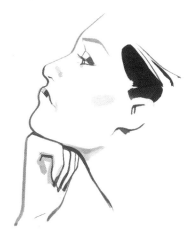

eyelid exercise

Look straight ahead into the mirror throughout this exercise.

1 Curve index (first) fingers under each eyebrow and gently push up – then hold against your brow-bone. Keep your fingers in that position.

2 Now close your eyes in five to ten very small downward movements. You should feel a gentle stretch in the upper lids.

3 Keep lids stretched downwards for a count of six.

4 Release the stretch slowly for three counts.

5 Open lids. Relax. Breathe deeply.

Repeat three times.

to eliminate lines on the bridge of the nose

1 Place pads of middle fingers firmly on the top of the bridge of your nose, just below any lines or bumps.

2 Place your index fingers each side of the bridge of your nose. Hold firmly.

3 Gradually move the muscles under your finger-hold in the direction of the arrow in five tiny, slow upwards movements.

4 Hold for a count of five, then slowly return in five movements.

5 Do this three times.

6 Stay relaxed, keep breathing and do not scowl!

NB The finger resistance must be held gently but firmly throughout.

turkey neck eliminator

1 With a straight spine, look straight ahead and tilt head up.

2 Then gently jut out your chin. At the same time, draw lower lip over top lip. DO NOT SMILE UP WITH MOUTH CORNERS.

3 For extra resistance, place first lightly under chin.

4 Now press tongue firmly against lower teeth in a forwards, upwards thrust. Feel the movement under the chin.

5 Hold for a count of five.

6 Slowly release the pressure.

7 Stay relaxed and breathe. Repeat three times.

Women who do facial workouts should see great improvements in just six weeks, says Eva. (See below for what one client thought.) Here are her other anti-sag secrets...

• 'Sleep with one pillow, not two, to avoid a double chin.'

• 'If you must read in bed – and I try to advise clients not to – then lie with your head on a single pillow and hold the book above you. If you lie propped up with the book balanced on your tummy, it's just asking for a double chin.'

• 'If you work on a computer, bring it up to eye level, for the same reason.'

• 'Improve your posture; if you stand straight, your face is less likely to sag. Imagine that at all times you are being pulled up by a piece of string from the centre of the top of your head.'

• 'I'm a big fan of Frownies* – which have been used by beautiful women for improving the lines on the forehead since 1898. They are small, skin-coloured adhesive papers that you stick onto the forehead so that you can't frown. Used regularly, they really do help frowns to disappear, making the forehead smoother.'

what Eva Fraser's facial exercises did for me...

AGE: 50-ISH • PROFESSION: INTERIORS CONSULTANT

'I started doing facial exercises because I wanted to look as good as I feel – which is terribly well. My particular problems were the lines going from either side of my nose to the corners of my mouth and my jawline slackening. I have a superstitious fear of the surgeon's knife so I wanted to try anything else first – but with no expectation of miracles. I had heard about Eva Fraser's programme from a friend and it seemed absolutely logical to me that if you work out your body and look quite different, then the same thing could happen to your face.

'I started off with the book; that was helpful but I wanted individual attention and analysis so I went to Eva's studio in London for a course of four private lessons.

'The first lesson takes one and a half hours, the next three are an hour long. During the first and second you learn all the basic movements, then the third and fourth you work the muscles against resistance – you have to hold on to each muscle at one end and work the other to make the muscle springier and shorter. You have to leave at least two weeks between lessons for the muscles to get strong enough to go on to the next stage.

'There are exercises for every part of your face – brow, nose, foreheads, the apple of your cheeks, around your eyes and mouth, jawline. Eva explains all the time which muscles she is working with and why. I understood immediately why it would work: for instance, if you do an exercise to tighten your cheek muscles, you can see it lifting the lower bit of your face.

'It takes at least 20 minutes a day for the first three months: you sit in front of the mirror with your own personalised set of drawings, trying to do things like wiggling one side of your nose up towards your outer eye in six movements. But you do feel your muscles getting stronger and you realise how few you use ordinarily. For the next three months, you do 20 minutes every other day, then you advance to about ten minutes on alternate days.

'Eva's programme is simple and sensible. The worst things are what you see in the mirror and the horrendous white cotton gloves which you have to wear to stop your fingers slipping when you do the exercises inside your mouth.

'After about two weeks, people started to say "you look awfully well" and I suddenly realised I was looking good and the only thing in my life that had changed was that I was now going to Eva. It has helped my face enormously. I don't know if it makes me look younger but it does retard the "Newton Effect" – everything falling down. The exercises to lift my cheek muscles have made the lines from my nose to mouth enormously better, and my jawline is more defined. Also my skin glows much more and is much smoother, probably because the exercises increase blood flow to the skin. The course is very good value and, as a bonus, I hardly ever need to use night creams now – Eva says your skin will balance itself in three days and she's right. I think external creams can give you a lift but they can't work as well as exercises like these. But facial exercises are like any other sort, if you give up everything starts going right back so you do have to keep on the maintenance programme.'

(See Directory for details of Eva's books, video and courses.)

fabulous facials for older faces

We go behind the masks, steaming, sloughing and pampering to find out which facials are best for older faces...

Facials are a luxury. For some women, they're a luxury they 'can't live without', to brighten dull and dingy skin – or to plump it up before an important event. Right now, there's a beauty salon boom in facials for older women. In mid-life, we're supposed to have more money – and (allegedly) more leisure – to indulge ourselves. And when we look in the mirror on a bad day and start to fret about lines that didn't seem to be there last week, a time-defying salon treatment can be extremely seductive. But not all facials are created equal. And not every mature skin will benefit. So here's what you should know before you put yourself in a beauty therapist's hands.

First of all, remember that no once-in-a-while treatment can make a significant long-term impact – although it can whisk away drab-looking dead skin cells, leaving your skin looking brighter and (depending on the ingredients) temporarily 'tighter', or 'lifted'. It's what you do to your skin on a daily basis – religiously cleansing, very lightly exfoliating (*see p.22*), moisturising and applying sun protection – which makes the long-term difference.

However, in a mature skincare regime, 'There is a place for facials,' believes Nelson Lee Novick, MD, associate clinical professor of dermatology at New York's Mount Sinai School of Medicine. 'If people want a nice, pampered experience and they have fairly normal skin, I don't have a problem with them having a facial.' But even people with normal skin are advised to wait six weeks between facials, warns Dr Novick – simply because too much of anything – like intense cleansing or even too-vigorous massage – can irritate the skin. Anyone with inflamed acne, rosacea (characterised by redness, pimples or enlarged blood vessels, *see p.62*) or skin conditions like eczema and psoriasis, should avoid facials, as they may aggravate the condition. If you're suffering an infection – such as impetigo or herpes – you should also forego a facial, for the time being.

According to Mary Lupo, MD, associate clinical professor of dermatology at Tulane Medical School in New Orleans, 'I've seen patients with flat warts that were manipulated and actually spread on their face.'

Susan Harmsworth, spa consultant and founder of the aromatherapy-based beauty therapy and skincare range E'SPA, says that women with sensitive skin – which is often a problem for menopausal women – should also be very cautious about facials. 'My advice, if you have sensitive skin, is to arrange for a "patch test" in the salon, before your facial. They can apply the products they're going to use on your face to an out-of-the-way area behind your ear, to establish there is no reaction.' If a salon won't accommodate this perfectly reasonable request, she says, go elsewhere.

The vast majority of mature skins, adds Susan Harmsworth, should not be steamed – a procedure which is still integral to many facials. 'Ask before your facial if there's steaming involved and say you want to skip that step,' she says. 'Don't let a beauty therapist try to persuade you; steaming can lead to broken capillaries.' (And in women suffering hot flushes, it can be extremely uncomfortable.) The only

our own favourite facials

Eve Lom (facialist to the rich and famous)
Decleor Aromaplasty Facial
Thalgomarine Collagen Facial
Aromatherapy Associates Rose Facial
Dr Hauschka Facial (which starts with your feet – because the state of your feet affects your face)
E'SPA Luxury Facial for mature/dry/dehydrated skins
Anne Sémonin (only available in Paris – but almost worth the pilgrimage)
Bliss Spa High Herbie (in which your feet, body and scalp get treated, too)

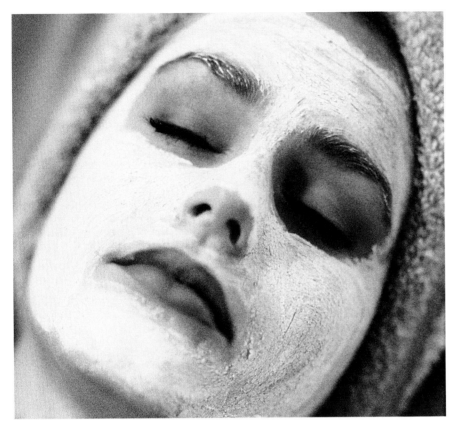

mature skins which can be safely steamed, she explains, 'are the 2 per cent of the population with sallow, tough, Mediterranean-type skin, which needs stimulation.'

Most facials consist of cleansing, exfoliation, massage, extraction, a mask and a finishing dab of moisturiser, before you go out into the world. If you use Retin-A or Retinova, make sure to tell the therapist beforehand; these skins should not be exfoliated at all as they have already been thinned by these prescription creams (see pp.30–31). Anyone with a tendency to broken capillaries should also ask for exfoliation to be skipped, according to Dr Lupo. AHAs – alpha-hydroxy fruit acids – can also be used as chemical exfoliants, as an alternative to the 'grainy' kind of scrub; again, these should all be avoided by any

woman with sensitive skin. (If in doubt, have the patch test, as recommended by Susan Harmsworth.)

One step that makes many of us particularly uncomfortable is 'extraction', or squeezing of the pores to remove blackheads and clean out clogged pores.

This should only ever be done to warmed skin, and manual squeezing, which is commonplace, makes dermatologists blanch. 'Sterilised implements are by far superior to the two-finger technique,' says Dr Lupo. If you squeeze in only two directions – with fingers – you can rupture the pore and send sebaceous material into the surrounding skin. By applying pressure with a "comedone extractor", the only way the stuff inside can go is up.'

Marcia Kilgore, meanwhile – who has an eighteen-month waiting list for

her facials at her Bliss Spa in Manhattan – advises women also to ensure that the right type of mask will be used on the face. 'Mature skins almost always need a hydrating mask, except in rare cases of oily skin,' she explains. 'Ask the facialist if the mask sets on the face – in which case it will be too drying for the skin; as the mud or clay dries out, it strips away the vital oils. Instead, you want a mask that stays moist throughout.' Marcia's favourite ingredient for mature skin masks is seaweed, although she warns it's not appropriate for anyone with an iodine allergy. (E'SPA's mud-mask facial, meanwhile, gets round the problem of over-dehydration by applying the mask over a layer of aromatherapy oil.)

Above all, the experts tell us, don't be bossed around (especially by a beautician who's probably young enough to be your daughter). So if, during any part of the treatment, you don't like what's being done to your face – or you feel claustrophobic – communicate that to the facialist and ask her to move right along to the next step. If you follow these guidelines you should emerge glowing beautifully. Not looking (and feeling) like you're having a hot flush...

KEY WORDS TO LOOK FOR IN A FACIAL

Mature
Moisturising
Replenishing
Hydrating
De-sensitising
Anti-ageing (although this may imply the use of AHAs, which are not suitable for women with sensitive skin).

TRIED & TESTED

─NON-SURGICAL FACELIFTS─

Non-surgical facelifts, using electrical tools, to stimulate the skin, are often trumpeted as the alternative to going under the knife. In our experience, they are terrific before an important meeting or a glam evening out – but trying to fit the prescribed series of regular frequent appointments in order to see any lasting 'anti-ageing' benefits would send most women's diaries into meltdown.

The bottom line is: can they really make a difference? We recruited a panel of willing volunteers with nothing to lose but their wrinkles – and were truly amazed by some of the results. Due to the high cost of treatments, the companies only felt able to offer two testers a full course of treatments or a machine to use at home. But when even two testers give a 10/10 mark, you know there's something good going on. Here are their experiences...

Integra Plus Facecare System
10 MARKS OUT OF 10
In this at-home treatment, probes glide over the face.
Improvements after the first treatment:
Tester 1: 'my skin looked very refreshed and felt very soft and smooth.'
Tester 2: 'my skin looked fresh, felt extremely soft, looked very smooth.'
Improvements after the second treatment:
Tester 1: 'skin looked clear and firmer and progressively better over the course; overall the machine was excellent.'
Tester 2: 'my skin looked smooth and clear and firmer.'
After the course was completed:
Tester 1: 'my face looked firmer and smooth, felt very soft and cleansed. I got comments from friends about how good my skin looked.'
Tester 2: 'my skin looked clearer, fresher, firmer and felt great; I very much enjoyed using this machine – my skin felt wonderful after each treatment and my friends commented.'
DOWNSIDE: **Tester 1:** 'I would have preferred to have someone else do it to me, as it would have been more relaxing.'
Tester 2: 'the time factor – each treatment takes 30 minutes to one hour and you're recommended to have one every three days for sixteen treatments, then one a week.'

SALON TREATMENTS

Medi-Wave 10
10 MARKS OUT OF 10
The advantage of this treatment over some others, according to our testers, was that it takes just ten minutes at a time.
Improvements after the first treatment:
Tester 1: 'skin felt softer and certainly looked clearer.'
Tester 2: 'skin and face felt "alive."'
Improvements after the second treatment:
Tester 1: 'as above, plus my cheeks felt tighter; my daughter said my jawline didn't look so flabby!'
Tester 2: 'much the same, but face felt less "tired".'
After the course was completed:
Tester 1: 'huge improvement; skin firmer and seems thicker! Cheeks, jawline and jowls tighter. It's taken ten years off my face; friends who hadn't seen me for a while said I was looking good for my age. I am now using the home treatment (Medi-Wave 5) to maintain the improvements; I would recommend it to anyone – better than buying a lot of expensive face creams and cheaper than surgery.'
Tester 2: 'at 60, I started at a disadvantage but can now see the difference. I don't think the evidence of where lines used to be will ever completely disappear, but my jawline is firmer and cheeks fuller. I am completely convinced of its anti-ageing effects.'
DOWNSIDE: **Tester 1:** 'none.'
Tester 2: 'slight pain in fillings which can be alleviated by using a gumshield; after every session, the pads left red marks but these disappeared after one hour.'

C.A.C.I.
9.5 MARKS OUT OF 10
Improvements after the first treatment:
Tester 1: 'skin looked visibly firmer; noticeable uplift.'
Tester 2: 'better! Smoother! Lifted! Skin felt softer, some fine lines were reduced a friend said my face looked "ironed out".'
Improvements after the second treatment:
Tester 1: 'on the next two to six visits, skin felt softer, as well as maintaining uplift; general improvement noticeable'.
Tester 2: 'I had an early appointment which

left me looking sleepy and tired for the rest of the day, but 24 hours later I could notice a definite improvement and my skin looked lifted and rested.'
After the course was completed:
Tester 1: 'definite improvement; my whole face looked firmer and the outline tighter; deep lines – including frown-line – are reduced. Right from the beginning, friends commented on improvements. It really boosted my confidence and took five years off my face.'
DOWNSIDE: **Tester 1:** 'none.'
Tester 2: 'none, other than the time involved.'

O-Lys Light Therapy
8.5 MARKS OUT OF 10
Improvements after the first treatment:
Tester 1: 'amazing! I look fresher, more awake and my face was visibly lifted'.
Tester 2: 'unrelaxing vile-smelling peel, too harsh for my skin (which has never minded anything); apparently most people sleep through it but I simply didn't enjoy it. Skin looked the same after treatment as before.'
Improvements after the second treatment:
Tester 1: 'there was quite a gap between my first and second visit so my face had "dropped"; afterwards, it was firmer, smoother, plumper – virtually restructured.'
Tester 2: 'the second treatment was more pleasant. Skin looked possibly fresher.'
After the course was completed:
Tester 1: 'my face and neck are firmer and younger-looking; my best friend said she had never seen my face look like this. The whole treatment is a real pleasure and the creams and serums used are non-allergic. A tremendous confidence-booster.'
Tester 2: 'definitely fresher. Can't do any harm and may do some good.'
DOWNSIDE: **Tester 1:** 'it's like finding the elixir of youth – but unfortunately the cost is a bit prohibitive for ordinary mortals. Also, the efficacy of the treatment is down to the practitioner's skills.'
Tester 2: 'the previously mentioned "disgusting" peel on my first visit; also, my nose and mouth peeled for four days afterwards.'

THE MAGIC OF MANUAL LYMPHATIC DRAINAGE...

Manual Lymphatic Drainage*, a form of massage, can be wonderful for tired-looking faces. MLD, as it's known, was developed in the 1930s by a couple called Emil and Astrid Vodder. It's a very light, rhythmic form of massage that works on the superficial lymph system, just underneath the skin – you may hardly feel the movements and wonder whether anything at all is going on!

Lymph is the clear fluid that oozes from a graze or a burn; it moves protein, water, white blood cells and electrolytes round the body. The more efficiently your lymph is flowing, the healthier your body - and the less puffy your face. Lymph also has a detoxing effect as it moves toxins to the lymph nodes, where they're pushed back into the bloodstream or out of the body, often via sweat in the armpit or groin.

In fact, some women report that MLD is a bit of an all-round wonder treatment: it not only gives the face a boost, but may have an effect on improving cellulite (*see p.182*) – and also, we've been told, can gradually fade scars and stretch marks. But there are some cautions: MLD may not be recommended in the case of active cancers, thrombosis, some cardiac problems or where there is a risk of embolism. Although therapists take a medical history before your first treatment, it's wise to mention if you have asthma, thrombosis, low blood pressure or thyroid problems.

salon safety

Don't take salons at face value, warns Barbara Simpson-Birks, a lecturer in beauty therapy and salon-owner, who is so concerned about the standards in some salons that she has established the Institut Distingué, to give a 'star' rating to beauty salons, covering staff, treatments, client-care, etc. Her advice is:

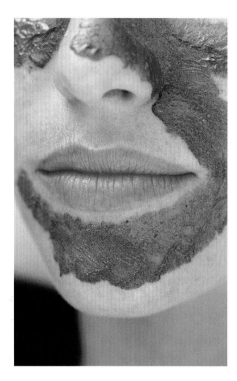

• 'Ask if the beauticians you will be seeing are qualified, how long they trained for (and what in); also ask how often they've carried out a particular treatment you're interested in. My experience is that good beauty therapists need to have been trained for at least two years – and practice makes perfect.'

• 'Check that the salon is adequately insured for public liability; many will display their certificate of insurance – usually for £1,000,000 up – on the walls; if not, you are perfectly within your rights to ask to see it.'

• 'Assess the overall hygiene of the salon. Are the floors clean? Is each customer given fresh towels? Ideally, there should be evidence of some form of sterilisation, for tweezers, cuticle clippers, etc. In the case of electrolysis, a new needle should be used for each client – so ask, to make sure. If there is a steaming machine, ask how often the water is changed (at least once daily is ideal, to prevent bacterial growth).'

• 'The staff themselves should look clean, tidy and presentable. Personally, I'm even happier if I see them wearing a uniform or protective white gown.'

lie back and relax

Eve Lom, top London facialist, prescribes facials every six to seven weeks – and believes they're not only good for skins, but for stress levels. 'A facial is a wonderful opportunity to take time for yourself to relax,' she says. To enhance the relaxing experience, she suggests using the facial to take time to meditate (she's a long-term devotee of Transcendental Meditation), or just to breathe deeply and rhythmically, from the abdomen. (See p.162 for the optimum breathing technique.) 'For many of us, it isn't practical to meditate daily, and we go through life not breathing to full capacity. A facial gives you time out to breathe perfectly for an hour or so.' And oxygenate your skin – from the inside out...

skin s.o.s.

Age spots, rosacea and sensitivity – resulting in redness and flare-ups –

are skin woes that can potentially trouble women more as the years roll by. More than

fine lines and wrinkles ever can, they often lead to feelings of vulnerability and anxiety.

So when your skin's sending out an S.O.S., here are the solutions...

ROSACEA – AND WHAT TO DO ABOUT IT...

The red patches of acne rosacea, which most often occur on cheeks and nose, can be a misery for women, causing immense emotional distress. thirty-plus women (and sometimes men) are most likely to be affected. There are four different phases in rosacea, according to leading cosmetic dermatologist Prof Nicholas Lowe**: the first is flushing and/or blushing; the second acne-like pustules and papules (small, raised red lumps); thirdly, permanently enlarged blood vessels (spider veins); finally, red, lumpy, bulbous enlargement of the noses (medically called rhinophyma). In rosacea keratitis, pustules and acne-like rashes can affect eyes and eyelids.

The underlying cause is a mystery, although different factors, including hormonal changes, can make it worse. Various triggers, particularly sunlight or heat, seem to stimulate chemicals in the body which cause the blood vessels to enlarge. Some foods, particularly coffee, chocolate, oranges, spices and alcohol may also act as triggers. Cosmetics including AHA-based creams may also make rosacea worse.

Camouflage make-up can work wonders. Several Hollywood stars rely on Laura Mercier's brilliant cover-up Secret Camouflage*. (*For tips on how to cover up rosacea, see p.74*).

Drug therapy includes antibiotics (usually tetracycline, which is safe for most people, even over long periods) or Rosex gel, Dr Lowe's preferred treatment. In the last extreme, Dr Lowe puts patients (though never women of childbearing age) on a very low dose of the drug Roaccutane.

Any redness, flushing and spider veins left after treatment can be removed by laser. Kathryn Marsden also suggests taking vitamins B1 and 2, and soothing skin with Bach Flower Rescue Cream*. She also suggests consulting a reputable nutritionist in case of digestive problems. Qualified Chinese herbal medicine practitioners also have a very good track record with skin conditions in general.

SUN SPOTS – AND WHAT TO DO ABOUT THEM...

Hyperpigmentation, an umbrella term for sun spots, age and brown/ liver spots, is a major skin woe for women. In lay terms, hyperpigmentation is an over-production of melanin, usually from cumulative over-exposure to the sun. If you spit-roasted in your twenties, sun spots – as we'll call them all – are almost a given. (Melasma is another type of hyperpigmentation usually triggered by pregnancy, the use of oral contraceptives, or in some women by hormone replacement.) Facially, it can range from a freckle to diffuse, all-over discoloration. By our forties, there's a 50 per cent probability that we'll develop at least one or two 'sun spots', which also appear on the hands, décolletage and the tops of the feet. Darker-skinned individuals are more susceptible to sun spots, say experts, than naturally fair people.

Zealous sun protection can protect against sun spots. And it's never too late to start. How to get rid of existing ones is a challenge that the cosmetic world is currently trying to overcome. Some attempted treatments have been drastic. According to Barbara Salamone, educational director of skincare company BioElements, 'Harmful ingredients like mercury have been used in skin bleaching products - and only recently banned worldwide because of their toxicity. People were poisoning themselves because they were unhappy with their skin colour.'

If you feel self-conscious about sun spots, good camouflage makeup (e.g. Laura Mercier's Secret Camouflage*) should be your first step. Safer lightening creams with ingredients such as fruit acids (AHAs and BHAs) may reduce sun spots, exfoliating the top skin layers while a bleaching agent, such as hydroquinone, a synthetic chemical, lightens the newly forming cells. But be aware that even the over-the-counter skin lighteners are potent creams – and have to be used *forever* to maintain results, so weigh that up in your mind before you go down the 'skin-bleaching' route...

High-dose hydroquinone creams are

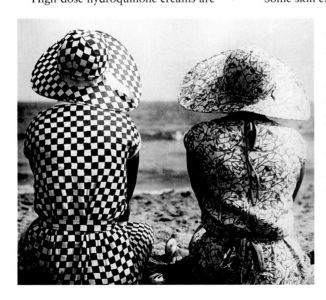

available only through dermatologists, but many over-the-counter formulations contain lower percentages. However, it can take two or three months of daily application for colour to fade noticeably. Naomi Lawrence, MD, assistant clinical professor of medicine in the division of dermatologist at the University of Medicine and Dentistry of New Jersey, advises creams should be applied using a magnifying mirror and a Q-Tip, to avoid bleaching the surrounding area.

Hydroquinone has downsides, too. Dr Daniel Maes, of Estée Lauder, says bluntly: 'It kills the skin cells.' Lydia Sarfati, chief executive officer and founder of Repêchage Skin Care, feels that chemicals such as hydroquinone 'assault the skin and are too harsh for use on the face.' The ultra-strict US Food and Drug Administration has approved it for cosmetic use but is now reviewing studies suggesting carcinogenicity when large quantities are fed to rats. Remember: a lot of what we put on our skin is absorbed into the bloodstream, so this isn't a concern to be instantly dismissed.

Some skin experts, meanwhile, are excited about an alternative, gentler fading agent from the Orient: kojic acid, derived from mushrooms. Unlike hydroquinone, kojic acid can be used all over the face. According to Jan Marini, who has a signature skincare line, it will lighten dark areas but not bleach normal skin colour. 'Kojic acid also helps over-pigmented areas left by

acne lesions,' she adds. We recommend patch testing any skin lightening cream on the inner forearm, and waiting 24 hours to see if there is any redness, itching, burning or irritation, before applying to the face.

Confusingly, products are now appearing on the market labelled 'Whitening' or 'Brightening'; they aren't intended to bleach or whiten the skin at all but to enhance translucency and luminosity. (Most contain vitamin C derivatives or, in some cases, extracts from sheep or cow placentas.) So, if you specifically want to fade sun spots, make sure you get the right product.

Unfortunately, the effects of any of these treatments for sun spots will only last as long as you use the product. And be aware: maintenance means a serious daily commitment to SPF plus sunscreen, outdoors *and* in, because the skin becomes 'photosensitized', i.e. susceptible to UV rays. If lightened skin is exposed to the sun, it produces even more melanin and you could end up worse off than you started.' (Prof Nicholas Lowe maintains that this applies even if you're not going outdoors; 'If you don't apply a sunscreen every day your skin will respond to the sun and start to go darker – even if the sunlight is coming through a glass windowpane...')

Retin-A and Retinova can both help to fade sun spots and, more drastically, skin peels and laser treatments (*see pp.30 and 145*). But remember, whatever technique you resort to, sun spots will return – unless you stay away from the sun.

We would also urge a little self-acceptance. We like the philosophy of BioElements' Barbara Salamone. 'Love those sun freckles,' she says. 'Love the skin you're in...'

SENSITIVE SKIN – AND WHAT TO DO ABOUT IT...

63 per cent of all women report having sensitive skin. For many of us, the problem becomes worse as we get older because the skin's ability to keep the outside world *out* and the inside world *in* is increasingly reduced. Three factors influence this: tiny cracks appear on the surface which, literally, open the door to irritants; skin thins – due to sun damage and/or ageing; and dryness, a natural side-effect of ageing, compounds the problem.

Sensitive skin is most reactive when a woman is aged about 45–50, according to Dr Daniel Maes**; skin is thinner and there are also the hormonal challenges of menopause to cope with. This touchy skin scenario isn't helped by the fact that, as we get older, we tend to use more products and increasingly heavy formulations to make up for what our skin's losing: ultra-rich night creams, heavy-duty exfoliants, fruit acids, strong cleansers, as well as a wide range of spot-targeted cosmetics for everything from necks to heels, designed to fight the ravages of time.

Although we believe more is more when it comes to moisturising, surveys reveal that by mid life, the average American woman is using 15–20 products – containing as many as 200 different chemicals – on her skin every single day. The average British woman probably isn't far behind. And as Manhattan dermatologist Dr Debra Jaliman, MD observes: 'When skin encounters so many chemicals the chance of developing a reaction is increased.'

Sensitivity is linked to a disruption of the skin's 'barrier function' – the primary job performed by the dead cells and lipids (fatty, moisturising natural ingredients in the skin) which constitute the outermost 'barrier' layer of skin. Harsh cleansing, too much exfoliation, or not enough moisturiser during a brutal winter can all affect the barrier. Minute cracks develop that are not usually visible to the eye, allowing hostile irritants to penetrate down into the dermis.

Unfortunately, scientists now believe that sensitive skin actually ages faster. Faced with an irritant, two things happen to your skin. The first is immediate – and visible – itching, burning, stinging and redness. The second may be invisible until too late.

Trying to defend itself, the body releases substances that destroy collagen and elastin, the vital proteins which support the skin. The new wrinkle-busting 'resurfacing' treatments used by dermatologists and some anti-ageing skincare products (which work by triggering inflammation) can also contribute to sensitivity, leaving skin even more vulnerable to pollutants such as UV rays and smoking.

The silver lining to this cloud is that, in Dr Maes's experience, skin sensitivity often calms down of its own accord after the menopause. In the meantime, avoid aggressive skincare, limit exposure to potential irritants, concentrate on protecting the skin from future damage – and consider exercising caution when it comes to anti-ageing products...

sensitive skin checklist

▷ **Keep it simple: use a minimum of products and avoid those that weaken the skin's barrier function, i.e. exfoliants and AHA creams**

▷ **Stay out of the sun – minimising the risk of an irritating interaction between chemicals in skin products and the sun**

▷ **Look for products that are labelled fragrance-free, or hypo-allergenic – although this is no guarantee that they won't trigger a reaction**

▷ **Protect the skin with an SPF15 reflective sunscreen (look for the words titanium dioxide high up the ingredients list)**

▷ **If you are really sensitive, patch test new products before using them on your face – either on your forearm or behind your ear, where it won't show; be alert for itching, stinging, redness or a feeling of heat. (You can do this using an in-store tester, rather than invest in the cream itself)**

▷ **Never change your entire skincare regime all at once; introduce products one by one so that you can establish what you're reacting to**

▷ **If you boost your overall health – through eating well and exercising – you may find that skin becomes more tolerant as your overall immunity improves**

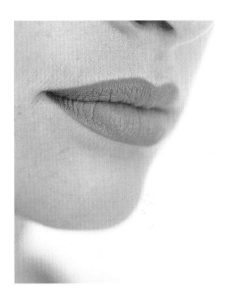

FACIAL HAIR – AND WHAT TO DO

Do you live in dread of turning into a bearded old lady? Well, so do we.....
One of life's cruel tricks is to send facial fluff production haywire around menopause. Even women who've never been bothered before can find hairs start sprouting more noticeably - particularly on the upper lip. Then there are those single, wiry hairs which make a break for freedom...
The reason? 'Hairs usually have a hormonally controlled, natural growing cycle, with a cut-out mechanism,' explains Dr Andrew Markey*. 'At menopause, the cut-out mechanism in some hairs fails to kick in so they go on getting longer.' (Annoyingly, excess facial hair in women, like men, can go in tandem with thinning scalp hair.)

Single stray hairs can be plucked with an efficient pair of tweezers. (We swear by Tweezerman's and Rubis tweezers*.) If you're too short-sighted to spot them, make a pact with your nearest and dearest friend, or a trusted beauty therapist, to tell you if you're sprouting.

Options for removing facial hair:

Bleaching Jolen Cream Bleach is the DIY favourite; however, excessive use of bleaching products containing hydrogen peroxide can irritate sensitive skin.

Depilatories Notorious for itchy itches and odorous odours but new formulations have reduced problems by adding soothing ingredients and masking chemical smell. These products may still be perilous for those with truly sensitive skin – so again, do a patch–test, use a product specially targeted at facial hair, for recommended time only. You will stay smoother for around two weeks.

Waxing Salon or home waxing will keep you smoother longer; fine hairs appear in around two weeks, thicker growth in four to six weeks. But remember, you need around 5mm–1cm regrowth before you can wax again.

Threading Two intertwined threads roll across the skin catching hair and pulling from the root. Painful! and only available at a few beauty salons. Same regrowth as plucking.

Electrolysis Fine needles conduct a very low electric diathermy current to destroy hair. There's a high pain factor and since up to 30 per cent of hairs are dormant at any one time and won't be affected by the treatment, you will need a series of treatments. Duration and frequency of sessions vary widely depending on the size of area to be treated, number of follicles and any previous treatment – if you have recently waxed or tweezed, it takes longer. Make sure you consult a qualified electrolysist*; if electrolysis is done badly, it may create scarring. Destroying the follicle by galvanic tweezer removal is another form of electrolysis as is transdermal electrolysis, which uses a probe and an ionised gel (rather than a needle) to transmit the current via the skin to the hair follicles. It claims to avoid swelling, bruising, scabbing or scarring, but as yet is only in limited distribution. All forms of electrical hair removal can leave red marks which may last for some days.

Epil-Pro* A new and very successful technique where tweezers grab the hair as thousands of sound waves pass through it in a fraction of a second. There is minimal pain, irritation and damage to surrounding tissues.

Laser hair removal Various different laser-type systems are now in use, including the Ruby laser (Prof Nicholas Lowe's laser-of-choice), PhotoDerm and SofLight, the first laser to get FDA approval in the US for hair removal. The best results with Ruby and PhotoDerm are in women with dark, coarse hair against pale skin; grey, white, ginger and fine downy hairs respond poorly because there is not enough pigment for the laser to focus on. Coloured women are generally advised not to have laser treatment as it could affect their pigmentation but the manufacturers of SoftLight claim that because its laser beam doesn't target melanin, unlike Ruby and PhotoDerm, it can be used on all skin and hair colours.

But – Prof Lowe suggests being very cautious. 'You can set up a laser hair-removal clinic with one day's training; there are virtually no studies of long-term effects and initial promises of permanent hair removal are already being rewritten, as it emerges that about 30 per cent of hairs grow back.'

Always follow manufacturers instructions for at-home treatment.
If you are anxious, consult your doctor and ask for a referral to an appropriate dermatologist.

how to win the war against the big wrinkler

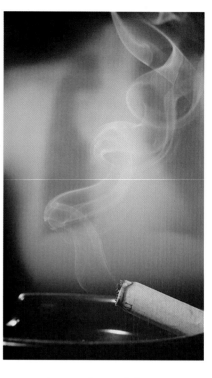

Most smokers know there's nothing good to be said about the habit. It can make the smoker – and other people ill – very ill. It's very expensive. And when it comes to beauty, it's Public Enemy No. 1, causing almost as many wrinkles as the sun.

FACTS TO TELL YOUR SMOKING MIND

- Smoking increases the likelihood of your getting lung cancer, breast cancer, pneumonia, stomach cancer, oesophageal cancer (gullet), myeloid leukaemia, artherosclerosis (clogging of the arteries) and osteoporosis.
- The death toll globally due to cigarettes is greater than both World Wars, estimate experts.
- Five women in the UK die every hour from smoking related diseases – that's one woman every 12 minutes, 42,500 every year.
- Women who smoke 20 cigarettes a day could be quadrupling their risk of breast cancer.
- Lung cancer is set to overtake breast cancer as the biggest cancer killer of women.

Problem is that although most smokers really want to give up, nicotine is a highly addictive substance – just like cocaine or heroin. Most people become physically dependent on nicotine within a few weeks of starting smoking. Nicotine hits your brain rapidly (within seven seconds) and because it leaves the body quicker, smokers reinforce the habit with tens, and more often hundreds, of puffs every day.

Nicotine makes smokers psychologically as well as physically dependent. It's a friend against the world, pepping you up or calming you down. And, totally illogically, it gives insecure people the illusion of self-confidence. 'My cigarette was my emotional breastplate against a frightening world – even though I knew it was really just a handful of chopped up, dried plants in a paper wrapper,' one ex-smoker told us.

The key to giving up, according to experts, is to understand that your mind thinks about smoking on two levels – which can be totally contradictory. Although the conscious mind can know and respect all the bad things about smoking, the powerful pre-conscious mind – the one targeted by tobacco advertisers – can override all your best intentions. With the help of advertisements and, of course, other smokers' examples – from parents long ago to friends and role models now – it can reassure you smoking is just fine. Of course, you need it – to relax, keep thin, be social. Of course, you will give it up. But not just yet.

Kicking the habit is seldom easy but it is possible. (Sarah used to smoke three to four packs a day, but stopped puffing more than fifteen years ago. What's more, she didn't put on weight.)

Remember, however seductive it may feel, smoking is the biggest enemy ever to health, wrinkles and well-being. Here's how to wage war on the weed.

THE QUIT CAMPAIGN

1 Set the date, make it the No. 1 priority in your life. Pick a mid-cycle date if you can – PMS seems to exacerbate withdrawal symptoms.

2 Rehearse the arguments for giving up, write them down as emotionally as you can, then tape them on a cassette recorder so you can play it back when you're feeling tempted. Be honest about your feelings about cigarettes – then ask yourself whether they make sense.

3 Make a list of the benefits, e.g. helping your skin, stopping a smoker's cough, spending less on dry cleaning, having fresh breath, getting on better with non-smoking friends, not having to dive out first thing in the morning or last thing at night for emergency supplies. Estimate how much it will save you and list how you will spend that money.

4 Keep a smoking diary so you can identify your personal cues for a puff (e.g. coffee time, talking on the phone, after a meal, having an argument, in a bar) and then avoid them if possible, when you first give up. (Later, you can challenge yourself by exposing yourself to cue situations.)

5 If you can't avoid cues, plan diversions or activities which are incompatible with smoking, e.g. drinking fruit juice (cigarettes taste vile afterwards), taking exercise, or confine yourself to no-smoking zones.

6 Give your fingers something to fiddle with e.g. worry beads, tapestry or executive toys.

7 Tell friends, family, work colleagues. Ask them for positive feedback when you get to the end of each smoke-free day, week, month.

8 Consider joining a support group such as Nicotine Anonymous where you can share the experience with fellow addicts.

9 Ask your doctor, health practitioner or pharmacist about nicotine replacement therapy (patches, gum, inhalator or nasal spray). It can't give motivation but it can aid giving up. But remember, it's still nicotine so don't continue longer than you need.

10 Explore smoking cessation therapy, e.g. hypnotherapy, cognitive behavioural therapy, acupuncture.

Last thing on the evening before, get rid of all your cigarettes, ashtrays and any smoking trophies such as lighters. (Use your global match book collection to light soothing scented candles...)

TIP

'If you're going through a particularly stressful period when you're quitting cigarettes, take a herbal stress remedy such as Bach Flower Remedies Rescue Remedy,' advises Robert Brynin, director of the British-based National Health Association, a medical research company that runs stop-smoking clinics countrywide.

GIVING UP

1 On the day, quit completely. Chances of success go up ten times if you don't smoke at all on the first day.

2 Drink plenty of fluids to get rid of the toxins, particularly pure water and fruit juices.

3 Remember you're giving up one day at a time. You only have to get through to midnight. If you're tempted, tell yourself that if you want to smoke tomorrow, you can chain smoke a whole pack. Then replay your tape.

4 If you do lapse, don't beat yourself up. Treat it as a lesson to be learnt: ask yourself 'why did I do it? what was going on in my mind? what can I do differently?' Tell yourself that one cigarette doesn't mean you have to be a smoker again. Get rid of all the evidence, air the room, change your clothes and play your tape.

5 At the end of every smoke-free day, revel in the fact that you've kicked it a day at a time and you're on your way to a clean bill of health, a fatter purse and a smoother, fresher-looking face.

the good news about giving up smoking

• After 48 hours, your taste buds and sense of smell will work much more keenly – food, wine, your favourite scent will take on a new delight

• After 72 hours, you will breathe more easily – wheezes will evaporate – and your energy levels will zoom upwards

• After two to twelve weeks, your circulation will improve and walking and running will require less effort

• After a year, your chances of heart disease will go down by half

• After ten years, your risk of suffering from (potentially fatal) lung cancer will be reduced by between 30 and 50 per cent.

glossary

For advanced readers only! If you just want to find out which creams our testers judged the best, keep turning the page. But every week, it seems, we hear about baffling new 'wonder' ingredients. Making sense of it all requires more than a heartfelt wish to get rid of wrinkles: it sometimes feels like you need a science degree. (And a sense of humour.) For label-hounds and anyone as fascinated as we are by what makes today's skincare more effective than ever, here's a run-down of the key ingredients in today's 'wonder creams'.

AHAs (also known as alpha-hydroxy acids, a family of skincare ingredients that includes lactic, citric, malic, glycolic and tartaric acids) These brighten the complexion by loosening the bonds in the skin, helping to get rid of the flaky 'dead' top layer and speeding up cell renewal. The key here is to think 'acid': these are generally too harsh for sensitive complexions. (*For more on AHAs, see p.34.*)

Antioxidants (*See p.13 for the low-down on antioxidants.*)

BHAs (also known as beta-hydroxy acids) First cousins to AHAs, these also brighten skin by speeding up exfoliation. Many dermatologists say they're gentler on the skin than AHAs.

Blue copper So far vitamins have dominated the skincare scene but dermatologists are now looking at the anti-ageing potential of minerals, too. Osmotics were the first company to introduce blue copper (in a moisturiser of the same name), which helps to prevent free radical damage by activating an antioxidant skin enzyme superoxide dismutase – aka SOD! Blue copper also seems to stimulate collagen production and is used in hospitals for wound healing.

Ceramides These lipids, made in the lab to a natural blueprint (and sometimes genetically engineered) help stabilise skin structure by retaining moisture in the skin – making them a valuable anti-ageing ingredient.

Collagen If only skincare was as simple as slapping on collagen to top up your skin's own natural supply. Alas, it doesn't work like that; using a collagen cream certainly won't add to your own supplies. However, collagen is an efficient humectant – it actually attracts water to the skin – so it is a highly effective moisturising ingredient.

Elastin Like collagen, elastin is a vital part of the skin's connective tissue network but, again, putting elastin in a moisturiser won't top up the skin's reserves although it creates a good barrier for locking in vital moisture.

Emu oil Another case of 'watch this space': emu oil – rich in collagen, linolenic and oleic acids – has been used by the Australian Aborigines for centuries and is now being trialled as a skin-rejuvenator. At Boston University Medical Centre, studies on animals found the oil produced a 20 per cent increase in skin production, 80 per cent in hair production. According to Michael Horlick, professor of medicine, physiology and dermatology at Boston University Medical Centre, 'This is the first real evidence to suggest the oil could stimulate skin and hair growth. Skin cell reproduction rose dramatically, which meant the skin became thicker and hair follicles became more robust.'

Enzymes In washing powder and contact lens cleaners, enzymes are used to break down dirt and oil, but inside every human body there are thousands of these proteins which act as kick-starts to, for instance, digestion of food and the metabolism of stored fat. Recently, the beauty industry has woken up to what enzymes can do for skin. Some skincare actually incorporates botanically derived enzymes, such as ingredients from papaya (papain) and pineapple (bromelian) which exfoliate and brighten skin. Other creams are formulated to have an enzymatic activity. Today, skincare is incorporating enzyme activators designed to quench the production of natural 'bad-guy' enzymes, collagenase and elastase which damage collagen and elastin. According to David Adhoot, technical director of D-D Chemi-co, a supplier of raw materials to the cosmetics industry, 'Influencing enzymes is going to be the next big trend – one with tremendous scope, including everything from skin firming to slimming to protecting.'

Humectants Valuable ingredients in moisturisers or facial sprays which attract moisture from the air to the surface of the skin. Commonly used humectants includes glycerine, sorbitol, squalene and urea. (Yes, that's right.)

Liposomes High-tech skincare 'rockets' which can be launched into the epidermis to deliver their moisturising cargo deeper than would otherwise be possible, so helping to fill in the gaps between the intercellular cement.

Lycopene Coming up fast in the antioxidant stakes, lycopene is an exceptionally strong free-radical scavenger, extracted from tomatoes, pink grapefruit, red guava, watermelon and the skin of red grapes. One study has found that lycopene deficiency is associated with skin changes, including acne and dermatitis. It was first spotted by European pharmacists, who observed that Hungarian girls achieved radiant skin by rubbing tomato pulp on their face and bodies, but it has taken until now for lycopene's potential to be realised by the cosmetic industry as a weapon against photo damage.

Milk proteins Expect to hear more about ingredients derived from your daily pinta. Milk proteins have been discovered to smooth and firm while inhibiting irritation. (This is the equivalent to the dermatologist's Holy Grail, since many potentially effective ingredients are ruled out because in trials they have caused rashes, redness or irritation.)

Nanospheres A fancy term for minute, rounded particles.

Oxygen Will oxygen turn out to be the Next Big Thing in Saving Our Skins? We say: don't hold your breath. (*See p.36 for more on oxygen creams.*)

pH This is a term often seen on packaging, denoting acid balance. Your skin is naturally slightly acid, with a pH between 4.5 and 5.5. The correct balance can be disturbed by the use of soaps (most of which are strongly alkaline) and some cosmetics which are not acid-balanced, potentially triggering irritation. If you see the term 'pH-balanced' on packaging, it often denotes that it is designed for sensitive skins.

Poly-hydroxy acid (aka glyconolactone, or G4) Yet another of the fruit acid family, recently introduced by the same scientist who had the first patent on AHAs, Eugene Van Scott, MD, who says that the ingredient can be tolerated even by people with rosacea or atopic dermatitis (who are extremely poor candidates for other acids). The molecule is smaller than an AHA molecule, so is absorbed into the skin at a slower rate, reducing the potential for tingling or burning on application. (Once in the skin, the molecule is converted into acid, which dissolves the 'glue' that attaches dead cells to the skin's surface. Hence its skin-brightening effect.)

Proanthocyanidins (grapeseed extract, pine bark extract, bilberry extract) These are super-potent antioxidants (*see p.13*) and causing a lot of excitement in the beauty world. French researchers started tracking these proanthocyanidins in the fifties, as they looked at a scurvy cure dating back four centuries, when a crew of landlocked explorers who'd run out of food managed to beat scurvy with a tea made from the needles and bark of nearby pine needles. Applied topically to the skin, they are powerful neutralisers of free radicals; expect these mega-

antioxidants to turn up in more and more creams soon.

Pycnogenol This French maritime pine bark extract contains antioxidant elements which neutralise the free radicals that attack the body's cells, helping to prevent the breakdown of collagen and elastin. Pycnogenol can also strengthen capillaries.

Retinyls/retinols Ingredients derived from vitamin A are now widely used in anti-ageing products (*see p.32 for more information*); they can be helpful in enhancing skin radiance and maintaining the complexion's smoothness.

Salicylic acid A 'beta-hydroxy acid' (BHA), which was first synthetically produced in 1860 as a treatment to reduce aches and pains, later used as a wart-removing cream – and since the 1980s has been incorporated into anti-ageing skincare.

Tea (black tea, green tea) The key ingredient in tea is polyphenolic acid, which acts on the skin as a powerful free-radical scavenger – meaning that tea is yet another ingredient in the armoury of antioxidants being used in high-tech skincare. Preliminary studies have shown that topical and ingested doses of either green or black tea extracts protect against sunburn and skin cancer induced by sunlight; scientists are currently trying to identify the specific mechanisms that provide this protection. Green tea also acts as a skin-calming ingredient, which is why you may find it teamed with others that have a potentially irritating effect to 'balance' the formulation.

the make-up facelift

'More women should explore what make-up can do for them before taking a leap into the world of cosmetic surgery. Get a makeover, have some fun with colour, learn some techniques that can make you look wellgroomed and colour coordinated. You can spend a few pounds on make-up and a great haircut – and maybe save yourself thousands on a facelift.'

DR ANDREW MARKEY, DIRECTOR OF DERMATOLOGICAL SURGERY AND LASER UNIT
AT ST JOHN'S INSTITUTE OF DERMATOLOGY, LONDON

FOUNDATION COURSE

We asked the world's leading make-up artists for their secrets of the flawless finish – because great-looking skin needn't be the preserve of fresh-faced teenagers...

When it comes to make-up guidelines for older faces, most make-up artists come up with three words: Less Is More. 'Foundation isn't plaster,' says Kevyn Aucoin. 'It can't be used to fill in lines and wrinkles. In fact, if you try to apply foundation, concealer and powder over laughter lines in the hope of camouflaging them, the opposite happens. You draw attention to them.'

However, foundation and powder can 'lift' older skin in a few seconds. 'If you're looking for one product that makes a huge difference to older women, it's foundation,' says Trish McEvoy. 'Skintone naturally becomes more uneven as we age. Perfectly applied, foundation smooths the complexion, so making it look younger and fresher again...'

STEP-BY-STEP GUIDE TO FLAWLESS FOUNDATION

Great faces, the professionals all agree, start with the 'perfect canvas'. So here are the insider secrets on how to create a flawless base...

1 Wash your hands. Never apply make-up with dirty hands; you spread grime – and germs – over your face.

2 Moisturise, then ideally wait ten minutes or more before applying foundation, or you'll find that it disappears very quickly. (The exception is if you use an oil-free foundation formulation, which can go straight over moisturiser without slipping.)

3 The golden rule with foundation is: get exactly the right colour and apply it where you need it most. (*See p.72, Finding Your Perfect Match.*) You might think you need it all over, from hairline to jawline. 'That's *never* true,' according to Laura Mercier. 'Older skins only need foundation where there are shadows, darkness or broken veins. That may include: the inner-most corner of the eye on the "nose-bone" (which most women overlook), the inner half-circle under the eye, on broken veins either side of the nose, and just under the corners of the mouth, which can be shadowy in some women. These are the key places that foundation can make the face look instantly younger. The rule is: what is dark, make light.' (Where you do *not* usually need to apply foundation is to the laugh lines at the outer corner of the eyes and upper cheek. 'The reason for applying foundation or concealer is to disguise discoloration – and the laugh lines usually aren't discoloured,' observes Laura.) Mary Greenwell's advice for disguising dark circles, meanwhile, is to lighten them – but not to obscure them completely. 'I find that if you totally disguise them, it takes the character out of the face – and it can look like a mask.'

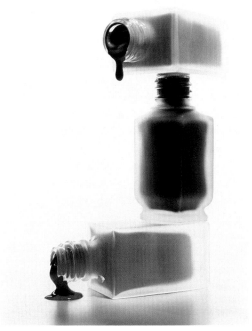

4 Trish McEvoy believes in using a Q-Tip to dot the foundation on the skin. (She makes special longstemmed versions*, which can reach easily to the bottom of a foundation bottle). This makes it easier to get the foundation exactly where you need it, and to apply just the right amount; if you tip foundation from the bottle onto your fingers, it's easy to get too much foundation – and then be tempted to rub it all into your skin...

5 Blend foundation into skin using fingers or a damp, squeezed cosmetic sponge (available at make-up supply stores and from many beauty counters), whichever suits you best. (Many make-up artists actually like to work with their fingers, warming the make-up as they go.) 'If you use a sponge, work the foundation well into it before you put the sponge to your face, to ensure it goes on evenly,' advises Laura Mercier. Also apply foundation to the eyelids. 'Veins and blueness show up here as we age,' observes Trish McEvoy. Use foundation to create as smooth a base as possible for eyeshadow, then set the foundation with powder.

6 If you need extra coverage in some places, you can either layer on a little extra foundation where required – or use concealer. 'When applying make-up, think 'layers",' says Laura Mercier. 'You don't want one thick layer of foundation, but you can build it up where you need extra help.' Many make-up artists use a brush to apply concealer, then pat with a finger, warming the concealer on the skin and almost pressing it into the complexion. 'If you smear concealer on with your finger, you can wipe the foundation right off, at the same time,' points out Trish McEvoy.

7 Make sure the foundation is beautifully blended so that you can't see where your skin starts and the foundation ends. 'The biggest mistake, as we age, is not blending enough,' observes Mary Greenwell. 'You have to do your makeup in the best possible light – I prefer daylight, facing a window – and blend, blend, blend. And a magnifying mirror is a must if you can't see well.' (Actually, we suggest making up in the coldest, most northerly light that's available to you. If you look good there, you'll look good everywhere.) Once you've powdered, there's no more opportunity for blending.

8 Most make-up artists we know advise applying powder with a velours powder puff, rather than a brush – which can over-load the face and settle chalkily into fine lines. (Many make-up artists' lines – from M.A.C. to Trish McEvoy, Bobbi Brown to Vincent Longo – make velours puffs, which you can also find at beauty supply stores. These are not to be confused with old-fashioned swansdown puffs, which will deliver way too much powder – as do the big, fluffy powder brushes that you'll find in many make-up lines. Mary Greenwell, however, is one of the make-up artists who likes to apply powder with a brush – but she gets round the problem of overdoing it by using a small, 2cm (3/4 inch) brush (hers is by Shu Uemura*). 'This is small enough to make it easy to avoid getting it in any crinkles - and highlighting them.' If using a brush, always sweep powder lightly downwards on the face, never upwards – or you'll accentuate pores and hairs. (The same applies to blusher and foundation.)

9 Use loose powder, in preference to pressed powder, for morning make-up. (You can carry pressed powder with you for daytime touch-ups.) 'Press the *edge* of your puff into your loose powder,' advises Bobbi Brown. Then thwack the puff once or twice on a hard surface – like the edge of a washbasin, or the palm of your hand – to shake off any excess. 'Then press the powder into your foundation, again using the edge of the puff.'

10 Make-up artists all agree that excess powder – which tends to settle into lines – is extremely ageing. 'So if there's too much powder on the skin after applying with the velours puff, I use a bigger, fluffy brush to whisk away the excess,' explains Bobbi Brown. (NB Sometimes Trish McEvoy avoids the use of powder altogether on older skins. 'Experiment with just pressing the puff itself onto your foundation to absorb the extra oil,' she advises. 'You may find that's all you need to do to blot the shine.')

FINDING YOUR PERFECT MATCH

Most of us were raised in an era when you learned to test make-up on your hand. But hands are usually darker than our faces, because they get more UV exposure than almost anywhere else. So the best place to test foundation is on the jawline and the lowest part of your cheek. The perfect shade will 'disappear' into your skin, so that you almost can't see that it's there. 'Carry a mirror with you so that you can do the natural-light foundation test,' advises Bobbi Brown.

For broken veins, choose a shade that exactly matches your foundation – or layer on foundation, in very thin layers, until you've achieved the level of coverage you want. There are always fewer concealer colours to choose from than foundations. If you can't find the perfect colour, Vincent Longo recommends blending two shades on the back of your hand with a stiff brush, to get the right shade, then dabbing that onto the skin.

What most of us want to avoid, says Vincent Longo, is foundation with even a *hint* of pink in it, 'especially if you're prone to flushing'. Most foundation ranges today feature shades based on so-called 'yellow pigments', which are extremely natural-looking. If you're not sure, ask at the counter to see only the yellow-toned foundations – and focus on finding the best shade for you.

Bobbi is not a fan of translucent powders, preferring instead a shade perfectly matched to your foundation. (Most lines offer these options.) 'It's a myth that translucent powder is invisible; I find translucent powder makes a woman look pasty – and can be chalky on the skin.'

> *Attitude is more important to beauty than cosmetics ever can be. When you are at peace with who you are, you are beautiful. Work on the inside, as well as the outside.*
>
> BOBBI BROWN

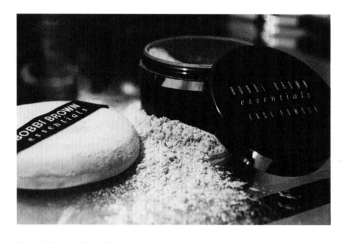

'Apply a couple of possible shades of foundation to the jawline in a downward stripe and leave a few seconds before blending. Then go to the nearest source of daylight to see how they look.' Artificial lights distort colours so that a shade which looked perfect in a marble beauty hall may be quite wrong when you get it home.

Don't rush selection. The skin's chemistry can make foundation change colour after a minute or two.

When choosing a concealer for under-eye circles, Bobbi Brown advises selecting a shade very slightly lighter than your foundation.

FOUNDATIONS – WHO USES WHAT...

Legendary TV interviewer **Barbara Walters** is a fan of Make Up For Ever's Pan Stick foundation (while **Cher** loves their Star Powder No. 900 – to add a touch of shimmer over skin). **Cheryl Tiegs** saves time with all-in-one Shiseido Compact Foundation, in Natural Deep Beige (and likes M.A.C. Pressed Powder, too). Great colours for dark skins are hard to find – but **Oprah Winfrey** swears by Bobbi Brown's Foundation Sticks in # 7, # 8 and # 9. Some of the celebrities who use Laura Mercier's foundations and concealers include **Sharon Stone, Madonna, Susan Sarandon, Angelica Huston, Glenn Close, Priscilla Presley, Meryl Streep** and **Catherine Deneuve** (who goes for the Oil-Free Foundation). Both **la Deneuve** and **Cher** go for Laura Mercier's under make-up base, Foundation Primer. **Jilly Cooper** loves Yardley foundations – 'Other brands always make me feel like I'm wearing foundation; with this, people just comment how well I look.' And for that sun-kissed look? According to colleagues, designer **Adrienne Vittadini** is always pulling Bobbi Brown's Bronzing Powder out of her bag...

more secrets of flawlessness

• 'You should spend twice as long on your foundation as any other element of your make-up. If you're giving it less time than that, you're skimping,' says Mary Greenwell. 'It makes such a huge difference that it's worth the extra time and effort.'

• If your skintone is still fairly even, in summer you can get away with tinted moisturiser for a light, natural coverage. But if you need a dab of concealer to cover flaws, apply it *before* the tinted moisturiser, for a natural look.

• Many women are self-conscious about freckles and sun spots – and want to even them out. When it comes to freckles, says Mary Greenwell, 'you have to accept that if you're going to cover them totally, it's going to look like a mask. So I'd advise a foundation that's mid-way between the colour of your freckles and the colour of your complexion, to play them down a bit – with concealer (or Estée Lauder's Maximum Cover), on the bigger age spots. The best way to apply concealer to a sun spot is with a 3mm ($1/8$ inch) brush. Dab it onto the affected area, then set with powder, applied with a velvet powder puff. The rule is: always start with a little product, then build up. It's easier to add than take away. Alternatively, use a cream-to-powder formulation, which is half-way between a foundation and a concealer, in terms of texture and coverage.' (Most leading beauty houses now make these foundations, which are also extremely convenient to carry around in a handbag. They go on smoothly, like foundation, then dry swiftly to a lightly powdered finish.)

• 'If you over-do foundation, lightly whisk off the excess with a very slightly damp cosmetic sponge,' advises Laura Mercier.

• 'As you touch up make-up during the day, don't over-powder – or make-up will look "caked",' cautions Vincent Longo.

• Kevyn Aucoin is a great believer in the minimalist approach for older faces. 'When I'm making up my mother – who's in her sixties – I find myself just using a little concealer, applied only where she needs it, with a little brush. A touch of powder over the top – and that's it. But she still looks fabulous – because at this age, less really is more.'

• One of the cleverest tricks we know for a younger-looking complexion comes from Trish McEvoy. To soften the appearance of laugh lines around the eye, she applies a dab of Trish McEvoy Refiner* there. (This is a portable wand of moisturiser, but you could experiment with a dab of eye cream.) 'It recreates the dewiness that young skins have, and counteracts the natural paperiness that women tend to have round their laugh lines, which is accentuated by powder.'

There is something to be said for acceptance. As make-up artist Pablo Manzoni points out, 'Look at Jeanne Moreau. She was a sex symbol with bags under her eyes. People just thought she looked like she was having a terrific time in the bedroom.' (And she probably was.)

FACE-SHAPING TRICKS

Most of the make-up artists we spoke to were agreed that face-shaping – using contouring powder to create shadows and re-shape features – is tricky, tricky stuff. Jenny Jordan, for instance, is sometimes asked by clients to help them re-shape a bumpy nose. 'And I have to say to them: what'll happen if you want to blow it? All the shading will come off on your Kleenex...' Embarrassing stuff.

For round cheeks, however, movie-star make-up artist and adviser to Max Factor Gary Liddiard, has a tip for creating contours that's worth a try. He suggests using two foundations – your usual shade for the whole face and then just a shade darker, for blending on the cheek under the bone to the jawline. (Be sure to blend, blend, blend at the jaw itself.) 'The new foundations are so easy to blend that the contouring is basically undetectable. If you then use blusher as you normally do, no one will know – but everyone will notice...'

If you have a thin face, meanwhile, Stephen Glass suggests using an under-makeup primer beneath your foundation, in a pale or white shade. (Lancôme, Dior and Chanel all offer them.) 'It makes the face glow and stand out more,' he explains. 'And be careful of blusher placement,' he adds. 'Blusher must go on the cheekbones, never underneath – or the cheeks will look hollow.' His last tip? 'Earrings make a tremendous difference to the impact a thin face has – but steer clear of anything too big, or they may swamp your face.'

camouflage make-up for rosacea and other problems

So popular is Laura Mercier's make-up range with rosacea sufferers that she was recently invited to speak at a conference on the subject, and her postbag bulges with letters from grateful women. The product they rave about is Laura's Secret Camouflage* concealer (which is also a favourite with Hollywood stars like **Priscilla Presley** and **Isabella Rossellini**). The reason, Laura explains, 'is that Camouflage has a very high level of pigmentation, so you get excellent coverage without having to put it on thickly'. The technique, she explains, is to dab the finger in Secret Camouflage, and apply to the affected area, building coverage layer-by-layer until the characteristic redness is completely disguised. 'Then set with a light covering of powder.'

Another product which gets top marks from make-up artists for its truly incredible covering powers is Estée Lauder Maximum Cover. Be warned: if you apply it straight from the tube, it goes on way too thick. The technique, explains Stephen Glass, 'is to invest in a small plastic spatula. Then squeeze around three pinhead-sized dots of Maximum Cover onto the spatula. Dip your ring finger in the foundation, then wipe your finger on the edge of the spatula. You'll be left with just a tiny amount of Maximum Cover on your finger – but because it covers so densely that's still enough to disguise some broken veins or an age spot. If you need more, do exactly the same again – and repeat until you've covered all the areas where you need the extra help.' (He recommends Maximum Cover only for areas affected by broken veins, dark circles, rosacea, birthmarks and port wine stains or age spots, not as a general foundation.)

NB If you have a birthmark, vitiligo (uneven pigmentation) or scarring (including burn scars), you might want to know about the British Red Cross's cosmetic camouflage programme. It's available on referral from your doctor only. The consultations offered – with specially trained volunteers who are all experienced therapists – are free, and most of the special creams (which are waterproof and contain a sunscreen) are available on prescription. Further information is available from the Beauty Care Officer at local Red Cross branches in the UK.

Advice is also available from the British Association of Skin Camouflage (BASC). The BASC will supply the name of your nearest member, who – for a modest fee – will discuss individual requirements and recommend products from the Dermablend, Dermacolour, Covermark, Veil and Keromask ranges. These are available on prescription and over-the-counter at Boots.

Stephen Glass also highly rates the Doreen Savage Trust* in Fife; Doreen herself has a port wine stain down the side of her face and provides information and help for people with birthmarks.

THE BEST ANTI-AGEING FOUNDATIONS WE'VE FOUND

The advent of 'light-reflecting' pigments – which work to create literally an optical illusion 'soft-focus' effect – are a real boon to older faces. Moisturising ingredients can also make a difference, time-releasing moisture into the skin to prevent skin looking dry as the day wears on. They're now being incorporated into foundations and powders. The two of us tried all the leading 'anti-ageing' and 'time-defying' foundations for this book. Our favourites were Futurist and Lucidity from Estée Lauder, Lancôme's Optim'âge, Helena Rubinstein Translucence and Lancaster's Oxygen Foundation. We also like Chanel's Double Teint – all-in-one powder-foundation – for on-the-go touch-ups. What was even more important than moisturisation or clever light-reflecting pigments, we discovered, was to find a shade that matched our own skin perfectly. That's what turned back the clock...

I apply make-up sparingly – and quickly. I play with bronzing powders and tinted moisturisers. It's important to be natural – but worked-at natural, which takes a lot of time! A face that's not overly made-up looks younger.

CATHERINE DENEUVE

THE ESSENTIAL TOOLKIT

Do you still put on blusher with the stubby brush that comes with the compact? Fiddle with those tiny eyeshadow applicators in an attempt to shade your eyes? Age-defying make-up relies on perfect application – and that means using the right tools. 'We need a bigger toolkit as we get older, because it makes for a more natural finish,' observes Barbara Daly. So we asked her to select the ultimate toolkit for the older face…

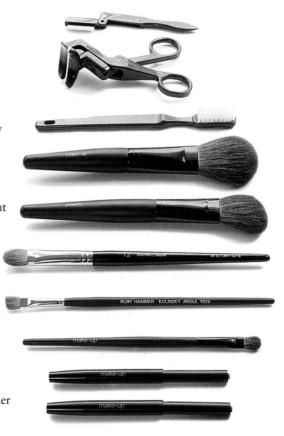

1 A lash comb. 'One of the most ageing make-up mistakes is clumpy lashes.'

2 An eyelash curler. 'They really do make a difference to older eyes…' (So we really do promise to learn how to use them this time, Barbara.)

3 An old, soft toothbrush. 'This is dual-purpose: it's brilliant for grooming brows into place – and for cleaning your lash-comb.'

4 A nice, fat blusher brush with a dome-shaped head. 'You don't want a spindly little one because that can make blusher go on in stripes.'

5 Although some make-up artists prefer velvet powder puffs, Barbara likes to apply powder with a brush. 'It should have a wide-ish head but not be as fat and fluffy as a blusher brush, so that you can apply powder just where you want it.' (NB If you do prefer to apply your powder with a puff – as many make-up artists suggest – a powder brush is still useful for whisking away the excess.)

6 An eyeshadow blender brush. 'The right size and shape will help you apply shadow to the socket and soften any hard lines.'

7 A slanted eyebrow brush. Stiff bristles are less likely to smudge, spread or smear pigment where you don't want it.

8 A smaller eyeshadow brush, for applying colour to the brow-bone.'

9 Two retractable lipbrushes – 'one for lip colour and one for applying concealer perfectly on broken veins and shadows. Then you can pat the concealer with your finger, warming it and pressing it into the skin.'

10 A soft, more pointed eyeliner brush, if you like to use eyeliner. (You can wet this and dip it in shadow for a more dramatic effect.)

brush notes

Invest in real hair brushes, rather than synthetic hair. Kevyn Aucoin says that 'artificial hair doesn't work as well. Synthetics tend to be stiff – and can even scratch your face.' (However, if you prefer synthetic brushes for ethical reasons, we recommend Origins' excellent range of brushes*.)

Good brushes are the key to a polished, professional look, but they're often too big to fit neatly into a compact make-up bag. The solution is either to opt for the travel size next time you buy: many ranges, like Bobbi Brown, Trish McEvoy and Shu Uemura, offer short-handled or long-handled options. Or adapt what you've got. 'I always cut down the handles on my brushes,' says Jenny Jordan. 'They fit into my kit more easily and they're better for fiddly application.'

blushing beauty

Women of a certain age should 'think pink'. Blusher can restore youth to a fading complexion, soften lines, blur sags – and give the skin a fresh (girlish) glow. But it's a fine line between healthily blushed and hotly flushed…

The great cosmetics legend Estée Lauder was evangelical about blusher. She used to keep a blusher compact in her handbag and apply it to the faces of women she met, to show them how 'glow' could transform them with the flick of a wrist. And it's true. As Bobbi Brown says, 'Nothing makes a woman look prettier than a shot of blush. And there is no faster "up" if you're flagging in the middle of an afternoon. It can instantly take ten years off you by making you look healthier.'

But where you apply your blusher today may not be where you wore it ten years ago. Natural changes in the shape of the face with age demand a shift in make-up application techniques. Until we're about 35, we can wear blusher high on the cheekbone. But because one of the first signs of an ageing face is the loss of fatty tissue and the formation of natural hollows, in most cases it becomes more flattering to place blusher towards the centre of the face and on the apple of the cheek, to soften it.

BLUSHER HOW-TO

1 Switching to a smaller blusher brush – a 2.5cm (1 inch) blusher brush, rather than a big fat version – makes for better control.

2 Dip the blusher brush in your chosen colour, then tap the handle of the brush smartly on a hard surface – like the edge of a table or a basin – several times, to ensure that you only have a whisper of colour left. ('Never blow on a brush,' warns Trish McEvoy, 'it just blows on germs…')

3 Where you put your blush depends on how plump your face still is. If you have developed hollows or sunkenness under the cheekbone, concentrate the blusher on the apples of your cheek. 'This gives a more youthful look,' says Mary Greenwell. 'To find the "apple" of your cheek, smile in an exaggerated way. The fatty area that sticks out is the apple. Using light, circular movements, apply just the very lightest dusting of blusher to the apples. With the same brush, blend, blend, blend at the edges until there are absolutely no harsh lines.' (If you overdo it, she advises, you can apply a touch of pressed powder with your velvet puff, to tone the colour down.)

4 If your face still has fullness you can apply blusher on the cheekbone as well as the apples. Again, make sure that your blusher brush only has the lightest amount of colour, by tapping the handle of the brush first. Then, advises Laura Mercier, 'Start at the ears and make an inward movement with the brush, as if you were going to draw an oval with it on the entire cheek. Break the oval, when you get to the apple of the cheek. Continue to make these ultralight broken-oval strokes until you have achieved the right depth of colour.' Then clean the last traces of blusher off the brush by drawing with it on a Kleenex, and use the brush to blur any edges, so that you can't see where it begins and ends. (Sweeping blusher in from the ears, explains Laura – rather than following cheekbones outwards – avoids putting too much pigment on the middle of the cheek.) 'Lastly, gently brush the cheek hairs down so they are lying in their usual direction.'

5 Trish McEvoy likes to whisk the lightest dusting of blusher around the temples and hairline, creating the lightest halo of warmth around the face. But again, the watchwords are 'softly, softly'…

NB To avoid the painted-lady effect, try applying blusher as the final step in a make-up – so that you can judge exactly how much you need, and not overdo it.

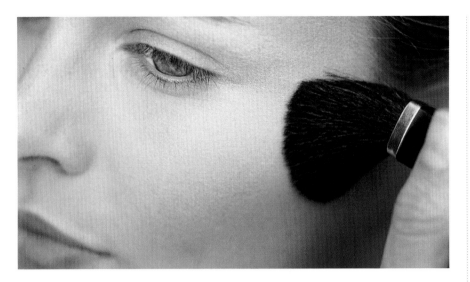

BLUSHER NOTES

• For emergencies: if you're out and about without a blusher and feel washed-out, reach for your lipstick, put a tiny dab on your finger – and apply to your cheeks. 'This works best with sheer lipsticks, which don't have too much pigment,' says Laura Mercier.

• If you have broken veins or high colour, Vincent Longo's advice is to 'avoid blusher that has any red in it – go for tawny or honey shades, instead, which create a peachy effect'.

• 'Don't be scared to wear blusher if you have a tendency to hot flushes,' says Laura Mercier. 'If you tone down the redness of your face with foundation, concealer and powder, you can add blush to look healthy and alive. But choose a tawny shade with a touch of brown in it, rather than fleshy pink or anything with blue undertones.'

cream versus powder blush

Many make-up artists suggest cream blusher for older faces. 'Cream blush is terrific if you're the sort of woman who feels she needs some help in the morning before facing the milkman or the postman, as it blends so beautifully on bare skin,' says Vincent Longo. 'It goes into the skin so it doesn't sit on the surface and look powdery, which is an advantage for older skins. And it's especially good in summer. Powder blusher can look dusty in intense light.' Cream blusher is, however, best applied over moisturiser on bare skin, or over foundation before powdering, otherwise it's hard to blend evenly.

THE BRUSH BATH

According to Bobbi Brown, it's essential to wash brushes at least every two months to get rid of skin-irritating oil, bacteria and mildew – and to ensure that colour glides on smoothly. To clean blusher, powder and eye brushes, gently swish (don't soak) bristles in sudsy water. (Use a mild shampoo, rather than soap.) Rinse immediately, squeeze out the water and rearrange the bristles in their normal shape. Then lay a towel on a flat surface with an edge and leave the brushes to dry with their heads hanging over the edge. For lip brushes, wipe bristles with a tissue, then dip them into a cup of non-oily eye make-up remover and tissue off the residue.

thinking pinker

Pink isn't just flattering as a blush shade – it also flatters older faces if you use it in the home. Sister Parish, who was America's favourite interior decorator, insisted that 'pink makes the rich look healthy'. Joan Crawford, too, couldn't get enough of pink: her three Manhattan apartments all had pink walls, pink lamps with flesh-toned shades, pink headboards and pink monograms on the sheets. Even Dorothy Parker – she of the wicked pen, who was so quick to skewer vanity in others – had a pink room in her Pennsylvania house that became a favourite because she felt its warm glow made her look younger. Which is worth seriously considering next time you're redecorating...

climbing out of a make-up rut

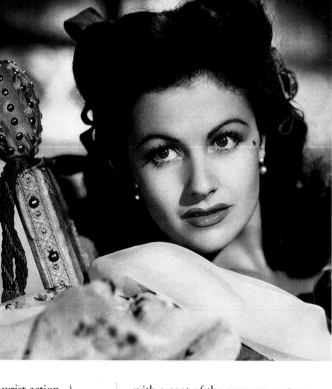

Old habits die hard. Especially when it comes to make-up. But one way that women inadvertently add years is by getting 'freeze-framed' with a particular look. Observes John Gustafson**, 'I think it's really sad to see an older woman who doesn't look her age – but her make-up does... I often meet women who are wearing the same make-up as when they were twenty. And all you see is the make-up. That was when that woman felt comfortable – so she stopped experimenting...'

Because our complexions change, tending to become drier and paler every year, too, make-up kits need to be adjusted to these new needs. The solution is to turn to insiders for help. John Gustafson goes so far as to suggest that 'You should get a department-store makeover – which is free, at make-up counters – at least twice, preferably four times a year. Mostly, you'll learn something. You might not like the results, but you should have acquired some new techniques to help you in future.'

But don't just sit there passively. Ask questions and in particular badger for how-to advice. New colours and textures call for new techniques, so ask about the equipment you'll need to recreate the look at home. Your best beauty investment is the right tools and

brushes for the job: Q-Tips and fingers just won't achieve the desired effect. But when you're next in a beauty hall, why not ask a make-up artist or counter consultant how to use these tools? (It really is all in the wrist action...)

'When it comes to makeovers, don't go in as a "blank canvas",' adds John. 'Wear your usual make-up, so the consultant gets an idea of the way you usually like to look, rather than projecting their own ideas onto you. And if you just want an update, rather than a whole new look, suggest that they work by adding colour to the make-up you usually wear – a sweep of one of the new colours on the lid, a touch of shimmer on the brow, but basically not straying too far from the make-up you feel comfortable with.'

He also has advice on how to wean yourself off a lipstick colour you're clinging to like a family heirloom. 'If you'd like to wear a brighter lipstick which you think would suit you but it's outside your usual "comfort zone", pick a bolder colour that appeals. Then wear one coat of your usual lipstick,

with a coat of the new one on top. After a few days, when you get used to that, add another coat of the new shade, until you're sure it suits you. Then you can move on to wearing the new shade on its own. And hey, presto – you've a new look...'

when less isn't more...

There's one exception to the 'Less Is More' rule, says Bobbi Brown. 'If you've never worn make-up, it's never too late to start. We tend to get washed-out looking as we age,' she observes. 'Make-up makes up for that...'

Happy is the woman who never makes a make-up mistake. Happy – and rare. As we age and complexions become washed-out, it's tempting to reach for the paintbox in the hope that it will instantly 'lift' the face. But if you make the wrong colour choices, what actually happens is that strangers and loved ones will see your make-up – not the 'you' underneath. 'Older women do need colour,' believes Bobbi Brown, 'but it's all about adding soft, flattering shades.'

analysis some years back, sub-dividing women into four categories – red, blue/red, yellow/orange and red/orange – then organising the cosmetic carousel so that you can pick the kind of colours you like – and the exact, most flattering tone is pre-selected for you.

To help show you how 'warm' or 'cool' shades can work best for you, we have put cool shades down the top of this page and warm shades below. Hold them up to your face. Look in the mirror and hold the book up in front of your face, then move the page

keep the palette neutral, sticking to smoky greys and browns. 'You can always use a touch of gold, pale pink or even lavender on the brow-bone. But don't go bold on the lid or in the socket.' Avoid burgundy, she warns, because it can bring out redness in bloodshot eyes. (Ditto pink on the brow if you are prone to red-eye.) 'In the same way, if you have a tendency to redness, examine brown eyeshadows carefully for any gingery notes, which will have a similar effect.'

Whatever you do, forget that old advice about matching your

cool

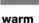

the colour code

When it comes to choosing colours, though, it's a minefield out there. Hard-and-fast rules are hard to come by. But some companies have set out to render make-up shopping mistake-proof, dividing the colours they offer into groups of shades most likely to suit, often by dividing us into 'warm' and 'cool' skintones.

If you are a 'warm', you are more likely to tan easily and have golden undertones. 'Cool' skins tend to have blue undertones, and to pick up colour in the sun less easily. (Classic English roses, for example, are 'cool'.)

This is where companies like Lancôme, Prescriptives and Estée Lauder all agree. Then it gets more complicated: they have their own way of sub-dividing the colours to steer you in the right direction.

Estée Lauder's system is called Colour Affinity and offers groups of colours in different intensities, matched to the cool or warm undertone of your complexion.

Prescriptives pioneered 'skin-tone'

so that first the warm, then the cool part, is just below mouth-level. It's amazing to see the difference: one will make you look vibrant and healthy – and the other, washed-out.

If you still can't tell, then the sales pros at most make-up counters are able to tell, at a glance, which grouping you fall into. You can then train your eye to spot the 'warm' and 'cool' shades in each colour family. 'There are even some "cool" browns,' explains John Gustafson. 'You can usually spot them, because in a sea of brown colours, they stand out as looking different. They're the ones that will suit "cool" skins.' ('Cool' browns are the taupe-y ones with blue/mauve undertones, rather than the bronzey red 'warm' browns.)

For foolproof eyes, stick to a palette of neutral, natural tones, and leave bright, funky colours to the teenagers. 'Don't get lured into wearing bright colours,' counsels Barbara Daly. 'Bright colour can be very ageing.' Barbara's advice is to

eyeshadow to your eyes. If you have brown eyes, try emphasising them with grey shadows; if you have blue or grey eyes, go for browns.

And for lips? Says Bobbi Brown: 'Steer clear of nudes – but don't go to the other extreme with fuchsia, either. You want colours that are softened – like soft rose, soft plum, soft apricot – but which are definitely *there*.'

There are also organisations like Color Me Beautiful, specifically set up to help pinpoint the elements of the spectrum – in cosmetics and fashion – most likely to flatter individuals. But do these colour consultations work? We are not convinced. Where they may score, however, is by helping rescue women from a 'colour rut'. If you've habitually bought virtually the same lipstick shade for years – and have 30 or so almost-identical shades languishing in your make-up kit to prove it – a 'colour consultation' may be worth a shot. But better, we feel, to try a department store makeover – or three – first...

warm

multi-cultural make-up

All skins are not alike: Oriental, Asian and black skins have distinct advantages when it comes to ageing. In Asian and black skins, extra melanin production makes skin much more resistant to sun damage, while in Japan, according to Noriko Okubo of Shiseido Europe, 'Sun protection is a must throughout life, because Japanese women like to maintain a very pale complexion. As a result, they don't suffer the wrinkling and crêpiness that Western women do.'

   Nevertheless, every woman everywhere faces beauty challenges. So we asked experts in Oriental, Asian and black make-up for some special tips...

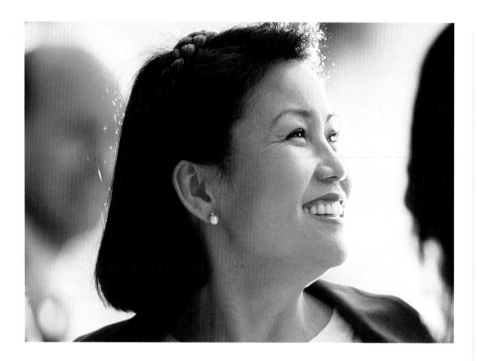

ORIENTAL

According to Noriko, Oriental faces age in one of two ways. 'Either they get plump – with marked sagging from jaw to neck – or become thinner, leading to hollow eyelids, cheeks and temples. Colour fades from all faces, giving a tired, "quiet" look, and circles under the eyes can become more prominent.'

◆ It's possible to 'correct' downward-drooping lines, says Noriko. 'You can't erase them, but you can minimise the sagging look by using upward strokes to finish the eyebrows, eye corners and lips.

◆ To make skin and features look more 'luminous', Noriko advises emphasising the definition of eyebrows, lips and eyes. 'But keep to a natural palette and avoid strong reds or dark black,' says Noriko, 'otherwise you can actually draw attention to wrinkles and sagging.'

◆ 'Hollow temples make eyes look closer-set,' explains Noriko, 'and lines between eyebrows or at the corners of the mouth create a stern look. For a serene, peaceful look, direct eyebrow and lip lines outwards.'

◆ For specific guidelines on how to shade Oriental eyes, *see p.85.*

◆ Sagging on the cheeks or the tip of the chin can create a plump, heavy look, so Noriko advises using two shades of base. First apply a base perfectly-matched to the face, wherever you need coverage. Then use a concealer that is very slightly lighter on hollow areas such as temples, eyelids and under-eye. Be sure to camouflage the dark circles around the hollow of the upper eyelid, which can be very draining.' And of course – the make-up artists' mantra – blend, blend, blend...

ASIAN

According to Ruby Hammer, whose family come from Bangladesh, 'Although Asian skins are resilient to sun damage – and stay wonderfully wrinkle-free in many cases – the real challenge is dark circles under the eyes.' Her suggestions for minimising/concealing the problem are:

◆ 'Tap, tap, tap away puffiness before you apply make-up; it really decongests the area. I also recommend a de-puffing cream, like Estée Lauder's Uncircle, which is also designed to get rid of darkness. Alternatively, rub an ice cube in your hands, then apply your cooled fingers to the area. You can even wrap an ice cube in a couple of tissues or some Cling Film and lightly run it around the puffy, dark area, without risking broken blood vessels.'

◆ 'Keeping the eyes themselves bright and sparkly – with a product such as Dr Harris's Eye Drops*, to get rid of redness – will distract from the circles.'

◆ 'Take the time to find a concealer that really matches your skintone, and use it on dark shadows on scars, which also go very dark. Many concealers are too pink or too light and just emphasise the problem in a quite different way. Aveda do a great Pecan shade that's good for many dark skins, and Nars* have good shades for dark skin – or you can get 'custom-blended' foundation at the Prescriptives counter, and they'll give you a matching concealer. Cosmetics A La Carte* also have a good range of dark colours.'

◆ 'Colour can really "lift" a face, and Asian skins can get away with bold tones – but make sure that your foundation is always perfectly matched to the skin on the jawline, and save the bright make-up shades for lips, eyes or nails. The foundation and blusher have to look natural, and it's better to emphasise just one feature strongly – eyes or lips, not both, to avoid looking overdone.'

◆ 'Asian women love nail polish. They also love to cook and it's hell on hands. My advice is to take the time to do a proper manicure, or have it regularly done professionally, because chipped nail polish looks so awful. Use base and top coat, and take time. Otherwise it'll be chipped before you've done the washing-up, and spoil your whole look.'

BLACK

Although black skins have the highest level of melanin – so are least vulnerable to the sun – Edith Poyer, Assistant Director of Product Development for leading black cosmetics brand Fashion Fair*, says it's a myth that black skins don't need protection. 'Under her make-up, every woman should be wearing a moisturiser with antioxidants and SPF in the formulation, that shields her skin from the environment,' she says.

◆ 'The specific problem of black skin is an increase in ashiness – a grey cast to the skin,' says Edith. 'You need a better moisturiser – i.e. a richer formulation – and perhaps to use an AHA-based product to exfoliate skin, at least once or twice a week, if not every night, to make it look brighter.'

◆ 'Although black skin stays relatively unlined, the last thing you want is for make-up to settle in any folds or creases. I always recommend a lightweight, oil-free formulation, which won't accentuate problems by settling into the lines. That way, you can avoid the use of powder – which again draws attention to fine lines and wrinkles.'

◆ 'Black skin can be very sensitive – more so as it ages,' explains Edith. 'And a pimple can turn into a black scar. You need a good concealer,

perfectly matched to your skintone.' (She recommends Fashion Fair's Cover Tone*, a maximum cover concealer.)

◆ 'To brighten the face, go for bold lipstick – plums, browns, oranges, purples. Dark skins can get away with these intense colours. But keep eyeshadows muted, otherwise you'll look overdone. A touch of purple or cranberry blusher can give a healthy glow, too – but use a very light hand. As with all make-up, less is more.'

◆ 'If brows are greying, use a dark charcoal pencil or a dark brown – not a true black – to colour them in, otherwise the look is too intense.'

◆ Remember: if you have healthy skin, you'll need less make-up – which will give you a younger look. Don't think of make-up as camouflage; work to improve the 'canvas' – your skin – underneath.'

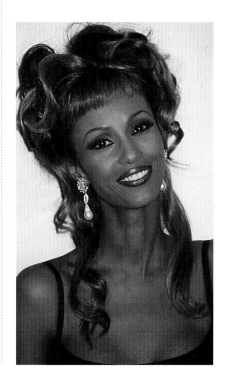

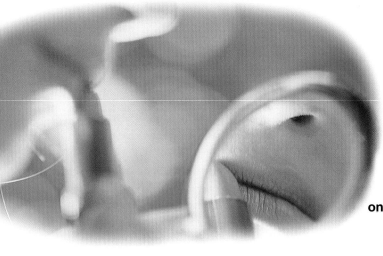

lips inc.

The world's top make-up artists share inside-track info on choosing and applying the perfect, age-defying lipstick…

We love shopping for lipstick. (Not least because you don't have to get undressed to try it on.) But ageing lips present challenges: feathery lines – which make lipstick 'bleed' – and dryness. As we age, the skin's barrier function becomes less efficient, meaning moisture escapes more easily. Lips are already super-vulnerable to dryness, because they start out with just three layers of skin, compared with 15 or so, elsewhere. What's more, over time, lips get thinner – because they lose fat – and paler in colour.

The good news is that lipstick – perfectly applied, in a flattering colour – can miraculously create the illusion of fuller, younger lips. The perfect lipstick also gives the face an instant 'lift', taking years off in a flash. But in our experience, there are certain basic rules that apply to older lips…

This is no longer a competition to see who can wear the most daring and outrageous lip colour; instead, it's time to find a shade that gives your complexion an immediate boost. The simplest trick? Hold a selection of colours up in front of your lips – and without even having to try a shade on your lips, you'll see which ones make your complexion look brighter and

your eyes sparkle. Then you can try the most flattering colour on the lips themselves, and see if it stays true on your lips – an important factor because as we age the body's chemistry can cause lipsticks to change colour on the skin. (That's why it's so important to wear a lipstick before you buy it.)

Another problem, we've found, is that lip colour disappears – seemingly into the ether – soon after application. We're not fans of most long-lasting formulations (neither are most make-up artists); they can turn lips as parched as the Sahara.

Instead, try our secrets for making lip colour stay put longer…

to frost or not to frost?

Super-frosted shades are not flattering to older lips because they can draw attention to lines and ridges. However, make-up artists are agreed that a sweep of light shimmer – or a 'dot' of a lightly frosted lipstick, blended into the middle of the bottom lip only – can be very flattering.

HOW TO MAKE YOUR LIPSTICK STAY PUT…

We really suggest steering clear of lipsticks which claim to be 'long-lasting'. In our experience, while they do deliver enduring colour, the formulations are also super-drying and leave lips parched. There are other ways to make your lipstick last longer…

Vincent Longo outlines the lips with a lip pencil, then draws all over the lips with the same colour. 'This creates an "undercoat" for your lipstick, which will last much longer.' (Vincent is also a fan of the special lip bases designed to help lipstick last longer; brands to look for include Estée Lauder, Guerlain and our favourite, BeneFit's Lip Plump.)

Using a lip brush to apply your lipstick, rather than slicking it on from the tube, always makes it last longer. (We advise buying a retractable lip brush, or one with its own cap, to stop it getting gungey.)

If you like to use gloss, meanwhile, be careful where you apply it. Says Laura Mercier: 'Confine this slippery substance to the middle of the lips. By applying all over the mouth, you'll cause the colour to "bleed" into fine lines.'

products we love...

If you ask us, BeneFit Lip Plump* is pretty much a miracle-worker: like a foundation for lips, it seems to plump out fine lines, as well as helping lipstick to stay on longer (and has optical diffusing ingredients to make lips look more generous); BeneFit also make a pencil called All Clear, a waxy pencil to outline the lips, creating a barrier so that lipstick doesn't bleed. Sarah also loves Guerlain's LipLift, while Jo favours Vincent Longo's Golden Lip Gloss.

what the stars love...

Goldie Hawn wears Vincent Longo's* Divine Flesh – and after dark goes for his Lavender (a glacé taupe-y shade). She also uses Prescriptives Eye Pencil, in Bronze, as lip-liner. Stila's* lipsticks have an equally devoted celebrity following: Susan Sarandon uses a shade called Loree – but also loves Nars Nude Lipliner*, under Nude and Raisin Lipsticks. (She obviously likes nearly natural shades because you'll find Bobbi Brown's Nude in her kit – which Michelle Pfeiffer chooses, too.) Tina Turner gets slick with Christian Dior's Saffron Lip Gloss, while Cybill Shepherd prefers to mix lipstick for a custom-blended shade – a hangover from modelling days. And what colour do Madonna and Joni Mitchell have in common? Estée Lauder Perfect Sheer Lipstick in Silent Red...

for a brighter smile...

Some lipsticks will make teeth look whiter than other colour choices. Barbara Daly tells us: 'What you want to create is contrast,' she suggests. 'Be careful with any colours with yellow or orange – including corals and brown-based shades. Pinks, reds and burgundies are often the best choices.'

LIPSTICK HOW-TO

• If your lips are prone to chapping or flaking, try this tip from New York make-up artist, Darac: slather on a thick coat of Kiehl's Lip Balm*. Leave for five minutes, then buff with a baby's ultra-soft toothbrush. The flakes will be gently whisked away, leaving lips smoother and 'prepped' for lipstick application.

• Make-up artists always apply foundation all over the lips before applying lipstick. Laura Mercier takes that one step further: when she's making up the rest of the face, Laura then lightly applies powder on top – using a velvet powder puff – before outlining with lip liner and adding lipstick and/or gloss.

• As we age, lips get 'blurry' and lose definition. That's where a lip pencil can be so valuable, outlining the lips and putting definition back.

Trish McEvoy has a secret for creating the optical illusion of a fuller pout. 'Using a lip-coloured pencil, draw just *outside* your natural lip line, using light, feathery strokes as you follow the line. (At the *corners* of your lips, however, make sure that the drawn line meets your own lip line perfectly – to avoid a "clown" effect.) When you're using the pencil to outline the cupid's bow – just above the middle of the top lip – draw in two soft "mountain peaks". Here, you can afford to go a little further away from the natural lip line. The effect is to make lips look plumper...'

• To avoid a harsh line when using a lip-liner, blunt the pencil slightly before using it on your lips, by drawing backwards and forwards several times on the back of your hand.

• When you've drawn on your lip line, use the pad of your middle finger to blur it very slightly. (Don't rub hard, or it'll smudge.)

If you still find that the line you draw is too obvious, Bobbi Brown suggests applying your lipstick *first*, then lip-liner over the top. 'It's sometimes easier to define lips this way,' Bobbi explains. 'The liner and the lipstick wear off together, so you're never left with an obvious outline around your mouth.'

• If shaky hands make it hard for you to apply lip-liner smoothly, hold the pencil near the pointed end, for maximum control.

• Don't try to match your lip-liner to your lipstick. Instead, advises Kevyn Aucoin, pick a shade of lip-liner that's closest to your own natural lip colour. That way, when your lipstick fades (or you've chewed it off), the line that's left looks natural – not unnaturally red, orange, burgundy or fuchsia...

• Puckered lips can create an uneven surface that lipstick often 'skips', making for uneven application. If this happens to you, stretch out your lips between your second and third fingers when applying colour.

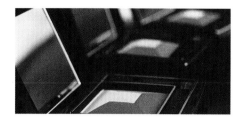

Eyes tend to present the biggest make-up challenge as we age: make-up just doesn't seem to work the way it used to, mainly because it settles into fine lines and wrinkles. 'But that's no reason to avoid it,' insists Vincent Longo. 'On the contrary, I think women of "a certain age" get a real looks boost from wearing glamorous eye make-up...'

getting your eyes right

Clever eye make-up can emphasise your eyes in the most flattering way. The first thing you need to do is learn to understand your eye shape. This makes perfect eye-shading easier. Once you've worked out your eye type – there are five basic shapes that dominate – follow the guidelines opposite. By using eyeshadow with care, you can modify the shape of your whole eye area and control emphasis. The time to practise this, however, is a rainy Saturday afternoon – not when you're heading off for a party...

Most eye-shading requires just three colours: a light 'base' colour – usually ivory, vanilla or almond; a medium tone; and a dark shade for eyelining and perhaps emphasising the outer corner of the upper lid. Choose muted colours in the same family – and remember, as with all make-up, the rule is blend, blend, blend.

first aid

• For puffy eyes, brush medium-toned eyeshadow over that part of the lid, to make it recede.

• For under eye circles, the trick is to keep the focus above the eye – so don't put on any make-up under the eye except concealer, patted on very lightly.

more tips for getting your eyes right

• Most make-up artists advise steering clear of frosted shadows, except on the brow-bone, 'which is rarely wrinkled', says John Gustafson. But the new, gently shimmering shades can open out eyes and be more flattering than matte. To see if a shimmer shadow will flatter you, says John Gustafson, apply a smear of shadow to the back of the hand. 'Then turn your hand sideways; the shimmeriness should go flat and more matte-looking. If it does, then it's suitable for older skins. If it stays shimmery *whichever* way you hold it to the light, don't buy it.'

• After dipping your brush in the eyeshadow pan, always tap the handle of the brush smartly on a hard surface to get rid of specks of excess shadow, which may shed onto your cheeks and spoil your foundation.

• Trish McEvoy's tricks is to apply eye make-up before base – so if you make mistakes, they're easy to remove with a Q-Tip dipped in eye make-up remover.

• There should never be any harsh demarcation lines with eyeshadow. An extra eyeshadow contour brush can 'blur' any harsh edges, but never rub with your finger in the hope that you can blend or soften colours. If you need to soften colour further, take a powder puff dipped in face powder (then 'thwacked', as usual), and press it on your eyelid to tone down colour.

• This is the time to wean yourself off liquid liner, which becomes increasingly hard to apply – thanks to wobblier older hands and crêpier lids. Make-up artists advise switching to a dark, powder shadow, applied with an eyeliner brush. Stephen Glass advises, 'If you like a more intense line, use a wetted eyeliner brush dipped in powder shadow – giving a much softer effect than liquid liner.' Or use a pencil, then 'set' and also soften the line with a matching powder shadow. A real trick is to work the liner carefully into the very base of the lashes, creating the illusion of much longer lashes when you then apply mascara.

If you follow these step-by-step guidelines and still can't seem to get your eyeshadow to work the way you want it to, consider one of the new cream-to-powder shadows. These glide onto the eyelid and then set to a powder finish, giving you a 'window' of about 30 seconds for perfect blending with your fingertip. We have had very good results with Revlon ColorStay Eyecolour and Almay Amazing Lasting Eye Colour, both of which come in a range of wearable, neutral shades. They are also great for weekends or casual days, when you don't want to wear full make-up but would like a little extra eye definition.

EYE SHAPES AND SHADOWS – HOW-TO

For all eye shapes, 'prime' the eye zone first with foundation and/or powder (*see pp.70–71*).

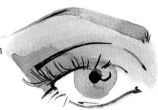

Deep-set eyes The goal here is to bring your eyelids out. Apply a light shade all over the lid, from brow to eye. Vincent Longo suggests using a slightly darker shadow along the lash-line from the centre to the outer corner, but not in the crease. This makes lashes look thicker and smokier, focusing attention on the eye, not on the recessive lid.

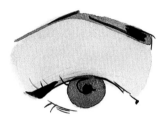

Almond This classic shape is easy to make up. Try applying a pale colour across the entire upper lid, from lashline to brow (if your eyelid is wrinkle-free you could try a whisper of shimmer). For extra emphasis, New York City make-up artist Liz Michael then takes a darker colour and creates a soft, horizontal V around the outer corner, just to outline the eyes. The line should end on both top and bottom lids at the pupil. 'I like to keep almond eyes looking fresh and simple,' says Liz.

Round You can use the same technique as for almond eyes. Alternatively, Vincent Longo suggests applying dark shadow on only the outer third of the lower eye area, which creates the optical illusion of 'stretching' the eye. For added drama and to 'lift' the eye, extend the dark shadow about 1cm (^{1}/2 inch) past the outer corner, in an upward direction, towards the temple.

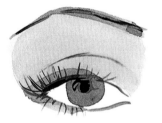

Droopy eye 1 (This same technique works brilliantly on Asian eyes, too.)
Trish McEvoy showed us a terrific trick for applying eye colour that is especially useful if you have droopy eyelids: when you apply eye colour/mascara to your top lid, hold your mirror at a 45° angle *below* eye level and tilt your head back so that you can see the entire lid and socket; the 'crease' disappears (even on very hooded eyes), so that it's easier to apply eye colour, liner and mascara. 'That way you can see the socket-bone. Often, if you have a droopy eyelid, the socket is invisible – but at this angle, it magically reappears on every woman.' For the bottom lid/lashes, hold the mirror slightly *above* eye level and tilt your head downward slightly, giving you the perfect view of the area you are making up. 'Clever shading can combat hooded eyelids,' continues Trish. Apply a light-coloured shadow to the lower eye area, and to the brow-bone, for emphasis,' she advises. 'Then, using a contour eyeshadow brush, use a mid-toned shade to shade the entire crease, in an arc. Don't apply eyeliner, because that will make the eyelid recede again. But add a coat of mascara to both top and bottom lashes.' When you open your eyes – and stare into a mirror straight ahead – your 'hooded' lid should be less obvious, thanks to the optical illusion created by your eyeshadow.

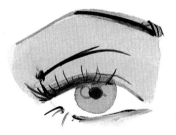

Droopy eye 2 If your eye droops at the outer edge, over the corner of the eye, follow the same instructions as above. In addition, line the lower eyelid with a fine eyeliner brush dipped in dark shadow, extending the line slightly beyond the corner of the eye, in an 'up' direction. (But don't line the top eyelid.)

brilliant brows

As we age, experts advise that it's vital to take into account brow shape – and what it does for a face that may be subtly changing...

According to make-up expert Kevyn Aucoin, 'There are women who know how to do make-up, hair and clothes – but their eyebrows just ruin their look.' Top of the list of brow challenges as the years roll on are thinning brows – as a side-effect of natural ageing, from over-plucking or an accident – and greying brows.

Eliza Petrescu – plucker-to-the-stars (whose clients at John Barrett's New York salon include **Vanessa Redgrave, Kirstie Alley, Cindy Crawford** and **Claudia Schiffer**) – believes the right brow shape can take ten years off a woman's age – by counterbalancing the natural 'droopiness' that affects lids as gravity kicks in. 'I curved Vanessa Redgrave's brows more because at a certain time in life, you need to have more of an arch, to create the illusion of an instant eye-lift,' she says.

So here's how to create the perfect, groomed brow...

★ Consider calling in a professional. Hollywood make-up artist Carol Shaw says: 'Having your brows shaped by a pro first helps get the perfect shape, so you can maintain the line at home.'

★ Buy good tweezers, which allow you to grasp each hair firmly and avoid unnecessary tugging. In common with most make-up artists, we are big fans of Tweezerman* tweezers and Swiss-made Rubis* tweezers.

★ Don't be brave. If you've a low 'ouch' threshold, Prescriptives' make-up artist Darac suggests using a toothache analgesic (e.g. Ambosol gel, from good pharmacies). Apply a few minutes before plucking, to numb it slightly.

★ Head for daylight. If your eyesight's not too good, use a magnifying mirror. (NB We swear that the ultimate place for brow-tweezing is in a parked car, during daytime.)

★ Try drawing in your brow, first. Use a brow pencil to draw on your ideal shape – then pluck everything that falls outside that line. (Blondes find this especially useful, using a taupe pencil.) But be particularly careful when tweezing the narrowest outer part of the brow; look at where the root of the hair is – and exactly where that hair lies – to make sure that you won't be creating a gap by tweezing it.

Actress Jaclyn Smith tweezes first thing in the morning, before her shower. 'That way, any puffiness or redness has a chance to subside before I get ready to put on make-up.'

★ Don't rush. Start by removing just the hairs above the nose. Your brow should start directly above the inner corner of your eye and extend as far as possible at the outer edge, to create the longest arch. Do a few hairs on one eye, then swap, to get a balanced look as you go along. Pull the skin taut, if you like, to minimise discomfort.

★ Accent the natural arch. The highest point of the arch underneath your eyebrows should line up with the outer edge of your iris. Tweeze any stray hairs that fall under that arch. And according to Laura Mercier, it's a myth that women shouldn't tweeze above the brows. 'I discovered that tweezing away some hairs at the top of my thick brows made my forehead look less heavy.' Go carefully, plucking a few hairs at a time – and standing back to analyse your reflection.

★ Swipe the area with a cotton bud, dipped in tea tree oil, after tweezing, to prevent infection.

★ Keep up the good work, with weekly – preferably twice-weekly – maintenance sessions. But be aware that continual plucking will eventually make the hairs grow more and more slowly, until they stop growing altogether. That's why it's so important not to over-tweeze.

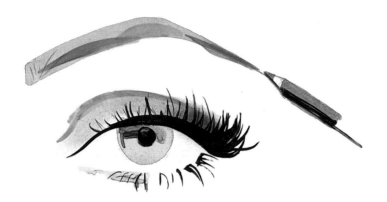

BROW ZING...

One of the commonest make-up mistakes we see on older women is brows that look drawn on. 'People shouldn't see your eyebrows coming before they see you,' points out Valerie Sarnelle, whose same-name salon in Hollywood is in many stars' Little Black Books.

For can't-tell-them-from-real brows, the options are: pencil, shadow (brow powders or eyeshadow) or pencil *and* shadow.

If you are simply enhancing the colour of your natural brows, eyeshadow alone is best. If, however, you are replacing any gaps in brows, we prefer pencil with shadow on top. NB Before you start, always brush brows downwards and then across with a small brush – an old, clean toothbrush is perfect, or an old mascara wand, cleaned up.

GETTING THE COLOUR RIGHT

• Our brows are not all one colour naturally – so consider using two slightly different shades of pencil, plus shadow, for the most realistic effect.
• Advice for grey-haired women from Mary Greenwell: 'Steer clear of blue-grey or charcoal-grey, which will look harsh.' Stephen Glass* recommends Kanebo's BR61, 'a really natural-looking taupe'.
• Be very careful to avoid brow pencils with even a hint of red – even if your hair colour is red. 'That ginger brow look is extremely fake,' says Mary. 'The make-up rule is: you should look like you've done something to your lips and your eyes – but not your skin or your brows.'
• If your hair's going white – or you've gone blonder, to disguise grey – make sure you're not using a too-intense brow colour. 'Too-dark brows can make you look like you're scowling,' says Mary Greenwell. Try going slightly lighter – to a light taupe, a shade that's usually 'specially for blondes'. This can soften the face.
• Some women with thinning brows believe semi-permanent make-up – literally, tattooing brows onto skin – can be the answer to their prayers. But we have never seen an example of this that didn't look unreal in both colour and shape. Far better to experiment with pencil and/or powder, we believe.

pencil how-to...

Most brow pencils give an effect that is way too obvious for most faces. But if you like pencil, test the texture on the back of your hand: it should be soft, and glide easily. Pencils are used either to enhance colour – in which case you're only trying to colour the hairs, *not* the skin – or to 'replace' lost hairs, drawing in the missing hairs onto the skin. After using pencil, gently use the brush again, to soften the line.

Even if you prefer a brow pencil, you will get a more realistic effect if you go over the lines afterwards with a toning powder shadow...

shadow how-to...

You need the right tool: a small, hard brush (*see The Essential Toolkit, p.75*), angled at the tip. Dip it in the colour and tap the handle of the brush smartly on the side of a basin, or on your wrist, to shake off excess.

Start at the thickest point in the brow and work outwards, using light, feathery short strokes – trying once again to get the colour onto the hairs, rather than the skin. At the outer edge, if your brows are naturally pale (or non-existent), you can apply colour to the skin to alter slightly your natural brow-line so that it flatters your face shape. You can also buy special brow powders (from Colourings, Chanel and Estée Lauder) with a slightly higher wax content than powder shadow, for staying power.

Comb the brows through afterwards again with a brow-brush to sleek them. If your brows are unruly, you can groom them in place with a brow gel – Body Shop make one, as do Estée Lauder and Trish McEvoy*.Or spritz a tiny bit of hairspray onto a brow brush and comb them into place.

Mascara is a true make-up miracle-worker – and it's the one make-up essential that most women would take to a desert island. However, while mascara can help turn back the clock, it can also advance it: tarantulas clinging to top and bottom lids are extremely ageing. (Much as we adore Barbara Cartland...) So, here are the secrets of age–defying mascara application...

mascara magic

- 'Emphasising the lashes gives amazing, instant definition to the face – especially if your lashes have lost their colour. Even if you don't wear any other eye make-up, opt for mascara,' says Mary Greenwell.
- Consider switching from black mascara to brown, suggests Barbara Daly. 'It gives a softer, more flattering look,' she explains.
- The perfect way to apply mascara is to work it well into the roots, 'then "shimmy" up the lashes using minute side-to-side movements,' advises Trish McEvoy.
- If you want to apply two coats, the trick for avoiding clumpiness is not to let the first coat dry before you apply the second.
- Barbara Daly advises all over-forties to invest in a lash comb, which will help comb out any clumps if you do get them. An old mascara wand, carefully cleansed (using lashings of eye make-up remover) will do the same job.
- Avoid clumpiness by changing your mascara at least every three months. In addition, 'Always wipe your mascara wand on a tissue, before applying it to your lashes,' advises Trish McEvoy. 'It gets rid of blobs and excess.'
- Never 'pump' the mascara wand in and out of the tube – this forces air into the tube and makes it dry out, fast-forwarding blobbiness.
- Lashes should be kept in optimum condition. Bobbi Brown finds waterproof mascaras dry out lashes – so recommends them only for sweatily hot days, weepy movies or emotionally charged encounters!
- If your lids have become droopy, use a light touch with your mascara – 'or do the outer lashes only,' advises Rex. 'A thick, dark veil of mascara only makes the eye area look heavier.'
- All the make-up artists we spoke to swear by the eye-opening effects of eyelash curlers – in fact, believes Ruby Hammer, 'if you use them regularly, they can actually give your lashes a permanent curl'. (Her favourites are Tweezerman*, which have non-stick silicone pads. Avoid metal curlers, as these can snap lashes.)
- Eyelash curlers always have to be used *before* mascara. Hold the curler from underneath; place it so that your upper lashes are in the gap between the two rims. Then squeeze for about five to ten seconds. Roll the curler slightly up and away as you remove it. For special occasions, consider false eyelashes. You can either buy them in strips, or in little clusters, packaged with their own rubber glue that ensures painless removal (with a little tugging). Stephen Glass recommends Eylure Natural Eyes* underlashes – used as top lashes. For a natural effect, cut them to fit before glueing into place. 'I apply eyeliner first, as a guideline, and then again after the lashes are in place, to disguise the glue.' Agrees Vincent Longo, 'They're useful as a boost – lashes often get more sparse as you age – and a must for special events. It isn't expensive to have false lashes applied in a salon, and they add a real elegance to any special evening.' (A salon session is also a good way of learning the secrets of truly professional eyelash application.) Alternatively, Eylure make One by One 'semi-permanent' lash clusters, which are particularly good for adding emphasis to the outer corner; at a pinch, they can even be left in place for a couple of days. (However, at any sign of sensitivity, remove the lashes – eye health is more important than lash length.)

MASCARAS WE LOVE

In the past, we looked for mascaras that pumped up the volume or dramatically lengthened our lashes. Not any more. What looks best at this age, we find, is a mascara that gives very natural results. We love Estée Lauder's Minimalist and Laura Mercier's Mascara*, both of which colour and separate lashes beautifully and realistically, rather than bulk them up. Maybelline Great Lash Mascara is a favourite with make-up artists everywhere as it doesn't dry quickly, giving plenty of 'play time' for clump-removal.

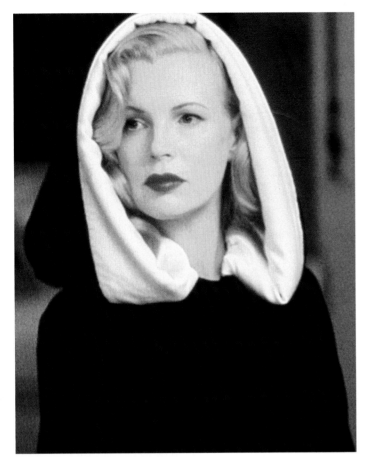

evening make-up

The art of after-dark make-up – for when the lights go down and the band strikes up…

Transforming your make-up for night is not a question of piling on extra layers. In fact, Barbara Daly's sage advice is: 'Don't stray too far from the make-up shades you wear for day. You want to look sophisticated – not like an entirely different person…' So we asked Barbara for her guidelines for after-dark make-up…

◆ 'You must always use the best possible light to make up in. By day, that's a mirror in front of a window. At night, if it's dark, I take the lampshade off a bright bedside lamp and make up in front of that. And I always use a magnifying mirror. The close-up view of the face is terrifying, to start with – but as the eyesight goes, a magnifying mirror becomes absolutely necessary…'

'Evening make-up isn't necessarily about using more products – it's about taking more time to put make-up on. If you've got plenty of time, do the whole works – and do it well. Otherwise, do only those elements of the make-up that you have time to do beautifully. It might mean you use fewer items – but you'll look better because they'll be more expertly applied. You can look a million dollars with immaculate skin, mascara and lipstick.

◆ 'Don't put too much coverage on the skin. You are not going to do yourself any favours by slapping make-up on all over. Sometimes women think that because it's evening light, they can get away with more base – but it's not true. Keep your base light – and keep it where you need it most. Use very fine layers of concealer to cover problem areas, rather than thick foundation.

◆ 'I am an advocate of loose powder for day and for evening. But slip a pressed powder compact in your bag for light touch–ups. Use it sparingly; if you keep powdering, it'll look caked – and ageing.

◆ 'This is the time when you can get away with a *touch* more blush. But I mean a whisper…' (You can also dust blush very, very lightly around the hairline, Barbara suggests.)

◆ 'I like creamy or shimmery highlights in the evening. Put them anywhere the skin would normally shine a little: the brow-bone, a touch on the lids, cheekbones, the middle of the bottom lip – but avoid any areas with fine lines or wrinkles. You want just enough to make you gleam – not to make you look sweaty.' (Stephen Glass recommends Lancôme's Maquilumine, a liquid highlighter that glides over the skin.) 'If you're unsure whether your facial skin can take shimmer, use a lightly shimmering powder on your shoulders and décolletage – in a gold or a glimmering rose – instead,' Barbara suggests.

◆ 'I am a big fan of lip gloss for evening – a sheeny product, on the middle of the bottom lip. But put it over a lip-liner and lipstick, as it tends to disappear easily. Otherwise, be prepared to touch it up regularly.

◆ 'You can use slightly smokier eye colours in the evening – but don't stray from your usual palette.'

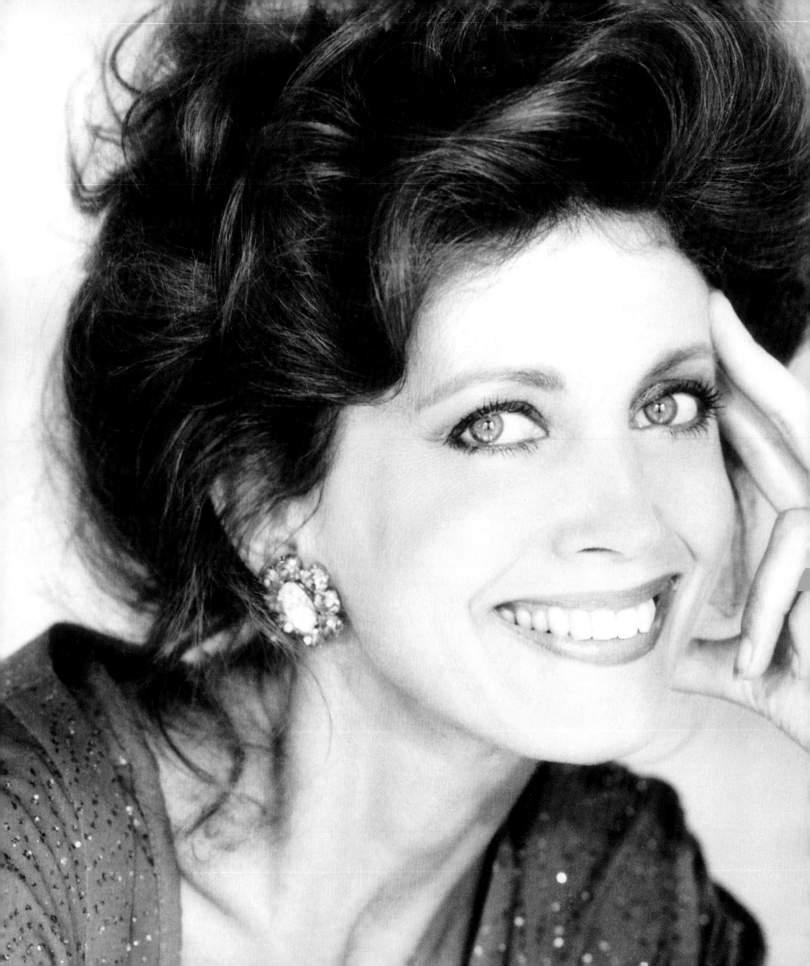

Gayle Hunnicutt

Texas-born actress Gayle Hunnicutt is in her mid-fifties. She lives in London and is married to journalist Simon Jenkins with whom she has a teenage son, Edward. Her son Nolan, in his early twenties, whose father is Gayle's first husband David Hemmings, drops in regularly, greeting her with 'Ciao, bella!'. We love Gayle's rollicking laugh, her zest for life and her determination not to be treated as a 'menopausal fruitcake'.

'I'm blooming now but I had four extremely difficult years health-wise in my early fifties and the lesson is that you must take responsibility for your health and fight your corner. I made a fundamentally wrong decision – to go back to work – six weeks after a radical hysterectomy, both ovaries and my womb out. I blame no one but myself but it would have been helpful if a doctor had said, "Think this through: you have just had a major operation and you need six months to recover".

'I worked solidly for nine months, then started rebuilding our house – another strenuous year. Afterwards, I couldn't rest because I was in so much pain – in my back, legs and pelvic area. Five eminent consultants suggested Prozac because I was so despondent. But I knew I was suffering from something physiological not psychological.

'I was beginning to despair when a very forceful aunt said: "None of these doctors are doing you any good: you gotta recast this play". I consulted a wonderful London GP, Dr Alison Joy, and a surgeon called Charles Akle. They agreed I was probably riddled with adhesions – little bits of scar tissue which kink or partially block the bowel – caused by not giving my body time to heal properly. Keyhole surgery relieved the pain immediately.

'It was chilling because if I hadn't been so determined, I would be on Prozac unnecessarily and still in pain.

'I also had a problem with HRT. I was given an oestrogen/testosterone implant after the hysterectomy. One year later, my oestrogen levels were extremely high, which knocked out my pituitary gland. I got very tired and my energy levels went right down. Unfortunately, you can't stop the therapy with implants because the hormones are in your system and it took another year for the oestrogen to be absorbed. Now I'm on natural progesterone plus a testosterone implant – at five months and ten days, I feel myself running out of gas – and an oestrogen patch.

'I've never been a great physical fitness person but I feel wonderful when I do it. I walk the dog every day, do yoga once a week and try to go to the gym. I also do Medau, a system of constant movement to music, with Lucy Jackson who is a grandmother with the figure of an 18 year old.

'You get very attuned to your body if you're not well so I do treat it as kindly as I can. I eat lots of pasta, rice, bread and veggies. Normally I only eat meat or fish every other day. I love fruit as a snack and I avoid alcohol because it just doesn't suit me.

'I don't pop a lot of vitamins but I do take buffered vitamin C, 1g a day, a multivitamin and mineral, calcium, zinc, and Udo's Choice oil*. And I love Green Magma, an extract of young barley from Japan which is marvellous for your gut. I take the herb echinacea to boost my immune system if I feel an infection coming. Homoeopathic Oscilloccinum is an excellent anti-cold and flu remedy.

'My two big beauty problems (other than ageing!) are ridgy, squidgy nails, which I've always had, and hair colour. I'm grey so I have my colour done every three weeks. I've found a wonderful browny red but even organic colour makes my scalp burn and itch. (*For our suggestions, see pp.114–119.*)

GAYLE'S BEAUTY ROUTINE
A good massage every three weeks; a facial after flying; **cleanser: Vaseline,** applied and wiped off three times before bed; **facial moisturising products** which Gayle rotates night by night: oils: **Clarins Orchidée Bleu, Cetuem Gold;** moisturisers and night creams: **Chanel Hydra-Système, Ponds Overnight Cream, Revlon Eterna 27, Clarins Multi-Regenerative System, Darphin Intral Balm** (when skin is really dry); **Givenchy Double Sequence ampoules;** before special occasions: **Clarins Beauty Flash Balm.**

fabulous fragrance-wearing — forever...

Fragrance can turbo-charge our pleasure in life. But a favourite scent won't always suit you forever – so here are the secrets that ensure you smell fabulous for a lifetime...

One day we may wake up – and our signature perfume won't smell the same any more. Our hormones can play tricks with our favourite fragrances, altering the way they interact with the skin. (That's why pregnant women are often nauseated by a fragrance they'd always loved.) Worryingly, though, our fragrance may change character without us even *realising* it – because we may also experience a gradual dwindling of our ability to smell, a natural process that begins in our fifties and can really become noticeable from 60-plus.

Jilly Fraysse, a fragrance expert who has worked at exclusive London perfume boutiques L'Artisan Parfumeur and Les Senteurs, has time and again seen customers experiencing this phenomenon. 'Whenever hormones go into overdrive – or into decline – it can interfere with fragrance-wearing,' explains Jilly. The first time she noticed the strange, chemical interaction between fragrance and menopausal skin was on her own mother-in-law. 'All her life she'd worn Arpège, because her husband bought it for her when they were engaged. But at about 50, it started to smell literally cheesy on her. And the worst thing of all was that she was unaware of it...' When Jilly herself hit the menopause, she found herself unable to wear Joy – a life-long favourite – because it made

her nauseous. 'But the silver lining to the cloud is that all this is usually temporary,' she says. 'Once the change of life is over, you can probably go back to wearing an old favourite without any problems.'

If your fave scent 'goes off' on the skin, all is not lost. 'You don't have to wear it on your skin,' says Jilly. Her alternatives: spritz it onto hems, cuffs and collars, or onto a cotton wool ball to be tucked into your bra. 'Be careful it isn't going to stain, if you're going to use it on fabric; spray it onto a white Kleenex, and if it doesn't leave a mark, it's safe on pale clothing.' She also suggests a voile of fragrance: 'Spray it into the air and walk through it, subtly perfuming your hair and your clothes.'

The white floral, jasmine-based scents tend to pose most problems, in Jilly's experience. 'Fruity and citrussy fragrances are usually "safer".'

Meanwhile – since our noses may be less sensitive – how can we tell whether we've overdone it? 'Nobody needs more than a single spritz either side of the neck, and one on the wrists and/or the back of the knees,' she advises.

Jilly's trick: spray fragrance on the outside of the wrists, rather than the inner pulse-points, 'because it subtly diffuses outwards when it's warmed by the body. And then,' she adds, 'there's the famous advice: wear fragrance wherever you want to be kissed...'

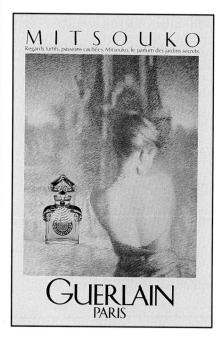

PS Our all-time favourite scent? Guerlain's Mitsouko. Rich, velvety – and irresistible...

FRAGRANCE – WHO WEARS WHAT...

★ **Sharon Stone:** Bulgari Eau Parfumée

★ **Kim Basinger:** Robert Piguet's Fracas and 'sweet, simple' Avon ones

★ **Suzanne Wyman (fashion designer wife of Bill Wyman):** Sunflowers by Elizabeth Arden

★ **Lady Weinberg (aka fashion designer Anouska Hempel):** Cabotine by Madame Grès

★ **Diana Ross:** fragrances by Knightsbridge perfumer Jo Malone (also a favourite of **Barbra Streisand**)

★ **Zsa Zsa Gabor:** Chanel No. 5

★ **Princess Michael of Kent:** Nina Ricci L'Air du Temps

★ **The late Jackie Kennedy Onassis:** always wore Guerlain Jicky...

★ **Shakira Caine:** Anaïs Anaïs

★ **Angelica Huston:** Jean Patou 1000

★ **Lauren Bacall:** fragrances by Provençale beauty company L'Occitane

★ **Melanie Griffith:** Must de Cartier

★ **HM The Queen:** Penhaligon's Bluebell

★ **Bianca Jagger:** Chopard Casmir

★ **Hillary Rodham Clinton:** Aveda Tantra

★ **Kate O'Mara:** Jardins de Bagatelle by Guerlain

★ **Valerie Campbell (Naomi's mum):** Angel by Thierry Mugler

★ **Sandra Bernhard:** Calèche by Hermès

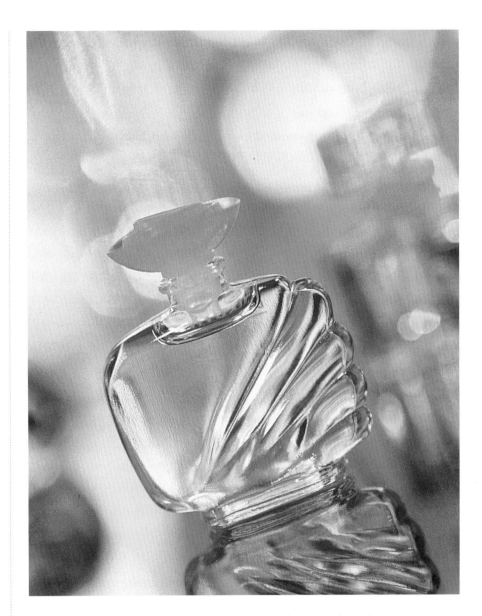

★ **Michelle Pfeiffer:** Donna Karan's Donna Karan New York

★ **Jane Asher:** Je Reviens by Worth

★ **Marie Helvin:** 'I change my fragrance all the time. I have a huge collection – everything that's on the market. I spray it all over my house and clothes.'

★ **Mary Wesley (novelist):** 'I always wear Mitsouko – have done since just after the War when I first encountered this delicious Oriental fragrance.'

★ **Rebecca Stephens (first woman up Everest):** 'I carried my Estée Lauder Alliage all the way to advanced base camp, and I remember it was appreciated by my fellow campers – especially the French. Perfume is the one luxury that goes everywhere with me!'

★ **Betty Boothroyd (Speaker of the House of Commons):** 'Guerlain's Mitsouko really is my favourite scent. It reminds me of holidays I had in Paris.'

make-up tips for the visually impaired

We applaud the crusade of make-up artist Jenny Jordan to introduce visually impaired women to the world of make-up and haircare, through special workshops organised by Action for Blind People. Through that work, she has pinpointed the key problem areas that visually impaired women face when it comes to applying make-up. 'Many of them shy away from make-up,' Jenny observes, 'yet they can get a terrific confidence-boost from wearing it.' She advises having a professional consultation with a make-up artist – in a department store, for instance – to pinpoint the right colours, and then following these guidelines...

◆ Use a good magnifying mirror – big enough to use but small enough to carry around in your bag.

◆ Keep your make-up simple.

◆ Try using cream-to-powder foundation, which is easier to apply than liquid foundation. Use a fresh sponge after five applications of foundation.

◆ If you have fairly good skin, use tinted moisturiser instead of foundation – it's easier to apply.

◆ Smile, then brush a soft shade of blusher onto the apples of your cheeks, using a soft, rounded blusher brush (or a ball of cotton wool approximately the size of a golf ball).

◆ You only need to put lipstick on the top lip and then rub your lips together.

◆ Use lip gloss, instead of lipstick.

◆ Cream eyeshadow – applied with your finger – is easier to manage than powder shadow.

◆ Have your eyelashes professionally dyed and then use colourless mascara (Max Factor, for instance), instead of trying to cope with a coloured wand. Applying five strokes of colourless mascara to the top and bottom lashes (moving from the inner corner to the outer corner of the eye) should give sufficient effect.

◆ Put Vaseline around your nails before you paint them; if you make a mistake and the polish gets on your finger, you can wipe it off without staining. Mistakes are less visible with clear or natural pink polish.

◆ Use eye make-up and nail polish remover in pad form. You have more control with them than liquids or creams.

◆ 2-in-1 cleanser-and-toner formulations save mixing up the bottles (and using toner before cleanser).

◆ Tidy your eyebrows by brushing them with a toothbrush, then stroking through with a dab of Vaseline, to keep them neat.

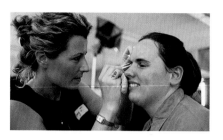

QUESTIONS TO ASK WHEN SHOPPING FOR MAKE-UP

Jenny also has these guidelines to follow when you're at the cosmetics counter. 'Don't be shy about asking for help,' she adds. 'In my experience, beauty consultants are just delighted to give advice to the visually impaired – but you can help steer them in the right direction with these questions...'

Foundation 'Please can you find me a cream-to-powder foundation that matches my skintone perfectly in daylight. And show me how many strokes of foundation I will need to make up my face.'

Blusher 'I want a blusher that gives me a healthy glow but also looks natural in the daytime. Please show me how many strokes of colour are enough. I would also like a soft, rounded powder brush to apply my blusher with.'

Lipstick 'Please pick me a long-lasting lipstick that brightens up my face.'

Eyeshadow 'I would like a cream eyeshadow that I can easily apply with my finger and suits my colouring.'

Look Good, Feel Better is the beauty industry's way of 'giving back' – funding a programme of workshops for women undergoing cancer therapy that's now operating in several countries. Volunteer professional beauty therapists and make-up artists teach ways with wigs and scarves – and a 12-stage programme for skincare and make-up. Among Look Good, Feel Better's supporters is make-up legend Barbara Daly, who says: 'I think what they're doing is absolutely sensational – giving women self confidence-boosting care at a time in their lives when they need it most. Because if you look good, you do feel better.' Liz Collinge has also worked with cancer patients, teaching them how to face special beauty challenges. So we asked Barbara and Liz for their look-good-feel-better tips for women undergoing cancer treatment...

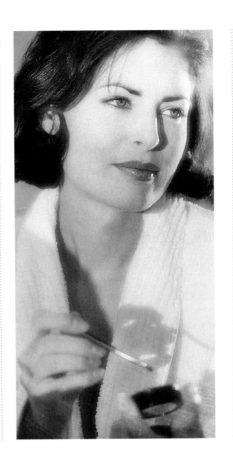

give additional depth, it gives you a guide while you're sticking on the lashes. Single lashes are another option if yours are simply sparse.

'Cancer treatment may make you very flushed – but don't be tempted to cover your whole face with foundation. Stand back and analyse where you need extra camouflage. First, apply your regular foundation but only where you really need it. Then if you're still too flushed, apply concealer – or try mixing it in on the back of your hand with a dot of one of those green under-make-up bases. Mixing the two makes for more natural results; the green concealer on its own is very draining,' says Barbara.

'If you're pale and washed out, don't think that a darker foundation is the answer – it will just look unnatural. Instead, choose a colour that matches your natural skintone, then add colour with blusher, or a

look good, feel better

'A common side-effect of chemotherapy is brow-loss, or lash-loss. The solution is to draw brows on to the skin with ultra-fine strokes using a pencil or brow make-up – preferably using two shades, since our natural brows are virtually never one colour. If your pencil has a brush at the end, use that to brush through the colour afterwards – otherwise, use an old soft toothbrush to soften the effect. I'd steer clear of tattooed eyebrows, because they can look false – and most women's brows do grow back, after treatment,' says Barbara.

'It looks more natural if you draw on the brows with the side of the pencil,

rather than the tip,' adds Liz. 'If the lashes have gone, I like to outline the eyes with a medium-to-dark eyeshadow, using a sponge applicator rather than a brush, for a more natural look. Avoid eyeliner pencils, which can give a too sharp line.'

'Lashes, if you have them, can be boosted with lash-thickening mascara. But if you've lost your lashes, I wouldn't use false lashes unless you're quite good with them,' warns Barbara. 'However, if you do have the knack, there are plenty of natural-looking lashes around and you don't have to look like Twiggy, circa 1968. Draw on a line with eyeliner, first – it'll not only

slightly rosy-toned under-make-up base. Alternatively, lightly dust on a slightly pink-toned powder during the day if your complexion needs a boost,' Barbara suggests.

'Try dusting just the tiniest touch of blusher around the temples, the hairline, onto the nose and chin if you're looking pale,' says Liz.

'Dry skin and lips can be a problem,' Barbara points out. 'Step up your moisturiser and keep a lip balm handy.'

And lastly, says Barbara: 'Lipstick is great medicine – so don't think twice about buying yourself a wardrobe of inexpensive new lipsticks as a way to cheer yourself up, fast!'

fabulous hair

It's simple: if our hair looks great, we feel great – but Bad Hair Days make for bad days. After 40, roller-coaster hormones and the onset of grey make for new hair challenges. The flipside is that these changes give us the opportunity to reinvent ourselves – with style and glamour. So we asked the world's leading hair experts – in cutting, colouring, styling (and even hair loss) – for their advice to ensure that hair looks and feels fabulous – forever. Here's everything you need to know to make every day a Good Hair Day...

hair shapes for older faces

Trading hairdressers is almost as much of a 'sister act' as swopping builders – or lovers. Many women feel that if their hairstyle is great, they can take on the world – if it's not, it's time to slink home with a paper bag on your head and wait until it grows again. Our expert line-up of world-famous hairdressers – John Barrett, John Frieda and Charles Worthington – all agree that the bottom-line key to a good cut is that it should complement your face shape. You don't know your face shape? And your hairdresser doesn't seem to either? Okay, here goes...

how to find your face shape

Tie your hair back off your face and wear something with a low neck. Stand or sit in front of a mirror, a little less than an arm's distance away. Grasp a lip-liner pencil (or anything like that, e.g. coloured eyeliner pencil) in your writing hand, close one eye and trace the outline of your face, round the hairline, jawline and back to hairline, on the glass. Now add in ears, neck and the outline of your head around the top and sides. There you have it. (Yes, it will come off with window cleaner!)

the experts' tips for cuts to suit your face shape

If you have a basically oval face (like the one on the left), you can wear almost any shape and cut, agree our experts. Since few of us can lay claim to that 'beautopia' shape, here are tips for styles to flatter different face shapes. We have taken the most common shapes. (Although not every woman will have exactly one outline; some are a variation of one or more.)

NB One of the most common problems with older faces is that they tend to get thinner – make sure always to balance this with softness and fullness rather than hard lines.

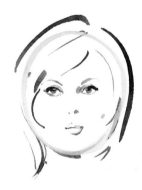

ROUND

Aim for:
- A slightly domed, pointy look at top of head to elongate head shape.
- A fringe cut on an angle, blending in slightly longer than the temple to create shadows under cheekbones.
- A sleek, rather than full, look at sides.
- Hair feathered at bottom onto neck to disguise a plump or short neck.

Plus: Use make-up to elongate eyebrows and eyes; miss out on blusher, but try highlighter on top of cheekbones and under brows; try lighter brighter lips.

I know haircuts can be traumatic for some women, but not for me. Hair grows back – and if you don't like it, you can always change it. Personally, I like short hair – it's me...

ISABELLA ROSSELLINI

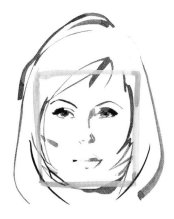

OBLONG

Aim for:
- A soft top of head.
- A slightly asymmetrical fringe, which graduates, blending and continuing the line into the body of your hair.
- Fullness behind the ears to widen face; this will also help if you have a long distance between nose and chin, or a long upper lip.
- A medium-length layered bob.

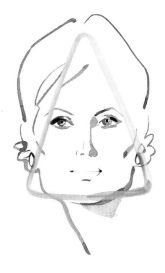

TRIANGLE

Aim for:
- Fullness at top on sides to balance head shape.
- A soft, slightly asymmetrical fringe to disguise hairline and shorten face.

Plus: Accentuate eyes; wear earrings to draw attention away from jaw.
(*See also square and oblong.*)

LONG JAWLINE

Aim for:
- Hair cut on an angle from chin to shoulder to soften line.

Avoid:
- Long straight hair or a short, e.g. ear-length, bob which will make the jawline look even longer.

Plus: Biggish earrings to distract eye from jawline.

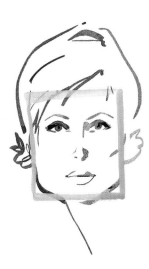

SQUARE

Aim for:
- A slightly domed, narrow look at top of head to elongate head shape.
- A slightly asymmetrical fringe.
- Short hair worn behind ears feathered down on neck to give length.
- Longer hair with fullness at top to balance jawline, soften outline and edges of hair and avoid hard lines.

Plus: Accentuate and lengthen brows and eyes, and use earrings to take attention from square jawline.

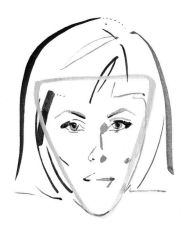

INVERTED TRIANGLE

Aim for:
- Gentle curves on the top of the head.
- A fringe which is longer in the middle and shorter at temples.
- A one-length bob to just below the ears.

PROMINENT NOSE

Aim for:
- A gentle curve at back of head to balance nose.

Avoid:
- The Mrs Thatcher look, which will make it worse.

the **long** versus **short** debate

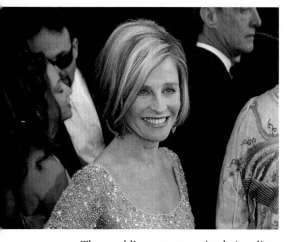

Once upon a time, the rule was: hit 40, buy a twinset, lop off your hair. But today – so long as your hair's healthy and shiny – the rule-book's been torn up...

The world's most expensive hairstylist, Nicky Clarke – who not so long ago actually turned down model Marie Helvin's request to cut her hair shorter – insists: 'I've got dozens of older clients with fabulous long hair. If it's in good condition, then who says it's got to go? The look might need adjusting a little – for instance, having it slightly layered, rather than just long and straight, or blown dry more regularly, or putting it up now and again so it has an air of elegance about it – but it's just ageist to lay down the law about long hair.'

Hollywood actress **René Russo** couldn't agree more. In fact, the suggestion that women ought to cut their hair in middle age has René

Remember hair will always 'lift' about 1cm (¹/₂ inch) shorter when it's dry – so if you want, for instance, a chin-length bob, it must be cut about 1cm (¹/₂ inch) longer.

insisting: 'It makes me want to grow it down to my toes, just to say go **** yourself.' Novelist **Jackie Collins** – who wouldn't dream of cutting off her trademark tresses – shares René's sentiments. 'Long hair's much sexier – I wear my hair up to keep it out of the way when I'm working, and down when I'm playing.'

Still, if you long to stay long, the one thing you don't want is to get freeze-framed with an outdated signature look. You know it's time to re-think your long hairstyle if you dust off your 20-year-old graduation photo or your wedding snaps to see that basically, your hairstyle was fossilised right there and then. If you're using your hair as some kind of security blanket to hide behind (*à la* Old English Sheepdog), it's probably also time for an update.

But if you want to avoid the 'time-warp' trap of long hair, the solutions are simple: have a few layers put in, texturise the ends with wax (creating a softer impression) – or learn how to put it up. 'For evening, there's nothing more elegant than a chignon,' insists Hugh, of Hugh & Stephen (who spends half the day 'up-do-ing' royals, aristocrats and stars of everything at his Pimlico salon). 'Long hair's much

more versatile than short hair – which is why women love it.' (*See p.102 for step-by-step instructions on how to put your hair up.*)

For longer-haired women who want to wear their hair down but off the face, John Barrett – who works out of Bergdorf Goodman, in New York – still believes that 'a thin black grosgrain head-band' is most chic. Donna Karan prefers to scoop her hair up into a mid-height pony-tail, 'which works like an instant face-lift,' she enthuses. Certainly, long hair lets you play around with the images you present to the world: you can put it up and feel professional for work, or let it down (literally') when it gets to Friday night. Alternatively you can loosely pin it up, so that – sexily – you can un-pin it in front of your partner.

But the downside, of course, is that long hair is old hair. Philip Kingsley, a leading international trichologist (who, insiders say, helps keep fortysomething **Jerry Hall's** bleached-to-high-heaven pony-tail as shiny as a racehorse), points out that hair which has reached 45cm (18 inches) long is actually around three years old. 'During that time, not only will it have been environmentally damaged – by hairdryers, for instance – but the

how short can you go?

An urchin cut works brilliantly on **Sharon Stone** – but you need to make sure a very short cut won't give you a pinhead. Before you commit to a cut, try scraping your hair right off your face and looking at yourself in a full-length glass, checking out your reflection from the sides as well as straight on. But according to John Frieda, a simple measurement can also tell you whether you can go for an **Audrey Hepburn** gamine look.

• Look straight ahead into a mirror, chin absolutely straight – not tipped up or down at all.
• Use your finger to follow a line on your neck, directly down from your earlobe. Stop when your finger is perfectly in line with the tip of your chin – or the lowest part of the chin, if yours happens to be double...
• Measure the distance using a tape measure or a ruler.

'If the distance is more than 5.5cm ($2^{1}/4$ inches),' says John Frieda, 'then short hair probably won't suit you and you'll need extra length, or extra layers cut into the neck, to soften the look. If that distance is less than 5.5cm ($2^{1}/4$ inches), short hair should flatter you.'

chances are, if you're over 40, it's coloured, too, so it may have taken a beating. And as you get older, the hair shaft actually becomes a little thinner in diameter – which makes it more likely to break.' Acknowledges John Frieda, 'If hair is fine or tatty, there's no point hanging on to it – it'll look better and have more oomph if it's short.'

The first, essential step to being a post-40 Rapunzel, believes Nicky Clarke, is to have it regularly trimmed. 'Every six to eight weeks is a must to keep it looking good. Women run away with the idea that because it doesn't need trimming to keep its *shape*, they can leave it longer between

cuts.' Then split ends become a problem.

Condition is also crucial. One reason why long hair was always a no-no for the over-forties is that hair conditioners didn't even exist until a couple of decades ago – so long hair was simply tatty hair. But the good news is that high-tech haircare – which enables us to keep our hair in glorious, gleaming condition even when it's way past our shoulders – has now green-lighted long hair for the over-forties. 'If you give hair plenty of TLC, there's no reason you shouldn't keep it – or grow it – long,' insists Philip Kingsley. **Jane Seymour**, for instance, gets away with

almost waist-length hair because it's always alluringly super-shiny.

Nicky Clarke points out that 'Long hair is also prone to static – it gathers a lot of electricity, especially in winter, which makes hair look flat and flyaway.' Leave-in conditioners help combat the problem.

Keeping hair well moisturised, explains Kingsley, also prevents premature breakage. Poor condition is often outwardly apparent when it's too late – when strands are already split and breaking off. So prevention is better than cure. And every expert we spoke to advised occasional deep-conditioning treatments as the ultimate maintenance option for long hair. 'Use them at least once a month – preferably once a week,' advises Nicky Clarke. (NB The hair masks voted tops by the testing panel for our previous book, *The Beauty Bible*, included Estée Lauder Herbal Hair Pack, Pantène Intensives Conditioner, St Ives Swiss Formula Mud Miracle and Lancôme Fluance Extra Rich Cream Conditioner.)

Over-drying – with a too-hot hairdryer – is bad news for long hair, however. Experiment with leaving hair to dry naturally until it's 80 per cent dry – or use your dryer on a lower setting, while you gently ruffle it – and try silicone-based serums, which help protect long hair from heat damage. Long hair's worst enemy, believes Kingsley, 'is Granny's prescribed 100 brush-strokes a night'. He prefers wide-toothed combs to brushes, which tug at hair.

For some women, giving up long hair is harder than giving up chocolate, sex or men. So why do it? With a little TLC, you can stay a glamorous Rapunzel forever...

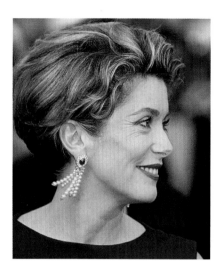

pump up the volume

Few of us go through life with a permanently thick and bouncy head of hair. Whether your hair always tends to be fine, thin and flat, or is just going through a bad phase, there are techniques which can improve the look by adding volume, curves and shape.

We asked former British Hairdresser of the Year, Charles Worthington – known for his expertise in creating big hair – for his advice on how to make more of what you've got.

'If your hair is usually bouncy but suddenly becomes flat, do look at whether you're taking care of yourself properly,' recommends Charles. 'I always know when regular clients are not eating well, or just not looking after themselves; their hair loses spring and bounce in the roots, and starts looking dull and lacklustre. And you must have exercise: cardiovascular exercise sends the blood rushing round your body, it feeds the hair follicle and everything just works better.'

Although some hairdressers say thinner hair is better short, Charles says just on the shoulders can be a good longer length because it will kick out when it hits your shoulders and you can also put it up easily. It's vital

not to let the hair drag itself down, he adds, so go for long layers to create shape, volume and curves. Both Charles and John Frieda agree that short layers, like shampoos and sets,

fluff It up

John Frieda has an amazing tip for volumising hair: rub the hair between your fingers, almost like rubbing butter into flour to make pastry. With wet hair, spray on your thickening product then get it to the point where it's almost dry, he says, and really rub it together – it fluffs out each individual cuticle. 'You can do it on dry hair when you want it to be really full: it's something I've often used in the studio for fashion shoots,' he says. (We tried it; it's extraordinary.)

are ageing (could someone please tell Her Majesty?). Have your style trimmed regularly, every five to seven weeks, depending on how fast it grows (remember that also will vary from season to season).

'For the fullest head of hair possible, use a regime of specially tailored products: shampoo, conditioner, styling spray and finally a fixing product,' says Charles. The key words to look for are 'volumising' and/or 'thickening'. Go for a good range; you get what you pay for. There may be a case for sticking to one brand because the products are formulated to work well together. Useful ingredients are panthenol, keratin-amino acids and brown sea algae (which you'll find in Charles's own range).

Hair condition will change with the seasons; for instance, as the central heating goes on, the scalp gets drier and you may need to shift to more moisturising products. If you're going grey, the hair texture changes and becomes dryer and more wiry, so it needs more nourishment and moisture.

Wash thin, fine hair every day if possible: 'It goes out of shape more easily than a thick mop; any warm atmosphere will make it limp and simply sleeping on it tends to crush the style.' But, as with make-up, less – overall – is more. 'Always use conditioner but use it sparingly or you risk making hair lank and droopy,' Charles recommends. You may find that volumising shampoos and conditioners seem to work better if you use them in the bath rather than the shower: 'The problem with power showers is that they can deliver such a jet of water that they strip the product out of the hair, whereas a bath tends to leave a residue.'

ROLLER CULTURE

Perms used to be the only big hair solution until Velcro rollers came along – and perms slunk out of the back door. A good thing too, according to all the hairdressers and colourists we talked to. Without exception, they rolled their eyes in horror at the damage wreaked by perms. Susan Baldwin of John Frieda says: 'They make hair dry, dull and basically dead-looking.'

Rollers are a godsend for fine, thin or flat hair but can be a mystery to the uninitiated. To decode The Big Roller Mystery, here are Charles Worthington's top tips:

◆ Go for easy-to-use Velcro self-grip rollers, secured with an extra Kirbigrip if you like.

◆ Put them into warm hair, then wait until the hair is cold before taking them out and styling. Warm hair is malleable; it 'sets' when cold.

◆ Roller size: hair needs to go round a roller a minimum of one and a half times. So start by measuring the length of hair on the different parts of your head that you want to lift. You need rollers with a diameter which is two-thirds the length of the hair; e.g. if your hair on the top is 7.5cm (3 inches) long, choose a roller 5cm (2 inches) in circumference – a good medium size to start with, by the way.

◆ You will probably need about 20 rollers in all. How many you need of each sort is usually a case of roll it and see: but start with at least six of each type.

◆ Putting in the roller: take a square section of hair, a little bit wider than the length of the roller. Put rollers in from the front top of your head and work back and down.

◆ Dry with a diffuser on a hand-dryer on a cool temperature to set the hair, or use a portable hood-dryer.

◆ When the hair is cold, take the rollers out, working from the bottom up.

◆ With your head upside down, spray a little fixing product onto the roots, before running your fingers or a brush through hair.

Heated rollers can be useful when you're in a hurry. Spray a little old-fashioned fixing spray (rather than a styling product) near roots. Only trial and error will tell you how long you need to leave the rollers in – so practise. If you're getting too curly, try letting them cool down a bit and only leave them in for a moment.

BACK IT UP

Fine hair is bound to droop a bit over the day, especially if you're hot, busy or hurried. It may sound a bit 1960s, but a little back-combing or back-brushing is marvellous for maintaining a style. Both techniques have a bad name for damaging hair but the trick is to do it very gently, says Charles. 'Hold the section of hair gently between finger and thumb, letting some strands escape, and tease the hair. If you hold the hair too tightly, you create too much tension. A natural bristle brush is the gentlest for back-combing hair and will fluff out a shape and give a little more volume with the least amount of tangles. To create volume just at the roots, back-comb them; then when you come to brush out the back-combing, use a brush with flexible bristles. Be gentle and don't pull at the hair shaft. If you want a lot of volume and staying power, turn your head upside down and spray with a styling or fixing product before back-combing.'

fringe benefits

If you have a furrowed or lined forehead, try a fringe before you try a brow-lift! John Frieda says that a fringe over the brow can be extremely de-ageing for older women, can soften a face, hiding a bad hairline and – if strategically styled – minimise facial flaws. 'Steer clear of heavy fringes, though,' he advises, 'as this look is too severe for women of practically any age. Go for something light and feathery.' (Think what a veil can do for a face. Well, a fringe achieves much the same glamorising, line-softening effect.)

more hair wisdom from john barrett

• Commit to a hairdresser you trust – one who does the hair of other women of your age, whose style you admire.

• Regularly look at photos of yourself and realistically analyse the pros and cons of your hair length with a good friend, as well as your hairdresser. Sometimes you can see yourself more objectively in a photo than a mirror.

• Talk to your hairdresser honestly and with an open mind. Most hairdressers will be as honest in giving you feedback as you are in seeking it. Repeat back what you've agreed to – to make sure communication is clear. Good communication is a two-way street and very necessary for something as important as your haircut, colour and styling.

• For Bad Hair Days, pull hair back wet – or use light conditioner to dress the hair, then pull it back with a very thin or a very wide head-band.

• Time emergency? Shampoo and blow-dry your fringe only. This can work with head-bands, pony-tails or simple, natural styles.

• Don't over-condition. Most people do – and it's just like over-watering houseplants, or orchids. Over-conditioning leads to problems like build-up, limp or hard-to-style hair. Use conditioner sparingly and focus on the ends.

put it up

Piling your hair on top is not only an answer for a Bad Hair Day, it can give you a whole new look – which is wonderful fun if nothing else. And a put-up job is incredibly useful if you've left your cut two weeks (or more) too late.

There are two main looks: sleek and smooth – think Audrey Hepburn in _Breakfast at Tiffany's_ – or soft and frothy. You can put up all sorts of different lengths of hair although the optimum length is just on your shoulders with long layers through your hair. Don't worry if hair is shorter, you can still get a lovely, casually elegant look by twisting it up and fanning out the ends (fix them in place with fixing spray). It doesn't even matter if the grips show, just look for ones with a pretty detail at the ends.

the steps

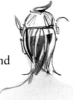

1 Divide the hair into four sections, back, top and two sides, using butterfly clips.

2 Starting with back section: if hair is long, brush horizontally to one side, then put a line of grips all the way from nape to top of section, criss-crossing them if you can to anchor the hair.

3 Fold hair back on itself in a pleat, tucking ends in and twisting upwards. Hold in place with the hairpins.

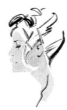

4 If hair is short, don't worry about tucking the ends in at the top, just fan them out casually and spray.

5 Now dress the sides. With the sides and the top you need to look at 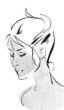 the overall proportion of your face and dress your hair to suit that (*see the section on face shapes, pp.96–97*). Either comb the sides back smoothly and pin into the pleat or let some or all of the hair drop casually down and around your face; use a heated roller or tongs to give shape if necessary.

6 Move on to the top: arrange fringe and hairline then back-comb or brush the rest if you wish, arrange gracefully over the sides, and smooth some back into the pleat; if your hair is short on top, either leave the top section as you would normally or pin some of it to the top of the pleat. Again secure with pretty pins if you have some wild bits.

7 As a final touch on this or any other style, try Charles' tip and 'polish' the surface of the hair with a serum product. Put a little tiny dab of serum – about the size of a five-pence piece or a dime – into your palm, then use a 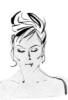 big floppy make-up brush to pick up some of the serum and brush it onto your hair. This also works brilliantly with long straight hair, giving it a glossy, almost glass-like finish.

the rules

◆ Always practise before trying to do this for an important event; allow hairdressing rehearsal time to play around, see what's easiest for you to do and what looks best.

◆ If possible, have your hair put up in a salon so you can see what the hairdresser does and she/he can give you some individual tips.

◆ The key to putting your hair up is to do it in sections: section off the back and start with that, then do the sides, then the top.

◆ A three-way mirror is very helpful.

◆ As well as styling and fixing products, you will need: matte Kirbigrips – if you're worried they'll show, look for ones with pretty details at the ends like a single tiny flower or rhinestone for evenings; small hairpins – bend one end into a fish tail beforehand so that they will stick there without sliding out.

◆ Rollers are not vital but hair that has been lifted in rollers is much easier to work with.

more hair wisdom from john frieda

• 'Always have a (free) consultation before booking an appointment with a new hairdresser. The relationship is all-important – you've got to feel comfortable. Ideally, you should visit two or three salons – and compare.'

• 'Don't be embarrassed to take pictures to give your hairdresser an idea of the look you want. It helps put you and your hairdresser on the same wavelength.'

• 'If you have a haircut you hate, wait a week before you rush off somewhere else so you're more rational. The eye takes time to adjust – after a week, you'll know if it's really bad.'

• 'To achieve body, blow-dry roots in the opposite direction to how your hair naturally grows. The secret is to imagine your head is a giant roller, and – with a blow-dryer in one hand – run your fingers through your hair, literally winding it around the head in one direction. Then, after a minute or so, switch hands; put the dryer in the other hand and wind it round the scalp the other way. Keep alternating, and as the hair gets closer to being dry, switch to a bristle brush or a Mason Pearson, instead of your fingers, for final sleeking and styling. Because the roots are being lifted and dried in opposite directions, the result is great body.'

Banana Reconditioning Treatment

Mash one ripe peeled banana with one tablespoon of sunflower oil and a half teaspoon of fresh lime juice. Mix well then apply generously to dry, well-combed hair. Leave for 30 minutes before shampooing as usual.

Why it works: Potassium in banana helps scalp health; natural sebum-like sunflower oil conditions dry scalp and hair; lime juice helps adjust scalp's acid/alkali balance and smooth cuticles to increase shine.

Lime Juice Perm Reviver

Mix a teaspoon of lime juice with 300ml ($\frac{1}{2}$ pint) cold water, rinse through the hair before washing.

▷ *Why it works:* lime juice contains citric acid and oils which contract the cortex of each hair strand to tighten curls without stripping natural oils.

Rum and Egg Conditioner

Mix together an egg yolk, a half teaspoonful of vitamin C powder and two teaspoons of dark rum. Apply to dry hair, leave for ten minutes then wash with a mild shampoo.

Why it works: albumen and lecithin in egg yolk revive hair, rum stimulates scalp, vitamin C helps adjust the scalp's acid/alkali balance, encouraging shine.

French Dressing for tangly hair

Mix one measure of vinegar to three of sunflower oil; work through hair and leave for five minutes before shampooing and conditioning as usual.

Why it works: acetic acid in vinegar encourages cuticles to lie flat and the oil moisturises the hair.

Tomato Sauce Colour Corrector

Chlorine in swimming pools often makes lightened hair khaki-ish. Apply a

kitchen magic

Your fridge and store-cupboard can yield as many goodies for your hair as for every other part of your face and body. Eat as many fruits as you can – but also mush them up and mulch them in!

Daniel Field, the leading London hairdresser, whose organic range is the favourite of stars like Gayle Hunnicutt (*see pp.90–91*), gave us the following recipes to feed your hair.

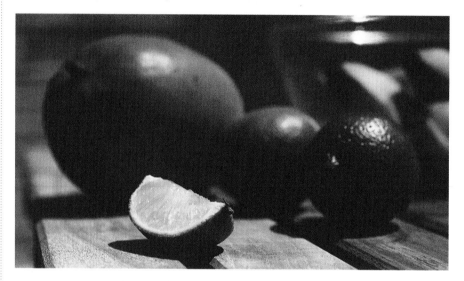

generous dollop of tomato sauce to well-combed, dry hair, massaging well. Leave for 30 minutes, then shampoo.

Why it works: the pink tones in the sauce neutralise the khaki.

Lemonade Detangler

Chemically treated hair can tangle easily. For a quick fix, pour some lemonade into a clean plant spray and spritz liberally over dry hair then leave for five minutes before shampooing and conditioning as usual.

Why it works: citric acid closes the cuticle layers and contracts the hair cortex back to its pre-damaged state.

Corn Oil for split ends and static prevention

Put a small amount of corn oil onto the palms of your hands and smooth down over dry hair, right to the tips. Shampoo as usual.

Why it works: the corn oil will protect the ends of the hair from the impact of the washing and drying.

Mango Winter Restorer

Chop a peeled ripe mango roughly into a clean bowl. Add a tablespoon of walnut oil and a squeeze of lemon juice. Mix well with a fork or blender until reasonably smooth. Wrap a bath towel round your neck before applying the mixture evenly all over dry, well-combed hair. Massage well into scalp and hair. After 30 minutes, rinse thoroughly – then shampoo as normal.

Why it works: the combination of minerals, vitamins and trace elements in the mango, plus concentrated scalp massage, stimulates scalp and follicles.

Léonor Greyl's tips for hair health

Madame Greyl is France's healthy hair guru; her Paris treatment centre* is a mecca for stars including, it's rumoured, Catherine Deneuve and Princess Caroline of Monaco. So we asked her to give us her tips for head-turning hair...

• 'If you've chosen a great quality shampoo and you're washing your hair quickly, you're wasting your money. Most women don't shampoo for long enough. Always comb the hair before you wet it, then put a blob of shampoo in the palm of your hand and add a little water, to dilute it. Apply evenly to the scalp and run your fingers through the hair. Gently work it into the scalp for ten minutes – then rinse for at least another five. Finish with a cold rinse, which is good for circulation.'

• 'Never use a fine-toothed comb on your hair; always use the widest-toothed comb you can find. Only use a brush when actually styling, to minimise wear and tear.'

• 'Visit a salon at least twice a year, spring and autumn, for a deep treatment "facial for your hair".'

• 'See a nutritionist for hair problems. Hair needs feeding from the inside-out as well as outside-in.'

• 'Wash your brushes and combs once a week in a mild shampoo.'

• 'Take two or three hours out of a busy schedule each week to make time for yourself: a massage, an exercise class, a walk. Hair health is a reflection of inner health and if you're under pressure, it shows up in your hair almost immediately.'

AT-HOME SCALP MASSAGE

Madame Greyl's prescription includes regular scalp massages. 'Women store a huge amount of tension in the scalp,' she explains. 'Sometimes, when I'm massaging a woman's head, the scalp is literally immovable – as if it's glued down – because the scalp muscles are so tense. Which, in turn, restricts blood and nutrient flow to follicles.' What we should aim for, through regular massage, is a scalp which moves easily over the bones of the skull.

• Ideally, she says, you should use borage oil (also known as starflower oil) for the massage; wheatgerm oil is also effective. (Both easily wash out again.) 'But if you prefer, you can also massage the scalp without using oil.'

• If you're using oil, part the hair in five or six places on the scalp, using a wide-toothed comb. Break open five or six capsules of borage or starflower oil, or drip wheatgerm oil from a dropper, and apply along partings.

• Lean forwards to boost circulation.

• Now bunch up the fingers of each hand and massage the temples, to release tension. Do this for at least a minute and try to feel the day's tensions ebb away.

• Then place the pads of the fingers of each hand on the front of your head, just behind the hairline, placed so that your little fingers are almost touching. Massage in strong, circular movements. You should be moving the scalp, not letting your fingers skim over the surface. Do this for a minute or so.

• Move your fingers back an inch or so, and repeat. After a minute, re-position the fingers, another inch back. Keep doing this until you reach the crown, and continue, massaging the back of the head down to the nape. Use all of your fingers and thumbs, applying even pressure.

• In all, devote a full three to five minutes to the head massage. (If it gets uncomfortable to lean forward for all that time, or you have neck problems, you can do the head massage in a sitting position; make a point of keeping your shoulders relaxed.)

• 'You should aim to do the massage three times a week,' believes Madame Greyl, who insists she has seen amazing improvements in hair health among women who pay attention to their scalps in this way.

plumping up your locks

Léonor's' spécialité de la maison is helping women with thinning hair. 'You need to feed the scalp,' insists Mme Greyl, who tailor-makes health-boosting, gloss-restoring hair masks for clients – using ingredients like wheatgerm, silk, chamomile, mimosa and borage oil – then prescribes an individual programme of products to maximise hair health back home.

thinning hair –
still a mystery after
all these years...

Hair loss isn't a men-only problem. One of the less engaging facts about getting older is that a significant number of women also experience thinning hair. According to biochemist Dr Hugh Rushton of Portsmouth University, one in three women in a recent survey reported some hair loss, compared with some 60 per cent of men. And alopecia, as it's called medically, tends to be an extremely traumatic event for women – who see losing hair as losing part of our femininity...

Genetic hair loss (alopecia androgenetica) and moult, or increased hair shedding (chronic telogen effluvium), account for by far the majority of all hair-loss complaints in women – up to 95 per cent, in fact, before menopause. Unlike men, who tend to lose a lot of hair in particular areas, like the temples and crown – 'male-pattern baldness' – women are more likely to thin diffusely from behind the front hairline to the crown. Alopecia areata (patchy hair loss) affects about 0.1 per cent of women. (The very rare scarring alopecias, caused by conditions such as lupus, may affect about 0.01 per cent but there are no precise figures.)

CHANGING HAIRLINES

Research suggests that at least 10 per cent of women suffer from genetic hair loss before the age of 50 (compared with 60 per cent of men), and the number increases at menopause. This is because the villain of the hair piece (sorry...) is believed to be a sidekick of the male hormone testosterone called dihydrotestosterone – or DHT for short. The female hormones, oestrogens, help protect women against the depredations of DHT but that protection fades at menopause as oestrogen levels fall and testosterone levels rise.

Underactive thyroid or hypothyroidism, a problem which is related to auto-immune disease (where the immune system, the body's police force, turns on itself) accounts for only 2 per cent of hair loss problems in women under 45. It makes a huge leap, however, to about 10 per cent as women approach and go through menopause. No one quite knows why, except that women are more prone to auto-immune problems. 'Increased weight gain but no comparable increase in appetite, plus tiredness and lethargy, and hair fall are potential signs of underactive thyroid,' says Dr Rushton. Unfortunately, this condition may also switch on genetic baldness in susceptible women by affecting the way testosterone (which women have as well) circulates in their bodies. 'It's totally treatable,' according to Dr Rushton. So it's vital to catch it early and get appropriate treatment. 'Don't be fobbed off by male doctors,' he insists.

genes or moult?

If you have one of the following...
◆ more hairs falling when shampooing and combing;
◆ less thickness of hair when you draw it back into a pony-tail;
◆ short hairs along your front hairline;
...but your parting is no wider and your hair looks the same to friends, then you're probably suffering from increased shedding rather than a genetic condition. (Beware that you don't think your parting is wider because the hair is grey.)

Unlike a genetic condition, a moult will correct itself eventually, usually within two to three months; if it goes on much beyond that, consult your family doctor who will probably refer you to a consultant dermatologist for investigation.

THE STRESS CONNECTION

What is now clear to hair-loss experts, however, is that stress not only exacerbates male-pattern baldness, both in women and men, but is also a direct cause of increased shedding or hair 'moults'. Stress events may cause hair loss but you may not always link cause and effect because the moult may not start until ten to twelve weeks later.

Dr Rushton says the most likely causes of non-genetic hair loss are:

■ Pregnancy: 50 per cent of women have post-natal hair loss, which usually re-grows without intervention.

■ Menopause: the reduction in oestrogen (female hormone) levels and a relative increase in male hormones may cause some hair loss which usually then grows back if the hormonal imbalance is put right.

■ Hormone replacement therapy (HRT): this has been reported, in some cases, to trigger hair loss similar to genetic hair loss; however these changes can be prevented with a well chosen HRT (i.e. one that does not contain an androgenic progestin).

■ Emotional shocks: acute stressors, from divorce to job loss, may affect hair.

■ Physical stressors: for example, a car accident, the aftermath of a heart attack, surgery.

■ Shallow breathing: hyperventilation, as it's called medically, can affect all your body systems.

■ Not enough rest and sleep.

■ Drug therapy: chemotherapy and radiotherapy for cancer, cortisone, sedatives, tranquillisers and barbiturates, amphetamines, antibiotics.

■ Immunisations: there is some evidence that immunisation in children may trigger temporary hair loss and this may also extend to some pre-travel immunisation.

■ Yo-yo dieting.

■ Poor diet and/or nutritional deficiencies: particularly iron, lysine, B12 and zinc.

■ Smoking: it robs the body of nutrients.

■ Eating disorders: for example, anorexia.

■ Misuse of hair: perming, colouring, using curling tongs or heated rollers, too much brushing with a sharp bristled brush and blow-drying at too high a temperature; these may all cause hair loss due to hair breakage.

■ Central heating.

■ Pollution.

■ Dandruff-like conditions: these may affect the rate of hair shedding.

■ Inadequate or infrequent shampooing: it's important not to reduce shampooing if you have hair loss.

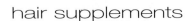

hair supplements

Naturopath Jan de Vries recommends MaxiHair by Nature's Best*, combined with Urticalcin homoeopathic calcium by Bioforce*. Dr Rushton formulated NutriHair for Nature's Best and has also written a useful booklet* about hair loss in women; NutriHair includes iron, lysine, vitamin C and vitamin B12 to help iron absorption. Or you could try brewer's yeast tablets – a cheap and simple option which is said to be good for the hair.

From starting a supplement, the average time before noticing a reduction in hair shedding is 16 weeks; since hair grows about 1cm ($^1/_2$ inch) a month, seeing the benefit in volume may take months.

drug treatments

When it comes to hair loss, there are few options from the pharmaceutical industry – and most experts agree their performance is fairly disappointing. Having said that, many people find that a small improvement is much better than nothing.

The treatment for genetic hair loss in women is usually a combination of hormone (anti-androgen) and topical drug therapy – but this must of course be prescribed and monitored constantly by a medical expert.

In addition, a prescription lotion, minoxidil (marketed as Regaine in the UK, Rogaine in the US), has been shown to stop hair loss in 60 per cent of women who used it, but only 19 per cent reported moderate hair re-growth and 41 per cent said there was no re-growth at all. However, the best therapy, in Dr Rushton's experience, is a combination of minoxidil, an anti-androgenic drug *plus* balanced nutritional support.

A new over-the-counter drug, Aminexil by L'Oréal (also based on the minoxidil formula), claims about 5 per cent more hair over a year, and no more hair loss during that period. However that figure is an average of those in the study, so some people have done better and some have seen no change at all, or possibly even a reduction in hair growth. (Bear in mind also that no form of hair counting, however high-tech, is 100 per cent accurate.)

The new anti-baldness prescription drug, finasteride (Propecia), which has been approved in America, is not suitable for women of childbearing age because it could theoretically cause birth defects (in 2 per cent of men, it can cause temporary loss of libido and impotence while the drug is taken). However, it may be possible for post-menopausal women (who have had no periods for two years) to be prescribed the drug. The downside is that no one is absolutely certain how effective finasteride is – or on whom.

The story behind the drug goes like this: finasteride was actually formulated as a drug therapy for prostate problems – and it was then discovered that it helped some cases of male-pattern baldness. It works by blocking the enzyme (5-alpha reductase) which converts testosterone, the male hormone, to DHT, the villain of the hair piece. However the snag is that there are two types of this enzyme involved; either Type 1 or Type 2 may be the dominant form of the enzyme in the scalp and hair follicle. Finasteride, however, only works on Type 2, the type predominantly involved in the prostate. At the moment, scientists simply don't know how many men's balding pates are controlled by Type 2 – and certainly not how many women's hair loss problems. What you might call a case of stale pate.

other options

If thinning hair is a problem, you may want to check out specific hair-restoring and thickening products by respected brands including Phytologie's Phytocyane* (in tandem with Phytologie's dietary supplement, Phytophanère), plus the ranges from Léonor Greyl* in Paris and from Jan Adams at Romanda Healthcare* in London. Some people have found help from Chinese herbal medicine; others are keen on Ayurvedic (Indian) head massage where practitioners massage shoulders and head with alternate firm and gentle strokes, using warm oil (coconut, sesame, almond or olive). Although massage and stimulation treatments are also often offered by well-known, bona fide trichology clinics, dermatologists tend to be sceptical of them – although they accept that they may be helpful in relieving stress.

feed your hair

Healthy hair responds to what you eat in the same way as your skin and the whole of the rest of your body.

Non-genetic hair loss, say experts, is much worse in women who are deficient in iron (vegetarians may need to supplement with chelated iron), have low levels of B group vitamins, including folic acid, or zinc, or have thyroid problems.

Iron is the biggest problem, according to experts. British figures show that about nine out of ten women between the ages of 16 and 50 are deficient in iron, and about one third of women between 51 and 64, despite the fact that they are not menstruating. A test for serum ferritin levels (not the haemoglobin level used to assess anaemia) can detect this type of iron deficiency.

According to Dr Rushton, who puts it down partly to the fact that many women prefer not to eat red meat, research has shown that if the iron stores are replenished to a certain 'trigger point' then hair growth will start. 'What happens is that the growing stage of the follicles is lengthened so there are, at any one time, more hairs in the growing stage.' But, he cautions, the whole process can take six to nine months – so you have to be patient.

For iron to be absorbed by the body, you need vitamin C and an amino acid called lysine (mostly found in meat). If you eat little red meat, it may be difficult to get enough iron in a form which your body can assimilate. In that case, consider a supplement.

Meanwhile, take care of your digestion with plenty of fresh vegetables and fruit and the foods in our chart below. Lots of pure still water is also vital – a sluggish digestive system can lead to dull, limp, oily hair. For more detailed individual advice, do consult a doctor with an interest and expertise in nutrition, a naturopath or a nutritionist.

hair food

Eat lots of:
Fresh vegetables, salads and fruit
Live yogurt
Cold-pressed oils *(olive, sunflower, sesame, flax)*
Pulses *(peas, beans, lentils)*
Whole grains *(brown rice, oats, buckwheat, millet)*
Seeds *(sunflower, pumpkin, sesame and linseeds)*
Almonds, figs and dates
Plus fresh oily fish, if you're not a vegetarian *(salmon, mackerel, tuna, sardines)*

Drink lots of: Water

Try to cut down on:
Cow's milk products
Caffeine *(coffee, tea, chocolate, cola)*
Sugar and salt

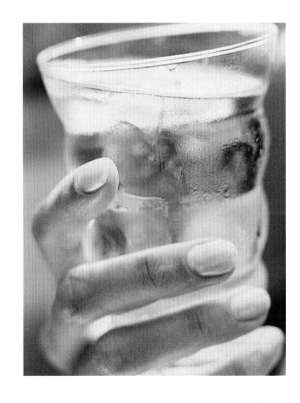

dandruff-busting

Good news first: true dandruff – a combination of flaking skin cells, a yeast called pityrosporum ovale and over-activity by the sebaceous glands – tends to die out as you get older. After 50, as the sebaceous gland activity dies down, dandruff should be just a memory.

Now for the bad news: you may experience the scaly drifts of 'shoulder snow' after 50 and the cause is likely to be a form of eczema or seborrheic dermatitis, triggered by dairy foods – and chocolate.

Here's how to tell the difference and what to do:

Step 1: Wash hair thoroughly every day with a mild medium-to-expensive shampoo (not a cheap one), which leaves your hair feeling clean and shiny. Soak your hair, apply a good blob of shampoo, rub into the scalp well, then rinse very thoroughly. If you can only wash your hair every other day, repeat the process. Put conditioner on ends only. Try this for four weeks and see if it makes a difference. If it doesn't, move on to...

Step 2: Consider your symptoms: if you have flaking, with or without itching or oiliness, you may have real dandruff. Try an anti-dandruff shampoo containing either octopirox (piroctone olamine) or zinc pyrithione (zinc omadine) for three to four weeks.

If, however, you have red patches on your scalp or eyebrows, or down the folds running from nose to mouth, possibly with some itching, you probably have a mild form of eczema (also known as seborrheic dermatitis). Try cutting out all dairy products for a month, particularly cheese, milk and also chocolate.

Step 3: If there is still no improvement, ask your family doctor to refer you to a specialist, either a dermatologist or a trichologist.

WHAT THE STARS USE...

Miami hairstylist Stefanie Galiardo uses Phytomousse S68 on **Ivana Trump**'s hair. 'It brings back all the moisture to sun-damaged hair,' he says. Roberto Ramos – hairstylist at LA's Estilo salon – uses René Furterer Carthame No-Rinse Protective Cream on **Bette Midler** and **Farrah Fawcett** – and, from the same range, **Raquel Welch** likes the Okara Rebalancing Shampoo for Color-Treated Hair. The Phytologie range is popular with stars including **Roseanne**, who puts oomph back in hers with Phyto-Volume Actif. **Sharon Stone** goes for Aveda's Deep Penetrating Hair Revitalizer – while

Valerie Perrine opts for Aveda's Pure Plant Shampoo Blue Malva, a colour-enhancer based on natural ingredients. **Jilly Cooper** likes the Botanical haircare collection, based on herbs and seaweed. As for **Emma Thompson**? She's a fan of Paul Mitchell's shampoos and conditioners. Rumour has it that **Madonna** likes Bumble & Bumble's gentle Seaweed Shampoo. **Sophia Loren**, meanwhile, is so hooked on Laurent D. Volumateur that she apparently bought ten bottles at a time. And to set her trademark blonde 'do', **Jane Fonda** reaches for Sebastian Laminates Hi-Gloss Spray.

haircare we love...

OK, we own up: our big indulgence is having regular blow-dries. We prefer to think of it as an investment in how we look. (The philosophy: it's better to spend money on great-looking hair than, say, a new jacket. Because we wear our hair every single day.) However, we are both very picky and tend to take our favourite hair products to the salon. They are...

Jo: I have a sensitive scalp, so I like L'Oréal Kérastase Sensitive Soothing Hair Bath, or Urtekram* all-natural Rose Shampoo and Rose Conditioner – like a walk through a rose garden. I also do regular deep treatments with what I consider to be the greatest hair conditioner in history, Estée Lauder Herbal Hair Pack. J-F. Lazartigue Energising Elixir* is also a miracle instant re-glosser. For styling, I like Aesop Wild Lime Hair Polish*, and a touch of John Frieda's Gloss & Groom Wax.

Sarah: I'm very keen on the Phytologie* range. I choose different products depending on how my hair feels at the time. As it's colour-treated and I live in a polluted environment, my hair is invariably dry and in need of TLC. My favourites are Phytojoba Intense Hydrating Shampoo, Phyto Fortifying Hair Serum and Phyto 9 Daily Ultra Nourishing Cream. I also love Aveda's PureFume Brilliant Spray On For Hair for a final spritz of super-gloss.

wig wisdom

The good news for anyone who's lost, losing or about to lose their hair is that wigs needn't look like wigs any more. Both real hair and synthetic wigs are now highly advanced – and even come with highlights, lowlights or salt-and-pepper shading, for ultra-real effects...

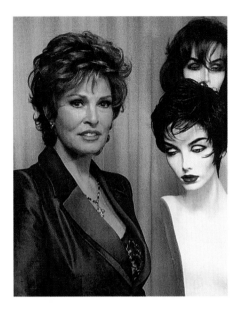

However, hairdresser Andrew Collinge advises that, if possible, 'The best time to buy a wig is before you need it – for instance, if you are scheduled to have chemotherapy or are suffering hair loss which might accelerate.' That way, he explains, it's easiest for the wig salon staff to direct you to the closest match to your natural colour and your style.

Few women, says Andrew, see hair loss as an opportunity for a radical makeover and a brand new 'do'. 'Most want to stay in the "comfort zone", as close as possible to their former look, because that way nobody but their nearest and dearest need know that anything has changed.' If you have long hair, or a very obvious parting, however, you may not be able to find a wig that looks like your natural hair. (Partings are the real giveaway with wigs; if you can't see the parting, it's often impossible to tell that a wig is a wig.) So Andrew's advice is to get your hair cut in a shorter style, or one that disguises your parting, if you know you are going to embark on a course of chemotherapy. 'Then choose a wig that recreates that shorter hairstyle.' If you have already lost your hair before you decide to invest in a wig, take along a selection of photographs to show the wig salon assistants, so that they can see how you want to look.

You might also want to consider taking your regular hairdresser along, for expert advice. 'Most women don't

think of it – but hairdressers are usually delighted to be of help,' says Andrew. 'If you've put your hair in the hands of your hairdresser in the past, he/she is probably the best person to advise you.' What's more, your hairdresser can 'customise' your wig.

Andrew recommends synthetic wigs, for their wash-and-wearability. 'Synthetic wigs no longer look like "dolly hair",' he explains. 'They're very realistic. And the price means that it's easier to afford two. You wouldn't wear a blouse day in, day out. Well, wigs need cleaning, too. But the synthetic type spring back into shape and don't need restyling.' If women are too sick to travel to a wig department for a fitting, meanwhile, a family can take along photographs or a lock of hair, and the staff will find the best possible match.

The other option is a real hair wig. Because hair is rarely one all-over colour, bespoke wig-makers can recreate your hair's appearance right down to the last, chunky streak. But maintenance can be a problem, unless you're flush enough to be able to afford two bespoke wigs. (Real hair wigs can 'drop', just like real hair, when they're washed – and may need professional restyling.) In many cases, they need to be mailed back to the maker for restyling – so you'll need to muddle through in the meantime with scarves. Also, warns Andrew Collinge: 'Real hair wigs only have a limited lifespan – probably about a year.' A question to

ask is whether or not the wig is made with European hair – the priciest option – or Chinese hair, which has been bleached to a lighter shade.

Several women who've undergone chemotherapy shared with us their approach to impending hair loss, which was to make the deliberate gesture of getting their head shaved. One breast cancer patient explained: 'I didn't want the trauma of having my hair fall out in handfuls. But by taking the very deliberate step of getting my hairdresser to shave my head before that happened, it put me in control of the situation – and I felt a lot better than if I'd just found clumps on the pillow.'

But nobody, the wig experts agree, should feel at all nervous about visiting a wig-maker, a wig shop or an in-store department. All appointments are carried out in private – offering not only tea, but sympathy. 'You may feel like the only woman in the world with this problem – but wig consultants understand that,' says Andrew Collinge, 'and they are there to help you feel better about yourself again...'

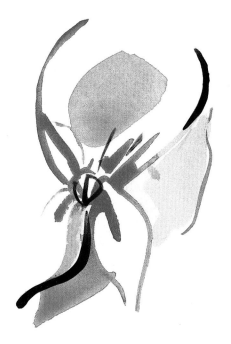

the art of the scarf

We are both keen supporters of Look Good, Feel Better, a programme which has dramatically boosted the self-esteem of thousands of women undergoing cancer treatment, through workshops at hospitals in the US and UK where they learn how to use make-up, scarves and wigs. Charles Worthington has produced a wonderful leaflet on how to cope with hair loss from cancer and its treatment (*see Directory for how to get hold of a copy*). Here are some of the tips and ideas it features...

• Headwraps and turbans offer a stylish and comfortable alternative to wearing a wig. Be daring and choose bright colours – they will lift your spirits. Cotton-knit turbans are great, as they don't slip. They help with the problem of heat loss from the scalp and also catch any falling hair. It is a good idea to wear them around the house, particularly when cooking, as wigs tend to make the scalp sweat. Cotton turbans also make a great base for tying a scarf. They keep it from slipping and help to give an appearance of fullness.

• When choosing scarves – those of 65–70cm (26–28 inches) square are best – opt for cotton rather than polyester or silk, which can slip.

A soft shoulder-pad placed on top of your head will give height and a more natural look.

• If you practise the basic tying techniques shown here, you will soon be confident enough to develop your own individual styles.

• Hats, of course, are another good way of disguising hair loss. Look for those with special gussets which are designed to hold the hat snugly on the head without slipping off. If you buy a straw hat, make sure the weave is close, so the scalp is properly protected from the burning rays of the sun.

• By combining headwraps with hats or berets, you can achieve a stylish effect and ensure your scalp is totally covered.

GET AN EXTENSION...

If you have fine hair, there is always the option of extensions. **Carly Simon** – she of the apparently lustrous mane – is said to be a fan of extensions, as are **Tina Turner** and **Pamela Stephenson**. There are two kinds: a temporary clip-in, clip-out extension, and a more permanent type with a plastic base which is bonded to the hair near the roots using heat; this bond is snapped when you want to have the extensions out – and the hair shouldn't be damaged.

These can both be colour-matched to provide low- or highlights, and then cut and styled with your own hair, in-salon. 'They can be quite effective volume-boosters for fine-haired women. But they aren't so appropriate if you're actually thinning on top,' explains John Frieda. 'The base of the hair extension needs to be hidden under layers of hair – and then it can look very realistic. But extensions are also quite high-maintenance: they grow out, along with your hair, so every few weeks you have to have the extensions replaced. A lot of women do it, though – and love the result.' However, John advises that it's important to locate a salon which specialises in extensions, to ensure they really know what they're doing. If your hair salon doesn't do extensions – and most don't – they should know (through the hairdressing grapevine) of a salon which is more experienced at this volume-boosting technique. But our advice is that it's certainly worth making an effort to find the right person. We've heard horror stories of extensions that were badly put in – and had to be cut out of the hair...

BASIC HEADWRAP 1

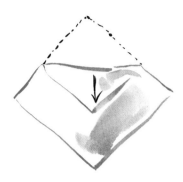

1 Lay scarf flat, wrong side up. Fold into triangle, leaving one point slightly longer than the other.

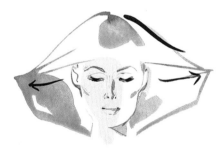

2 Drape scarf over your head with points in the back. Pull scarf down in front, 5–7 cm (2–3 inches) above your eyebrows.

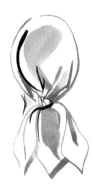

3 Tie the scarf ends in a half-knot behind your head, with flap anchored beneath the knot.

4 Tie the scarf ends into a square knot.

BASIC HEADWRAP 2

1 Follow steps for Basic Headwrap 1. Using both hands, spread lower flap under a half-knot, as close to the back of your ears as possible.

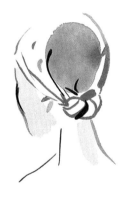

2 Carefully bring flap up over knot.

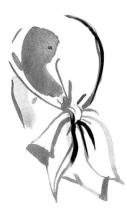

3 Or use this basis to play with interesting knots/bows.

BASIC SIDE TWIST

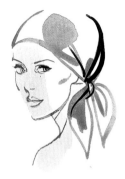

● Tie Headwrap 1, placing knot over one ear, instead of at the back of the head, letting the scarf ends hang loose.

CONTRASTING SIDE TWIST

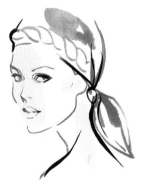

● Tie Headwrap 2. Twist a second oblong scarf. Knot and twist over headwrap, above ear.

TIP

*Sleeping on
a satin-like pillowcase
will minimise tugging of hair
at the scalp and wearing a
soft stretch cap at night
will keep your
head warm.*

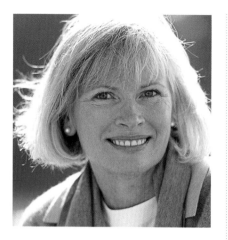

grey matters: the ultimate guide to haircolouring

Whether you've a few grey hairs, salt-and-pepper streaks or all-over white, there's an effective answer – and often many options, both salon and DIY. (Plus the choice of staying silver – but sensational...)

As life's landmarks go, the morning we notice our first grey hair isn't one that has most of us singing hallelujah from the rooftops. But today we can choose to play up the silver fox style – *and* look fabulous. Or colour it, and nobody (but our colourist) need know...

If you get it *right*, that is. According to the experts, that's really not so hard – provided you follow a few simple guidelines. The world's leading haircolouring experts are agreed: don't be tempted to make dramatic changes and stray too far from your natural, pre-grey haircolouring. Every woman has a 'buffer zone' of 'safe' shades – two or three either side, just lighter or just darker than her natural colour.

Be conscious, too, that nobody's hair is naturally all one colour. Consider having highlights or lowlights for a super-realistic effect. As Louis Licari (Manhattan's 'King of Colour') explains, 'A few lights are as good as a mini-lift for ageing women. If you put highlights above the temple, it automatically makes eyes lift upwards.'

For most of us, grey hair arrives just as we hit life's prime, when Nature plays a cruel trick and stops the production of melanin, the substance which gives hair its natural colour. Fifty per cent of the population is grey by the age of fifty. Studies have shown that more women are going grey – and sooner than ever before – as a result of pernicious anaemia (often linked to dieting), hormone treatments (including the Pill), and our frantic, stressful lives.

When grey hair sets in, it can make you look washed-out and pale. According to Louis Licari, 'When hair loses its colour, it loses its richness and lustre. And when this happens it tends to make skin colour look faded, too.'

We can all think of women who go grey gracefully, and look utterly chic. 'But they're the exceptions,' insists top London hairdresser, Nicky Clarke. 'And they tend to be fabulous, striking women, who'd look great whatever their hair colour.' Your skintone will determine how good you'd look if you decide to stick with grey. The sallow-skinned rarely find a silver frame flattering – nor do natural redheads, whose hair tends to turn a pale apricot when white mixes in. Classic silver-haired beauties tend to cluster at opposite ends of the skin spectrum: women with almost ebony colouring, or pale 'English rose' complexions. If you don't fall into those categories – or you just don't want grey hair, period – the fixes are quick and convincing.

Covering up the grey, meanwhile, restores not only the colour and rejuvenates the face – it makes hair glossy again. Hair texture actually changes as it goes grey; it may be wirier, coarser and/or dry. (Or even curlier.) 'Grey hair absorbs the light and looks flat,' says Jo Hansford, whose London salon is a mecca for the not-so-glad-to-be-grey. 'Put back the colour and the light picks up on it and automatically makes the hair appear healthier.' The good news is that today's high-tech colourants offer natural results – and boost hair health, to boot. So let us steer you through the colour maze...

make-up for grey hair

When you go grey, more colourful make-up is essential,' explains Bobbi Brown. 'Grey or white hair drains colour from the face, so you need the lift of make-up colour – soft shades, but not washed-out.' Bobbi's recommendations:

Lipstick: rose, red, apricot, peach (but not brown)
Blush: rose tones, pastels
If you have brown eyes: use a grey or brown shadow palette
If you have blue eyes: use a shadow trio of grey, slate and navy

YOUR PRODUCT OPTIONS?

A Few Grey Hairs

On dark blonde or fair hair, you could try **highlights** – lighter streaks which disguise the grey; up to three different tones may be used for natural-looking results. Highlights should be done by a pro. As there's no obvious regrowth at the roots, they only need to be touched up every eight to twelve weeks. On darkish hair, deeper blondes and redheads, try streaks of colour which tone down the grey only, bringing it back to your original shade; again, a good colourist is essential. 'Sometimes we use the grey hair as a third colour,' explains Jo Hansford, 'creating a tortoiseshell effect.' (Upkeep: every ten weeks, maximum.)

The other option – which you can try at home – is a vegetable rinse, mostly derived (as the name sounds) from vegetable sources (like henna or walnut). These are also known as veggie rinses, or just 'veg', in the trade. They increase the intensity of the original colour and restore glorious shine, gradually fading over six to eight washes. However, all the hairdressers we spoke to caution women to avoid henna like the plague, and to ask whether a vegetable rinse features henna 'Henna coats the hair in a colour that won't wash off and is impervious to other colours – so you can't change your mind,' says Christophe Robin, the Parisian haircolourist who looks after colour for **Catherine Deneuve** and **Kristin Scott Thomas**.

Another 'starter' option is **colour shampoos** and **colour conditioners**, which can also give a hint of colour. According to Jo Hansford, 'They can be a good way of building up colour gradually – helping you to decide whether you like a particular colour and want to go for a similar, semi-permanent colour. But beware of the warmer shades, as they can look a bit brassy.' (NB Top colourists tell us that they tend to prefer the colour conditioners to the shampoos.)

Up to 20 per cent Grey

Hide with a vegetable rinse (*see above*) or **semi-permanent colour** in the same shade as your natural hair. Semi-permanent colours, like veggie rinses, fade gradually without noticeable re-growth – and also last six to eight washes. Jo Hansford explains: 'I never say, "This will last X weeks" when I'm colouring women's hair, because if you wash your hair frequently, it'll need colouring more often.' Vegetable colour and semi-permanents are relatively low-maintenance options which coat the outer layer of hair with colour, rather than penetrating the hair shaft, which requires the use of stronger chemicals. Because they blend with the colour of grey hair, rather than cover your hair colour totally, the effects are very realistic.

Up to 50 per cent Grey

Cover with a **longer-lasting semi-permanent colour**, which stays for up to 24 washes, and gradually fades, meaning there is less obvious regrowth than with a permanent dye. (These are also sometimes known as **demi-permanent** or **tone-on-tone** colours.) There is no ammonia, so the colour molecules do not penetrate as deep as in permanent hair colours. However, longer-lasting semi-permanent colour does contain 1–2 per cent peroxide (the ingredient that opens the hair's cuticle, allowing colour molecules to enter the strand's cortex) – which is why the colour lasts longer than regular semi-permanents.

Up to 100 per cent Grey

Replace colour completely with a permanent dye; these are chemically based and so penetrate the hair shaft. Jo suggests adding professional highlights or lowlights first, to break up the colour and make it more natural-looking. Remember, roots will need retouching about every four to six weeks – but not always the whole head.

Fade to grey again...

So you've been covering up your grey – but now you want to go back to natural? According to Beth Minardi, of Manhattan's Minardi Salon, 'If you've been dying your hair, silver should evolve gradually. It's a matter of trimming off the old dye job, putting in lowlights, perhaps highlighting the re-growth – minimising the application of tint until there's less and less colour and more and more white.'

your colour options

John Barrett says that whatever your hair colour, you should take your cue from the base colour you are now – not the colour that you think you were fifteen years ago, or when you were a teenager…

BLONDE

Don't go too blonde; think of adding some lowlights or you may look too pale-all-over. As Louis Licari says, 'Your hair colour should give a contrast to your skintone so it defines your face.' Adds George at John Barrett in New York, 'Blondes tend to go too light and ashy. They should have some golden tones mixed in to keep the colour warm and natural.'

MEDIUM BROWN

According to Louis Licari, if this is your natural colour, 'You should go no lighter than light brown or light auburn.' George at John Barrett says that 'paper-bag brown' should have highlights, or lowlights. And try ash browns, rather than reds, which are very hard to take.'

BRUNETTES

Lighten up two or three shades from the colour you were naturally – preferably with extra highlights, for a more realistic effect. According to Louis Licari, 'Go no darker than chocolate brown or auburn.'

Explains Jo Hansford, 'When you go grey, the skin softens down and becomes paler. If you're greying and go back to your original brunette, the contrast may be too severe: you can end up looking like a witch.' Too-dark hair also emphasises wrinkles, undereye circles and sagging skin – another good reason to go slightly lighter. (If you need proof, 'Tie a black ribbon around a lemon,' suggests James Viera, senior vice president for L'Oréal, 'then try doing the same with a white ribbon. You'll see that the surface looks far smoother.'

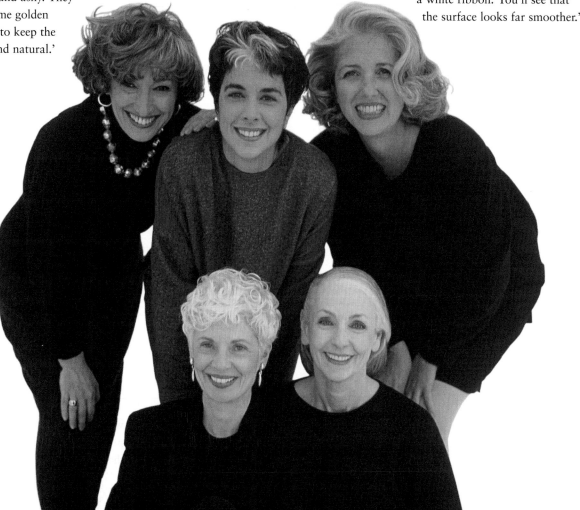

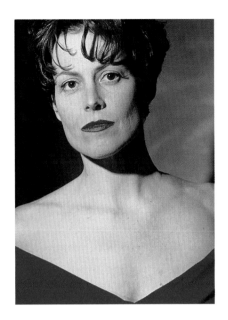

REDHEADS

According to Louis Licari, covering up grey hair with red colour is a tough one for greying women to carry off; red can turbo-charge any ruddiness in your complexion. 'You definitely need the right skintone and eyes for it to work,' he explains, adding that the pale colouring and freckled complexions of **Sigourney Weaver** and **Susan Sarandon**, for example – natural to many redheads – make them an exception to the don't-go-red rule.

Certainly, if you want to make a strong statement like covering grey with red, Louis advises: 'See a professional.'

SECRET: Don't ever be tempted to pluck a grey hair. 'Pulling won't kill the hair or make it grow back with its old colour,' explains Philip Kingsley. 'Plucking only distorts the hair follicle, making regrowth more wiry and obvious.'

TESTING TIME

Today's hair colourants are safe, effective and (mostly) fool-proof. But disasters still sometimes occur because people don't follow instructions on the pack. Take time to complete both of the recommended tests. To avoid having to re-mix ingredients, do the two tests at the same time – 48 hours before colouring – to allow for signs of allergy, i.e. itching, stinging, burning or redness. Be sure to have a patch test if you are having colour done in a salon, too.

A strand test

This is a colour test on a hair strand. The strand test should give you a good idea of the final colour result you will get, as well as the condition of the hair after colouring. Snip a small strip of hair (about 5mm/^{1}/4 inch wide) from an easily hidden area, such as the nape of your neck; apply the colour mixture. Be sure to note how much processing time was required to achieve the desired results.

A patch test (aka skin test)

This is conducted by applying a small amount of the mixed colour to a hidden area of your skin, usually the inside of the forearm, to determine if you're allergic to any of the components; watch for redness, stinging, itching or burning. Manufacturers recommend a skin test should be carried out every time a colour is used. Don't assume because you've used a colour safely in the past that you have the green light to go ahead without a patch test this time round. People have been known to use a product without any problems for many years and then develop a reaction.

HAIRCOLOURING – A RISKY BUSINESS?

As many women tell us, the use of hair dyes can trigger irritation – or even contact dermatitis – with symptoms ranging from mild itchiness to blisters and even hair loss.

But according to Marilyn Sherlock, consultant trichologist and member of the Academy of Expert Witnesses (who has frequently been called to give evidence in connection with hairdressing litigation), almost all hair dye-linked problems arise from misuse – not because of the formulations themselves. Her advice is always to do a patch test first – whether you're having your hair coloured in a salon, or doing it at home. (Allergies are more common with single-process colour; less so with the cap method of highlights or lowlights.) She also advises: 'Follow the instructions very carefully and time application; a lot of problems come from not reading the box – or leaving the colourant on the hair for too long.'

If you are experiencing scalp irritation and are re-colouring your hair frequently – say every three weeks – try leaving it for six weeks between treatments and touching up the hairline with a Tween-Time crayon*, to see if this helps.

In addition, if you have any cuts, sore spots or scratches on your scalp, it's wise to ensure that they are covered with a layer of Vaseline, to avoid penetration of the dye directly into the bloodstream.

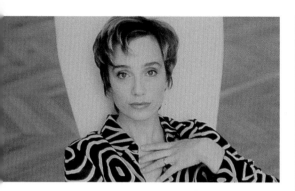

AT-HOME HAIRCOLOURING

If Martha Stewart coloured her hair at home, here's what she'd tell you. These rules apply to both permanent and semi-permanent colouring...

First of all...
• Read the instructions – preferably twice – before you start. (Do your skin and strand tests if advised on the packaging – *see p.117*).

• At the start of your colouring session, coat the frame of your face with Vaseline, to stop the haircolour 'taking' on the skin around your hairline.

• Put an (un-precious) towel around your shoulders, for protection.

• Take off all your jewellery so that you don't make holes in the plastic gloves.

• If the gloves provided with the kit are too loose, grip them on with a wide rubber band at your wrist. (If that's too tight, try sticky tape instead.) Otherwise, in our experience, the gloves tend to slip.

• Use a timer or an alarm clock to tell you when the time's up. It's all too easy to lose track of the minutes when you're immersed in a favourite TV show/book/phone call to a friend...

Then for semi-permanent haircolour...
• After protecting your hands and shoulders, dampen and towel-dry hair. Then open the applicator bottle, shake and apply.

• Work the colour into the hair, starting at the temples, but avoid actually rubbing into the scalp.

• Once applied, pile hair loosely on top of your head.

• Set a timer – even if the colour is designed to stop developing automatically.

• When the timer rings, rinse with water. Be thorough and keep rinsing until the water runs clear.

• Shampoo, style and/or blow-dry.

For permanent haircolour...
• Read the instructions very carefully, and do strand and patch tests some 48 hours before (*see p.117*).

• Mix, following the instructions carefully. Snip off the top of the developing solution bottle, open the bottle and pour in the colourant. Cover and shake.

• Having wrapped yourself in gloves and towels (and splatter-proofed your bathroom), apply haircolour evenly to all sections of dry, undampened hair.

• Time the process exactly, according to manufacturer's instructions.

• When the timer rings, dampen hair and work the mixture in, saturating the roots but being careful not to rub the colour into the scalp.

• Immediately rinse, shampoo and condition. (Many permanent dyes feature a conditioner in the kit; use this.)

• Style and/or blow-dry as usual...

home haircolouring timetable

Louis Licari – the haircolouring guru responsible for the colour of stars like Susan Sarandon – advises women to plan ahead if they want to achieve the best home haircolouring results. Here is his countdown to perfect colour – with maximum shine...

Seven days before
Treat hair with a deep-conditioner or hair mask; this strengthens the hair but allows enough time for the product to be fully rinsed out, ensuring that your haircolour will 'take' evenly.

On the day
Don't shampoo just before colouring. (The natural oils secreted by your scalp protect and hydrate it during haircolouring.)

The days after
Deep-condition with a hair mask once a week, beginning seven days after colouring. When it comes to day-to-day haircare, preserve your colour with shampoos and conditioners specifically created for colour-treated hair.
(NB Louis Licari – like John Barrett and many other top hairdressers around the world – swears by the gloss-restoring Phytologie* range of shampoos.

more haircolouring secrets

• Try on a selection of wigs in a department store to see how the different colours flatter you. (Or not.)

• Should you visit a salon or try home colouring? According to Manhattan colourist Brad Johns, 'Home and salon products contain the same formulas. In a salon you pay for expertise.'

• Ask friends for recommendations of colourists. Your regular salon may not specialise in haircolouring and you may get better results at one that does.

• If you can't afford salon colour on a regular visit, aim for a salon visit at least once a year for advice on the choice of tints to use at home.

• Standing at the home haircolouring fixture in a store is baffling. (We know, we've done it.) It is so hard to tell from the model's picture on a box what the results will be like. If in doubt when choosing permanent colour, go for one shade lighter; it will be easier to remedy than if it's too dark.

• Dramatic colour switches require far more maintenance as roots show faster. If you want to stray further from what Nature gave you (once upon a time), be prepared to spend extra time and money on touch-ups. Whereas picking a shade close to your natural colour will at least give the *impression* your colour is lasting longer.

• Be aware that active ingredients in dandruff shampoos may cause semi-permanent haircolour to fade more rapidly.

• If you live in a hard water area and colour your hair, use a deep-cleansing or 'clarifying' shampoo every few washes; when minerals build up on your hair, colouring (and perming agents) don't work as well.

• To extend the life of your semi-permanent haircolour, try a colour-enhancing conditioner between colour treatments. Pick a shade as close as possible to your coloured hair; a too-dark conditioner may 'stain' a shade that's lighter.

• After roots begin to show, you need to do a touch-up application. But don't apply colour to your whole head, as this will make the ends brittle and dry, creating 'stripes' in the hair as the colour is overloaded. Most packs include instructions for touch-ups; the difference is that you apply colour to roots only, working through to the ends for just a few minutes at the end of the treatment.

• If a home haircolouring treatment goes wrong, don't panic; check for a hotline number in the box. They may be able to tell you which shade will 'correct' the problem. With a semi-permanent colour, frequent use of a clarifying shampoo will speed up the rate at which it washes out again. But if a permanent colour has gone wrong, it's best to go to your salon, explain what's happened – and get them to put things right. Most salon professionals are highly experienced in fixing home haircolouring disasters.

• Consider a make-up makeover when you've had your haircolour done. Your old lipstick, blusher and eyeshadows may not work if you've had a haircolour overhaul.

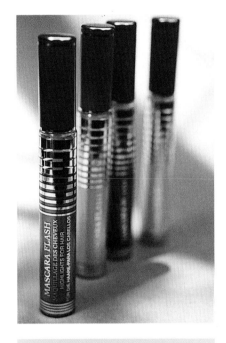

magic wands

Hair mascaras are the ultimate in no-commitment colour. These wands of colour brush or wash out when you're bored with them. They come in a wide range of colours – from bright blues to pinks via emerald – but we advise sticking to chic metallics like gold, bronze or the palest blonde. According to Susan Baldwin**, 'Hair mascaras are a brilliant cover-up for the odd grey hair.' Here's her how-to advice: 'Take tiny sections of the hair from around the face and apply the mascara from root to tip. Hair mascaras look great in fringes, but try streaking the side hair framing the face, too. They're also useful when your hair is coloured and the roots are coming through, if you stick to a colour that's closest to your natural shade.'

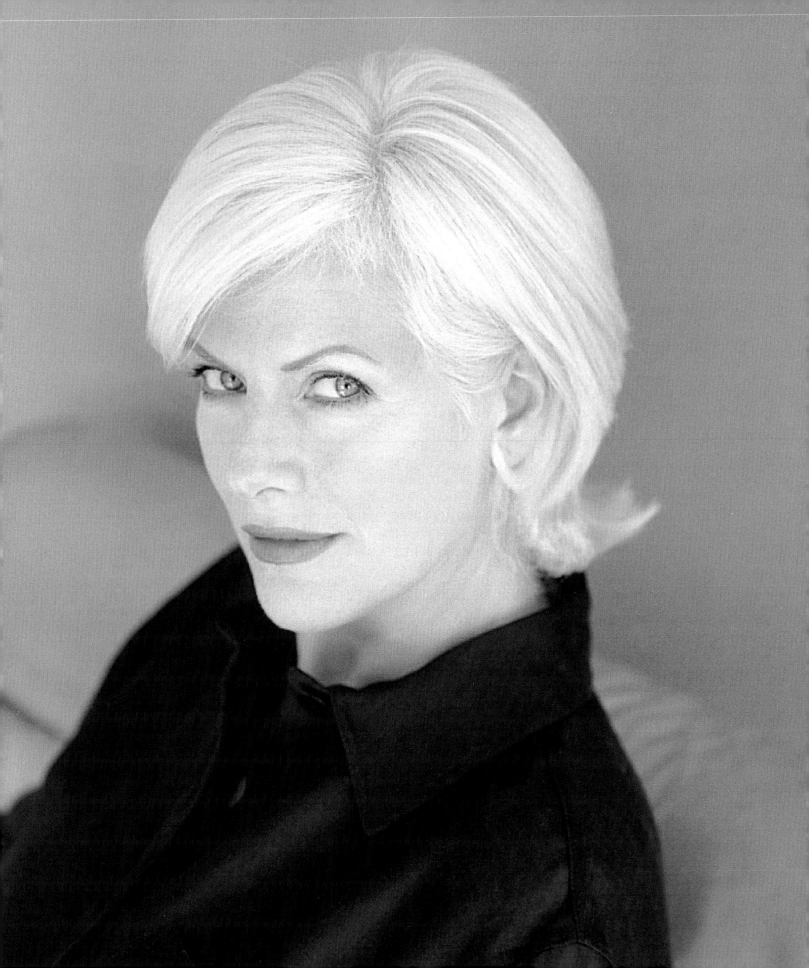

inspiring women

Jennifer Guerrini-Maraldi

We are inspired by Jennifer because of her *joie de vivre*, young-at-heart attitude and her wonderful style (she's Fashion Editor of *Country Life*. But middle-aged twinsets and pearls aren't Jennifer's fashion). And – not least – we're inspired because this Australian-born beauty, married to an Italian count, is a shining example of what sun protection and beauty care can do to keep a woman looking fabulous...

'Growing up in the harsh Melbourne sunlight with an outdoor lifestyle was the most fun – but not the best start in life for perfect skin. It was essential from an early age to take care of face and body. A strict rule, when we were growing up, was that no-one went outside in summer without a hat. To this day, I thank my father for enforcing that. All the sunblock in the world will never be as effective as a hat. In fact, you need both...

'My mother, Noelle Heathcote, is known for her flawless English rose complexion and never, never lay in the sun. Her strict beauty routine always intrigued me. I often sat on the edge of her dressing table watching my mother cleanse, moisturise and apply her make-up – the height of fifties and sixties glamour! I'm sure I drove her mad with questions. I remember her telling me that as a teenage girl, during and after the War, there were no luxuries like cosmetics – so she used Vaseline on her lips and eyes to get a healthy shine. This obviously worked wonders, as she has virtually no lines at 72 years old.

'The training stuck with me and I am addicted to the latest creams and cosmetics. I believe the big cosmetic houses produce the best of the latest beauty treats, because they pour so many millions into product development. I stick to the main brands – but I do also swear by Eve Lom's Cleansing Cream*.

'On the question of facelifts, I'm definitely anti. I would never voluntarily put myself through the torture of surgery, under anaesthetic, for reasons of vanity. I'm hoping the cosmetic industry will come up with the perfect, non-surgical way to iron out the wrinkles...

'I believe there are several key ingredients for looking good: fresh fruit and vegetables, exercise and plenty of sleep. (Obvious, and we're probably sick of being told them – but true.) But in my own life aren't always practical. Yes, I squeeze a few grapefruits or an orange in the morning, and I love vegetables and salad. It's the other things I also love – dessert and champagne – which counterbalance my intentions! But as long as I exercise regularly, it all works. For the past two years, I've had a personal trainer twice a week – but I get bored easily, so I'm constantly re-thinking the routine; I especially love kick-boxing.

'I love glamour and am married to an Italian who assumes women should always look glamorous. I think every woman should change her image every ten years. I call this "the Decade Dump". As the face matures, you need a different haircut, different make-up – and a change of style of what you wear. The Decade Dump focuses the mind on a youthful image. Keep it simple: the rules are neat, shiny hair, natural make-up and plain, well-cut clothes, with not too much jewellery in the daytime.

'Time is always a problem. And sleep is hugely variable; I tend to burn the candle at both ends, but make up for it by being a good cat-napper.

'But the most important ingredient for feeling and looking good is happiness. Growing up beside the sea was an idyllic childhood: free as a bird, breathing the purest air imaginable. While twenty years in England have been kind to the skin – it's the best climate for a beautiful complexion – I missed the sea. So my husband and I have found the perfect, stress-busting hideaway on the cliffs of Cornwall, overlooking beautiful beaches. We all need to switch off from our (increasingly) hectic lives, for the sake of good looks and well-being. If anything will contribute to feeling fabulous forever, it's going to be the return to the seaside and rejuvenating walks on the wild, wide open beaches. Just being by the sea again. Full circle from childhood...

'I never think about age. I'm too busy. Every hour of the week is accounted for, so no time to ponder the inevitable. And I plan to go on working my whole life. Retire? Never.'

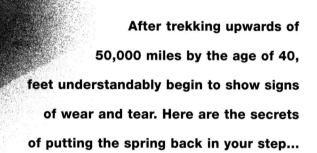

After trekking upwards of 50,000 miles by the age of 40, feet understandably begin to show signs of wear and tear. Here are the secrets of putting the spring back in your step...

feet, don't fail us now...

Blame our love of footwear, if you like, for the fact that women's feet age faster than men's. The glamorous, sexy shoes we love aren't designed for our natural wide-in-the-front, slim-at-the-heel shape – making foot faults commonplace: hammertoes, bunions and corns are all the result of crowded-toe conditions. Skin also changes with age; already the least lubricated on our body, skin on the feet becomes even drier – and prone to cracking and infection.

Of course, we tend to ignore our feet – until they start to hurt. According to Scholl, the footcare specialists, prevention is better than cure. 'However, it's never too late to get feet healthy, even if a woman has neglected her feet all her life,' insists

Scholl podiatrist, Katherine Royston-Airey. Ideally, she suggests, we should see a chiropodist or podiatrist every ten to twelve weeks for upkeep, more often with problems such as corns. The toenails will be trimmed (guarding against ingrown toenails), any hard skin build-up can be whisked away, and the chiropodist can warn you of any incipient problems – which can then be treated.

The state of your feet also shows on your face: pinched feet = pinched expression. And since walking is Nature's greatest anti-ageing exercise, happy feet are crucial to well-being. Caring for your feet with the same amount of TLC you'd lavish on your hands or your face can help you stay one jump ahead of foot problems...

NOTE: Twice as many women as men develop osteoarthritis. Be alert that signs of this disease can show up in the feet first; the symptoms are stiffness and pain in the joints; continued use of the joint makes it stiffen up until it refuses to move at all. Make an appointment with your doctor for a diagnosis and treatment; regular visits to a chiropodist/podiatrist will enable them to monitor the development of the disease and stop or reduce any deformity that may occur as a result of osteoarthritis.

FOOTNOTES

Just like our waistlines, feet can actually develop a kind of 'middle-aged spread': after years of being on the receiving end of pounding weight, the arch of the foot – which acts like a natural shock-absorber – may begin to fall. As that arch flattens, the foot is pushed forwards and outwards – and may actually become a whole size larger by the age of 45. Foot insiders recommend, then, that we should have an annual foot measurement – to track any changes. (Keeping a healthy weight helps, too: remember that every pound may exert three times its weight whenever your foot hits the floor.)

• As well as an annual measuring session in a shoe shop, you can determine your own foot length to make sure you're buying the right size of shoe. Stand barefoot on a piece of thin cardboard with the heel of your foot perfectly at one edge of the cardboard. Mark the place reached by the longest toe – for many people, this is the second toe, not the big toe. Cut a thin strip of cardboard from the edge to the point of the longest toe. When you insert this into a shoe, there should be 7–14 mm (^{3}/8–^{5}/8 inches) between the end of the cardboard and the heel of the shoe.

• The biggest favour that we can do our feet, according to the experts, is to whisk away hard skin – preferably every other day –with a foot file. Use the foot file on dry feet, before a bath or using a special foot scrub on wet feet. (We swear by Diamancel* foot files; they're expensive – but worth the investment in foot happiness.)

You *can* use a foot file on feet that have been in the bath or shower, but not if you've indulged in a long soak and feet have become 'spongey', as it's easy to remove too much skin.

• Scholl's advice is that feet should also be creamed – with a special foot cream – at least once (and preferably twice) a day. 'Use a special moisturiser, targeted at feet. Your regular body moisturiser isn't rich enough for the dry skin of feet, which get steadily drier after the age of 40,' says Katherine Royston-Airey. (The only exception to the daily foot-creaming rule is if you have sweaty feet, in which case, you'll only make them clammier.)

• By the age of 60, the padding under our feet starts to thin – making walking painful. Padded insoles can make up for that loss of natural cushioning...

• Poor circulation is another challenge as we age. Because feet are the furthest point from the heart, they can get short-changed when it comes to blood supply. But regular exercise – think walking, again – will boost blood flow to the feet, beating chills as well as helping any infections and cuts to heal faster.

• Soaking feet for 15 minutes in a roomy plastic basin is another swift soother (see over for suggestions of aromatherapy oils to use). If your feet are feeling particularly hot and prickly, add two drops of peppermint oil. Adding a handful of dried milk will make for a moisturising soak.

• Change your shoes every day and vary your heel height to keep the muscles in your feet and calves flexible. (In women who habitually wear high heels, for instance, the calf muscles may actually shorten so they can't put their heels to the ground.) Try to go barefoot often, too.

• If you like to wear open sandals, don't forget to slather your feet with an SPF in the mornings; feet are perfectly angled to pick up damaging UV rays, fast-forwarding ageing.

• Foot experts tell us that having corns removed by a professional chiropodist is far preferable to corn plasters, which don't discriminate between the skin of a corn and normal skin – so they may damage the surrounding tissue. (This could be particularly problematic for anyone with poor circulation, delicate skin or for diabetics.)

• Never buy shoes in the morning, when the feet are still rested; in the afternoon, you'll get a better fit.

• When out walking, take first-aid supplies – like plasters or antiseptic cream – with you, in case of accidents. If your toes chafe together, try a dab of Vaseline between them.

• That age-old advice – to put your feet up – really is the best way to combat swollen ankles and achy feet. Scholl's advice is to lie comfortably on the floor or on your bed with your feet propped at a 45° angle for ten minutes, so extra fluid can drain away.

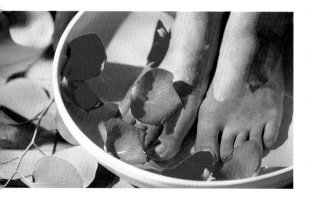

THE AROMA ZONE

Aromatherapy Associates gave us these aromatherapy suggestions for feet that have notched up plenty of miles. They prescribe regular foot baths, particularly for tired (or less-than-fragrant) feet and puffy ankles. Add up to 12 drops of cypress oil to warm water for smelly feet, and the same quantity of peppermint or lavender in cool water, on hot days. For cracked and super-dry feet, Aromatherapy Associates suggest concocting a special foot oil, made up of 90 per cent almond oil and 10 per cent wheatgerm oil, with 30 drops of healing frankincense oil per 50 ml (2 fl oz) of the base oil. Then massage it into feet on a nightly basis.

get fit feet fast

Exercising your feet will keep them flexible and strong (as well as beautiful), and will help you maintain your balance over the years to come. The Foot Health Council (an organisation founded to promote foot care) suggest these exercises for fabulously fit feet forever...

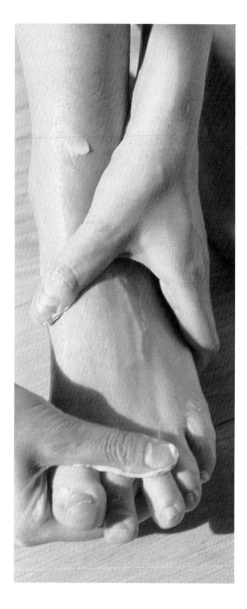

• Stand, feet slightly apart, and raise yourself slowly up, then down, with the weight on the toes. (If you have balance problems, hold on to a chair while you're doing this.)

• Stand on the bottom step of a staircase, toes extending over the edge. Bend the toes as if gripping the edge. Hold while counting to two, then flex the toes upwards and hold again to a count of two. Repeat several times, then reverse the way you're standing – this time dropping and raising the heels over the edge of the stair.

• Sit or lie with feet outstretched; arch one foot at a time and slowly sketch wide circles, first in one direction, then in the other. Repeat several times.

• Lie flat on the floor with the soles of your feet against the wall. Spread your toes wide as they grasp the surface and 'climb' the wall. (This is good for fighting cramp.)

• In addition, the Foot Health Council suggests standing and walking on tip-toe, as often as possible.

• We also like these suggestions from Gary Null and Dr Howard Robins, authors of *How to Keep Your Feet and Legs Healthy for a Lifetime**. To strengthen and increase flexibility of your toes, they suggest trying to pick up pencils or marbles from the floor. Another exercise (to strengthen toes, feet and legs) is to draw the alphabet on the ground with the toes. Then do it again in the air. Write each letter in capitals, or joined-up writing, whatever – and do it several times a day. Then every muscle in your feet will get a workout...

BE ALERT

Foot infections heal slowly in diabetics, so be very cautious about pedicures. In a salon, inform the staff you are diabetic; they will make sure not to use metal implements which may cut. In the same way, be especially careful using nail clippers, scissors, foot files or orange sticks if you are doing an at-home pedicure. Daily use of a tea tree oil-based foot lotion or a neat lavender oil massaged into your feet may help keep infections at bay.

AGEING FOOTCARE CHECKLIST

For healthy feet, do this at-home foot check-up once a month...

Examine your nails for...
• ingrown toenails
• fungal infection
• nail thickening

Examine the skin on your feet for...
• athlete's foot
• corns and callouses
• skin lesions or any changes in any moles (i.e. changes in colour, growth, itching, raised edges or bleeding)

Examine the skin on your legs for...
• varicose veins
• eczema
• skin lesions or mole changes

Check your footwear has...
• shock-absorbing soles
• uppers large enough to accommo-date deformities, i.e. bunions and/or hammertoes
• the right shoe size, as feet can change shape. (Shoes should grip the back of your foot, rather than flap.)

mature pedicure

If you can't get to a salon for regular pedicures, Clare Wolford, Education Director of Supernail of LA, offers this at-home treatment for older feet, to help prevent the build-up of hard skin or the development of ingrown toenails.

1 Soak the feet for five minutes in a bowl of warm-to-hot water, as this will soften the skin and nails. (Add a couple of drops of tea tree oil, if you like, as an antibacterial agent.)

2 Trim the toenails straight across and, to smooth them, buff lightly with a nail buffer (available at The Body Shop, at pharmacies or through nail salons). The buffing shouldn't be abrasive; leave anything more aggressive to a chiropodist. NB Ideally, toenails should be softly rounded at the edges. Unfortunately, it's awkward to get the right angle to cut them correctly. The at-home cut to aim for is straight across; lightly file down any sharp edges; don't clip the corners to round them, as this is what can lead to ingrown toenails.

3 Rub in cuticle remover and, ultra-gently, push back cuticles with an orange stick around which you've wrapped cotton wool, candy-floss-style.

4 Exfoliate and moisturise the skin with an exfoliant cream, to remove dry, dead and flaky skin cells.

5 Gently remove hard skin with a foot file, especially around the heels and on the ball of the foot.

6 Massage a light moisturiser all over the feet, making sure it's non-greasy.

7 If you like to wear polish, clean nails with soapy water and dry thoroughly before applying base coat, two coats of polish and a top coat.

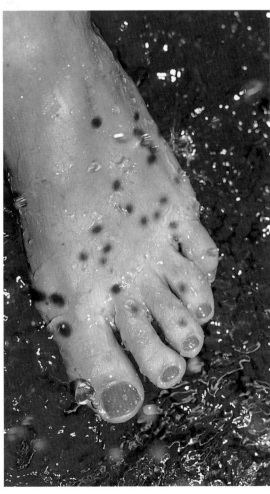

holding back the hands of time

Gentlemen may never reveal a woman's age – but our hands will often give it away for us. But it is possible to turn back the clock – with rejuvenating hand and nail care...

Hands go through hell. We subject them to daily dunkings in water, expose them to acidic household cleaners, endlessly handle pieces of paper (which strip vital oils from skin) – and forget that they're as vulnerable to sun damage as our faces. So even if our complexions get their daily slathering of UV protection, hands are left to the mercy of the elements, leading to 'age spots' – which form as the melanin (skin pigment) in unprotected skin reacts to sunlight.

Compared with the face, the hands have thinner skin, less fat to camouflage wrinkles and veins, and fewer oil glands and hair follicles the structures which moisturise naturally and generate new skin. All of that adds up to accelerated ageing. But if we treat hands regularly with lots of TLC, they will reward us well into our dotage...

age-defying manicure

After a certain age, 'nail guru' Robyn Opie – whose Chelsea Nail Studio, in London, is in many smart women's Little Black Books – believes that nails should go a little shorter. 'The most flattering shape is square with rounded edges,' she says. 'That's also the least vulnerable to breaking. Also beautiful are slightly oval nails that follow the natural nail line.'

Colour should be chosen to flatter, too. 'Women who are self-conscious of their hands often choose an opaque nude or biscuity shade, which actually makes pale-skinned hands look green or grey. Stronger colours – or 'pale brights' – are much more flattering. If you want to go pale, choose a strong sheer colour, like a pale pink or a sheer white.' (We love some of the funkier colours – like gold, or a pretty pale blue, which look good on hands of any age.) Robyn also gives the thumbs-up to the French manicure, where nails are clear rose and tips are painted

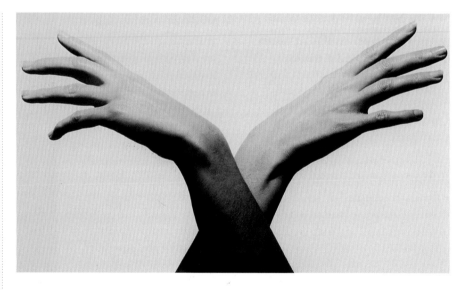

white – but only if nails are nipped shorter. (Leave the talons to **Barbra Streisand**, please.)

1 Remove nail polish; use an acetone-free polish remover, which is less drying. (The label should say 'acetone-free' or 'gentle'.)

2 File and shape nails, filing in one direction only, from the sides to the centre. Use a padded emery board,

now widely available from pharmacies and beauty supply stores, which is kinder to nails than old-fashioned metal files or 'sandpaper' boards.

NB Kathryn Marsden – who gave us the Nail Food suggestions on *p.128* – recommends to patients with fragile nails that they always file the nails *before* removing polish, to lessen the risk of breaking. So if your nails are vulnerable, swap steps 1 and 2.

3 Soak nails in a small dish: add a few drops of jojoba or almond oil to warm water, or create an 'oil bath' of slightly warmed olive oil on its own.

4 Apply an exfoliant to your hands and slough away dull, dead skin. (Or use a handful of fine salt, mixed with some of the oil from your soak.)

5 Wipe hands and apply a moisturising face mask to the entire 'glove' area. Rest your hands on a towel while the mask gets to work. Remove mask according to the instructions.

6 Cuticles will be softened by the mask and oil treatment, ready for pushing back. (Use a special cuticle remover, if you prefer.) Push them back with a rubber-tipped hoof stick or orange stick wrapped in cotton wool.

7 Scrub nails gently with a nail brush and clean, warm water. (Or swipe away the last traces of cream/mask with a pad soaked in facial astringent.)

8 Buff nails, using the soft side of a nail buffer from The Body Shop (or the old-fashioned chamois kind, available from some pharmacies). Rub gently to polish nails naturally and never allow nails to get hot while buffing.

9 Apply rich hand cream. Wipe over nails with a cotton pad soaked in soapy water, to remove the cream before polishing.

10 Apply base coat (to prevent staining by nail enamel), two coats of enamel and a protective top coat. (To prolong the life of your manicure, reapply top coat each day.)

more hand tips...

• Mara Caskin, manicurist at John Barrett's salon, suggests: 'To start you on a nail-improvement programme, invest in a manicure in the best salon available to you and watch and ask questions. If regular weekly manicures aren't within your budget or agenda, aim for at least four a year, for maintenance – and use them as a learning experience.'

• Frederick Brandt, associate professor of dermatology at the University of Miami, advises patients that fake tan can help camouflage obvious veins on the backs of hands.

• One of the biggest favours we can do hands is to keep hand cream by every set of taps in the house, on the desk and in the car. (Mara Caskin suggests keeping hand cream by a radiator. 'It feels better and absorbs faster,' she maintains.)

• Ideally, look for a hand cream with an SPF15 for daily use; research has found that age spots will actually fade somewhat if hands are no longer exposed to UV light.

• Most of us want hand creams that sink in fast. But Robyn Opie warns that, actually, these can have a drying effect on hands, because the alcohol in the formulation – which has a cooling action and makes the cream 'disappear' into hands fast – is actually dehydrating. 'So choose a rich, nourishing formulation that's a little stickier or greasier. It won't sink in quite so quickly, but your hands will love it...'

• Never submerge hands in water; even in the bath, try to keep them above the water-line. (Soaking nails will also shorten the life of your manicure.)

• Robyn Opie suggests rubbing left-over night cream into your hands.

• We both suffer fragile, flaky nails and have found that the best way to prevent breaks is to make sure that nails are never left 'naked', except during a manicure itself. (We also swear by Revlon's Calcium Gel Nail Revitalizer with Zinc, which is widely available, and Jessica Custom Nail Vitalizer* – it makes varnish last longer as well as glueing flakey nails back together.)

• Robyn Opie recommends this deep treatment at least once a week. 'Before you wash the dishes or do hand washing, slather oil all over your hands – anything from olive oil to hazelnut oil or almond oil. Then put Vaseline on top of the oil to seal it in. Put on a pair of disposable plastic gloves and slip your hands inside your rubber gloves while you do the dishes. The warmth of the water turbo-charges the treatment and once you wash away the gunk, hands will be super-smooth and silky.'

• Our tip is always to remember to take your own chosen polish to the salon when you have a professional manicure. Otherwise you a) have to buy theirs, or b) accept your manicure won't last as long, because you can't touch it up back home.

nail food

Nutrition has a terrific impact on nail strength; good growth depends on a healthy diet to nourish new cells developing from the base. Nutritionist Kathryn Marsden is a walking advertisement for her own philosophy of nail nutrition. 'Mine are so strong, my husband insists I could undo screws with them...'

As well as emphasising the importance of the best possible diet, Kathryn's vote goes to Essential Fatty Acids (EFAs). 'Evening primrose oil really does seem to have a significant effect on nails. My prescription is four to six capsules of Efamol Evening Primrose oil per day, or two capsules of mega-GLA by BioCare*. In addition, you should be taking a good multi-mineral tablet with B2, B3 and zinc in it.' The white spots we see on nails signal a lack of zinc – not calcium, as is often thought.

Kathryn's other secret nail-booster is to buff regularly using a Body Shop nail buffer. 'One side of the buffer is gentle enough to be used *over* polish, without causing damage to a manicure; the friction stimulates blood flow. I keep several buffers around the house, where I can be reminded to use them during the day...' (Do be careful with most other buffers which should only be used sparingly, if ever, on weak nails because they remove layers of nail, weakening them further over time.)

nail clinic

To Kathryn's diet prescription, Robyn Opie adds: 'Exercising regularly and taking time to de-stress has a hugely positive impact on nail health.' However, our experience is that even life-long tough nails take a pounding around menopause, with cracks and splits occurring right down the nail – and a healthy lifestyle alone can't always fix the problems. So we asked Robyn for her solutions to the common challenges to older nails...

Soft and peeling nails 'Nails bend and flake because they're too moist. Nail hardeners work by reducing excess moisture – but I only recommend them for a seven-day burst, or they start to over-dry the nails, making them brittle. For long-term improvements, massage the nail bed and the cuticle daily with oil, which will give you strong but flexible nails that resist breaking. Almond or hazelnut oil is perfect; add a drop of lavender oil to make it smell pretty.'

Dry, brittle nails 'If nails snap, rather than flake, it's because they're dehydrated. Over-exposure to water and sunshine (if nails are unprotected) can dry out nails. Brittle nails also respond to daily oil treatments.'

Ridges 'For longitudinal ridges, very lightly buff nails on a regular basis to smooth them. Then use a ridge-filling base coat to create a smooth base for polish.' (Ridges can sometimes be the result of a damaged nail bed, caused by a yeast infection, or from cuticles that have been cut or damaged; they can also be a sign of zinc deficiency.)

Lengthways splits 'Sometimes, nails start to split down a ridge, all the way down to the base of the nail. An acrylic nail will mend the split and allow the nail to grow out; at the same time, feeding the nail bed via oil massages will encourage healthy future growth.'

Dull, colourless nails 'A healthy nail is a pink nail. Dull, colourless nails may be a sign of a circulation problem. If you squeeze a nail, it will go white; if it takes more than three seconds for the pinkness to reappear, that's another sign of poor circulation. Daily nail massage will help – as will physical exercise.' (NB Smoking can stain nails brownish-yellow – another good reason to give up.)

Uneven skintone 'A big age giveaway is patchiness and dullness, as the skin starts to become more transparent. The fix: exfoliate skin regularly. Face masks, used on the hands, also brighten skin. And I've seen amazing, albeit temporary, results from electrical non-surgical facelift machines, used on the hands; they tighten the skin and improve circulation.

SEE YOUR DOCTOR IF YOU HAVE...

...thickening, crumbling or opaque nails; this may indicate a fungal infection.

...pitting, spotting and thickening – classic signs of nail psoriasis.

...darkening of the nail: a brown or black streak that begins at the base of the nail and extends to the tip could be a sign of melanoma (skin cancer), requiring urgent attention. Some antibiotics, such as tetracycline, may turn nails dark grey; this should fade once the drug is out of your system and the nail grows out.

And if nail problems continue for months rather than weeks, ask your GP for blood tests to determine any nutritional deficits.

WHAT THE STARS USE...

Ortiz, manicurist at LA's Privé salon, uses O.P.I. Nail Envy on **Candice Bergen** as an all-in-one base coat, top coat and treatment for weak nails. Meanwhile, Jessica Vartoughian, owner of West Hollywood's hot-hot-hot Jessica Nail Clinic* (and creator of the Jessica nail line), recommends Revlon emery boards: 'The grain is very soft, which is healthy for the nails.' Meanwhile, indulging her wild streak, **Jane Seymour** has taken Paint Job's 1956 Chevy Crocus Yellow nail enamel out for a spin...

high-tech hands

Cosmetic surgery for hands is fast growing in popularity. According to Professor Nicholas Lowe**, age spots (aka sun spots) on hands can now be removed by laser. Medical peels – using AHAs – are also being used to fade dark spots; they remove surface layers – revealing brighter skin underneath. Some doctors prescribe Retin-A to improve skin on prematurely aged hands, while others are now carrying out vein removal operations (like those for varicose veins on legs) to take out the prominent veins that make some women self-conscious (*see You're So Vein, p.142*). Because hands tend to get thinner as we age, some doctors have experimented with extracting fat from, for example, the buttocks, and injecting it into the hands – but this bruises badly and provides only short-term plumping. As with any cosmetic surgery procedure, these should never be undertaken lightly – no matter how self-conscious you are about your handshake...

hand workout

Exercising the hands regularly will help keep them youthful and supple. (Doctors actually prescribe knitting for arthritic hands.) Follow these simple exercises, to keep hands in tip-top condition...

- Stand upright with your hands by your sides. Raise them slowly, moving the hands back and forth from the wrist. Hold arms out at shoulder level. Then lower them, flexing the hands in the same way.

- Sit or stand with your arms by your sides. Turn the whole arm and hand so that the palms are facing backwards. Clench the fists and – with your arms straight – push them back as far as you can, several times.

- Lace your fingers in a prayer position, then turn them inside out so that palms are facing out, while straightening and pushing arms in front of you at chest level. Hold for 30 seconds and release. Repeat.

- To keep fingers flexible, stretch and separate your fingers. When you feel a good stretch, hold for five minutes. Follow with a thumb workout: hold your right hand outstretched, away from your body. With your left hand, very gently pull your right thumb back towards your body. Hold for five seconds. Switch hands. (These exercises will also help prevent RSI – Repetitive Strain Injury – so if you use a keyboard, take regular exercise breaks and give them this workout.)

- Look for squidgy 'stress balls' that offer a double-whammy: they exercise the muscles of the hands as well as busting stress.

- To help nails grow more quickly, improve circulation to fingertips and hands by drumming them on the table as if you were playing the piano.

- Or try piano lessons. According to a spokesman at the Royal Academy of Music, although the optimum age to begin piano lessons is between seven and ten, 'It's never too late to take up piano – which definitely promotes suppleness and strength. People can successfully play through their seventies and eighties, with great flexibility.' It may be too late to become a concert pianist. But belated piano-playing may mean that in future years we can still get the lid off a crusted-up honey jar...

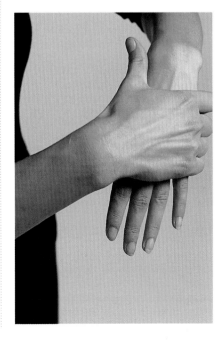

TRIED & TESTED

ANTI-AGEING HAND CREAMS

Until very recently, hands were left out of the anti-ageing arsenal. But the latest hand creams don't just re-moisturise: they may also protect the vulnerable hand skin against damaging UV rays, brighten the skin's appearance – and in some cases, claim even to fade age spots. Over a period of months, our panel of women testers rolled up their sleeves and tried the leading anti-ageing hand creams on the international market. They read what the manufacturers promised on the packaging – and reported back on the improvements they saw...

This was a very high scoring category with 11 creams scoring over eight marks. The lowest scoring hand cream that our testers tried notched up 5.62 marks out of 10.

Atrixo Regenerating Treatment
9.6 MARKS OUT OF 10 (£)
All of our testers said they would buy this product, commenting in particular on the pleasant smell, good dispenser and the fact that although the cream was rich and creamy, it was easily absorbed. This extremely inexpensive cream uses liposome technology to deliver active ingredients designed to soothe even rough, dry, chapped hands.
UPSIDE: 'improvement was immediate and long-term' ♦ 'feels good on application and makes age spots less noticeable' ♦ 'thick, creamy but easily and quickly absorbed' ♦ 'a real wonder cream with immediate results – the best hand cream I've used in years. It has even improved my nails and removed unsightly cuticles' ♦ 'I felt my hands were much softer and not as red and raw as usual' ♦ 'skin softer, lines less noticeable, no more dry skin' ♦ 'no more rough, dry, chapped hands – only smooth, soft, supple ones'.
DOWNSIDE: none of our testers had any negative comments about this product.

Chanel Douceur des Mains
9.3 MARKS OUT OF 10 (££)
This hand cream contains AHAs (fruit acids) to brighten skin and fade age spots, together with UVA and UVB filters plus antioxidant vitamins E and C; ceramides slow down the evaporation of water and strengthen the skin's barrier function. Two-thirds of the
testers said they would buy this, commenting that they liked the smell and the thick, creamy texture. (Not to mention the incredibly glamorous packaging.)
UPSIDE: 'the best hand cream I've ever used; initially my hands felt soft, silky and smooth, with continued improvements, making them look younger' ♦ 'improved texture and suppleness; hands felt cleaner and lighter – a super-hydrator for 'drained' hands that seems to beat the elements' ♦ 'more effective than ordinary hand products; hands are softer, wrinkles less noticeable – the difference in skin texture is quite visible' ♦ 'backs of my hands immediately looked smoother and brighter – like a 'beauty flash' product' ♦ 'the cream smooths in wonderfully and made my skin feel soft immediately'.
DOWNSIDE: 'Chanel's packaging is the best feature here – the fragrance could have been better; it's too strong a smell' ♦ 'hands felt nice and seemed soft but this was no better than a cheaper product'.

Estée Lauder Extra Rich Re-Nutriv for Hands and Arms
9 MARKS OUT OF 10 (£££)
This cream is designed not just to be smoothed into hands, but also the arms, right up to the elbows, suggest the manufacturers. It is water-resistant and features a sunscreen complex to reduce the potential for age spots. Three-quarters of the testers said they would buy this product, but as with several in the Re-Nutriv range, quite a few of our panelists said they didn't like the medicinal smell. On the other hand, some said it was 'lovely' – so we say: sniff before you buy.
UPSIDE: 'age spots seem to be less and less noticeable' ♦ 'both age spots and the texture on the back of my hands have improved – and I like everything about this product' ♦ 'makes my skin feel velvety-soft; cuticles and nails are a lot better' ♦ 'I am no longer ashamed or mildly depressed about hands and arms and have pushed up my sleeves, on occasion, without thinking; my body language is more expansive and I use my hands to illustrate points while talking with greater abandon than before using this product' ♦ 'the treatment really improved the skin texture of my hands and also seemed to

neutralise age spots somewhat' ♦ 'the improvement took two weeks to show up'.
DOWNSIDE: 'it works – but the packaging is very wasteful'.

Shiseido Benefiance Protective Hand Revitalizer
8.7 MARKS OUT OF 10 (£££)
Botanical and vitamin-derived ingredients (from saxifrage and vitamin C) are supposed to even out pigmentation and improve translucency and circulation, as well as providing a protective shield against future sun damage, say Shiseido. It has an SPF8. Three-quarters of the testers said they would buy this product.
UPSIDE: 'superb: cool feel and classy smell; hands are immediately softer, smoother and less dry and over time, age spots seem less noticeable' ♦ 'I love it: my hands really do look good; the skin is much improved, even though I looked after my hands before using this cream' ♦ 'my daughter noticed the lovely smell two hours after I first put it on. This cream has helped my nails, which were very dry – and it has reduced my age spots so noticeably that on one hand, they have almost disappeared' ♦ 'soft, silky and easily absorbed' ♦ 'I usually have very dry skin which snags tights but this cream sorted that' ♦ 'my hands, which I have felt for a long time gave my age away, are beginning to look more youthful' ♦ 'my partner commented that I have 'a young woman's hands''.
DOWNSIDE: 'washes off easily'.

Gatineau Vitamina Suractivée
8.5 MARKS OUT OF 10 (££)
Designed as a 'hand rescue remedy', for regular use morning and evening, this has a lightweight texture and acts as a barrier. It has antioxidant vitamins A and E, and a 'softening' complex with sugar-derived ingredients. Two-thirds of our testers said they would buy it.
UPSIDE: 'even when I only used the cream once a day on occasions, my hands still stayed smooth and soft, even though they are exposed to the weather for long periods' ♦ 'confession: I used it on my bum when I ran out of body lotion and it was excellent!' 'calloused knuckles softer' ♦ 'hands looked

less crêpey and cuticles softer' ♦ 'rough skin at ends of fingers disappeared; lasts for ages. I expect it's more expensive than my usual ordinary dry skin hand cream – but worth it' ♦ 'the overall colour of my hands seemed more even'.

DOWNSIDE: 'it was a good softener and smoother, but my hands look no younger' ♦ 'does not make skin firmer and softness only maintained through regular (daily) use'.

RoC Retinol Anti-Age Hand Treatment
8.5 MARKS OUT OF 10 (£)

Formulated to combat signs of ageing caused by sun and pollution, the cream is said to reduce skin looseness and wrinkles and remove brown spots. Ingredients include retinol, vitamin E, vitamin B5, glycerine and a UV filter (SPF8). Only one of the testers for this product said she wouldn't buy this cream.

UPSIDE: 'after ten days or so there was a significant improvement in crêpiness and this has continued, to my delight; I am absolutely thrilled with this product' ♦ 'quite a pleasant hand cream but no better or worse than any other' ♦ 'extremely pleasant hand cream – leaves no greasiness at all' ♦ 'my hands appeared to be lighter in colour and brown spots to disappear' ♦ 'soft fragrance that doesn't clash with my usual hand cream' ♦ 'my hands are definitely smoother and brighter in colour – more even, too; they're usually quite pink and mottled. This cream is quite simply fantastic!'

DOWNSIDE: 'did not live up to the manufacturers' claims to fade age spots; I am very disappointed and would love to know how they can make such a claim– will they give money back if customers bothered to complain?'

Dr Hauschka Hand Cream
8.37 MARKS OUT OF 10 (££)

This entirely natural product is made from organic and bio-dynamically grown ingredients and avoids chemical preservatives; it is based on pure plant oils, extract of marshmallow and extract of carrot, to heal cracks and fissures. The packaging certainly makes no medical claims but as with other Dr Haushcka products, our testers found impressive results with skin problems. Several testers were initially put off by the strong smell but all said they got used to it. Again, only one of the testers for this cream said she wouldn't buy it in future.

UPSIDE: 'I have used loads of hand creams as I suffer badly in winter and this is the best

ever; it leaves hands smoother, softer and less taut; after constant use, hands stayed soft even after working in the kitchen' ♦ 'I suffer from eczema on my hands but have had no occurrence of this since using the cream; my brittle nail texture has also improved' ♦ 'my hands had less wrinkles and were very supple and not at all dry, even during very cold weather' ♦ 'I am now seventy-one and my hands were very discoloured and wrinkled due to lack of care over the years, so this did present a challenge; there is definflitely a marked lessening in age spots; the condition generally is improved and even if I omitted to use it for a weekend, one application gave instant improvement'.

DOWNSIDE: 'it had no effect whatsoever on my age spots – a big disappointment'.

L'Occitane 20% Shea Butter
8.1 MARKS OUT OF 10 (££)

Shea butter – not so much a butter, more a tree nut oil – is a legendary natural remedy in ethnic communities, because of its intensely moisturising and protective qualities. The company who make this product works directly with several African communities in the manufacturing of their shea butter range, as a commitment to ethical business. Two-thirds of the testers said they would buy it.

UPSIDE: 'absorbed immediately; skin on the back of my hands immediately seemed much smoother and thicker (I have quite thin skin); you only need a small amount and it was absorbed immediately so I was able to do housework/letters etc.' ♦ 'age spots started to fade after two weeks' ♦ 'I had a very irritating patch of skin on my foot which has been driving me mad for eight months, scratching it till it bled; in desperation I put this hand cream on it and the relief was amazing; I use it on my feet every night; the initial problem has cleared up and I have the most wonderful soft skin on my feet' ♦ 'incredible – lumps of hard skin, brought about by gardening, have gone completely; skin looks and feels fantastic, no 'quicks' and no dragged cuticles' ♦ 'lent this to a male friend who had badly cracked skin on his finger; he saw a great improvement after three or four days';

DOWNSIDE: 'took several minutes to absorb completely, with a 'sticky' feel, so therefore didn't use when I was in a hurry to do hair or make-up – but as a result very economical as only a little is needed' ♦ 'not packaged very appealingly – like a tube of oil paint'.

Decleor Hand Care Cream
8 MARKS OUT OF 10 (££)

From this increasingly popular French company which bases its recipes on the art of aromatherapy, Hand Care Cream features shea nut butter, vitamin E, essential oil of cypress and parsley extract; massaging it regularly into the nails is said to protect them and to reinforce growth. Seven out of ten testers said they would buy this cream.

UPSIDE: 'within two days my hands were lovely and soft so I thought I would try the cream on my feet; they now feel as soft as a baby's and my hands as soft as when I was a teenager' ♦ 'hands looked younger, plumped up and less papery; within a week they looked less wrinkly' ♦ 'this is the best hand cream I've ever used' ♦ 'the best hand cream I have ever used – particularly noticeable as I wash my hands a lot' ♦ 'left an immediate glow and hydration, even to some dry patches on my knuckles' ♦ 'liked the shape of the tube and ease of application; it was easy to get the correct amount every time and the lid screws on and off easily'.

DOWNSIDE: 'I hated the smell and have used other hand creams I liked much more, but my cuticles are now in excellent condition and my nails look great' ♦ 'left the palms of the hands tacky and needed wiping before any other task; on going outside to play hockey, I had dust clinging to me. Ugh!'

La Prairie Cellular Hand Cream
8 MARKS OUT OF 10 (££££)

Meant to be used morning and evening over hands and cuticles, this rapidly-penetrating lightweight cream has a barrier function to keep hands moist even if you wash them frequently. In addition to La Prairie's 'cellular complex', it contains calming allantoin, witch hazel and chamomile. Half our testers said they would buy this product.

UPSIDE: 'after a week, the skin on my hands – which was dreadful after constant washing with five children to care for – was much softer and hydrated, and after two months of using this light, fluffy cream, my hands and my cuticles had improved dramatically' ♦ 'immediate improvement in age spots – but not complete banishment, and at this price, one expects miracles' ♦ 'plumped up the skin and faded age spots' ♦ 'dark liver spots lightened and crêpiness visibly improved' ♦ 'the skin was smoother and I liked the smell; my skin/hands were not greasy – unlike some creams. Would recommend it to friends'.

DOWNSIDE: 'not a lot of difference to hands and nails'.

eyes

Even if you've had perfect vision all your life, there's a moment somewhere in your forties when you realise your vision is changing. The print in newspapers seems to be getting smaller. Or your arms are getting shorter...

Presbyopia – middle-aged eye spread – is the first sign of ageing eyes for most of us. What happens is that because the lens of the eye, like the whole of your body, begins to lose elasticity, it loses its ability to adjust (accommodate, in medical terminology) to objects near to your eye. So reading, especially small newsprint, becomes increasingly difficult. Long-distance vision, however, can be unaffected. (Sarah has presbyopia but 20/20 vision otherwise.) Reading glasses are the easy answer – but remembering where you've put them can be a perennial problem.

Although little can be done about presbyopia, there is evidence that some other ageing eye problems, including cataracts (opacity of the lens resulting in blurred vision), age-related macular degeneration (AMD, the leading cause of irreversible blindness in elderly people which affects the central and most important part of the retina) and glaucoma, can be prevented – or helped – by good nutrition. The chief culprit once again appears to be oxidative stress, the process where free radical molecules cause damage to the cells (*see p.13*). An increasing number of studies show that both cataracts and AMD are helped by an antioxidant-rich diet and supplementation.

In one American study, women who had religiously taken vitamin C in daily doses ranging from 400mg to 1g for at least a decade were 77 per cent less likely to develop cataracts than others who got relatively little vitamin C in their diets. Vitamin E has also been shown to help cataracts. Another study found that the highest dietary intake of two carotenoid antioxidants – lutein and zeaxanthin, found naturally in spinach, kale and corn – was linked to a 57 per cent lower risk of AMD.

Supplementation may also have a therapeutic effect: in one study of 102 patients who had had AMD for seven to twelve years, treatment with 500mg per day of vitamin C, 400mg of vitamin E, 9mg of beta-carotene and 250 micrograms (mcg) selenium successfully halted or improved the degenerative changes in 60 per cent of participants.

Glaucoma (where vision is impaired because of abnormally high pressure on the eye) may also be helped by supplementation with antioxidants, ginkgo biloba extract plus fish oil. Research is on-going in these areas, worldwide – so watch this space.

There are also an increasing number of high-tech options for vision problems. Consult your family doctor and optometrist for details.

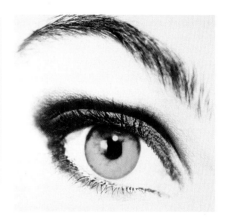

LOOKING BETTER...

Whatever comes out of your mouth, your eyes speak the truth about how you feel. And they give the game away about your age...

The skin surrounding the eyes is the thinnest on the body, so the moisture evaporates easily – and precisely because eyes are so expressive, the skin around them forms wrinkles faster than elsewhere on the face. Then there's the barrage of abuse that eyes are subjected to: contact lenses, mascara, eyeliner, marathon sessions at the computer, smoke-filled rooms and sunlight. 'But the good news is that everybody can improve eye appearance, to some degree,' says US dermatologist Debra Jaliman. Although we're generally fans of the simplest possible skincare, there is definitely a case for using a special eye zone product, particularly if you have sensitive eyes. We love Green People's Eye Gel* and Eye Cream. (Key words to look for, if you have sensitive eyes and aren't sure whether a product will suit you, are 'hypo-allergenic', 'fragrance-free' and/or 'ophthalmologically tested').

(*Also see Getting Rid of Milia p.136.*)

how to protect your eyes

◆ Eat an antioxidant-rich diet, with lots of fresh foods and oil-rich fish if you're not a vegetarian; consider supplements.

◆ Exercise regularly to reduce stress and eye pressure.

◆ Don't smoke – it robs the body of nutrients, is a major risk factor for eye diseases and makes your eyes look red and feel gritty.

◆ Protect your eyes from UV rays with big sunglasses, particularly when the sun's rays are strongest between 10 a.m. and 3 p.m. Unprotected 35-year-old eyes can have the vision problems of a 50-year-old.

◆ Have regular eye checks, yearly if you wear glasses or contact lenses. Check out symptoms such as increased dryness, redness, itching, burning or watering.

◆ Be aware that some medications e.g. antidepressants, steroids, blood pressure lowering drugs, antihistamines and some antibiotics may affect your eye health.

Unpack Your Eye Bags

Some mornings we wake up with eye bags we could put our shopping in. Here are our favourite low-tech de-baggers:

• Exercise. Eye bags are due to fluid retention; bags are usually worse in the morning because fluid collects overnight. Any load-bearing exercise where gravity is pulling the fluid down, e.g. jogging or bouncing on a mini-trampoline, even running up and down stairs, makes bags disappear swiftly south.

• Apply ice or 'frozen' teaspoons. Wrap a cube of ice in clingfilm, smooth round and over your bags – supermodel Linda Evangelista's favourite trick – or do the same with teaspoons (stainless steel rather than family silver) chilled in the freezer.

• Lie down with slices of cucumber or raw potato over your eyes.

• With your middle fingers, tap the under-eye area lightly and swiftly, moving from the inner to outer corner of your eye and back, for a minute or two.

• Track your bags: are they worse when you've eaten certain foods, e.g. wheat or salty foods, after you drink alcohol, in smoky rooms? If so, you could be sensitive to that substance. Try avoiding it and see if that makes a difference.

• Try switching brands of products you use daily, e.g. eye make-up remover, contact lens solution or mascara, in case you are sensitive to one of those.

• Try substituting an eye gel for your regular skin cream, night and morning; the lighter gel on the eye zone may help puffiness.

• If you still want to use a cream at night, make sure it stays out of your eyes by using a very thin layer; pat along the bony ridge beneath your eye, not right under the lashes, then lightly dot cream along brow-bone, under the brow.

WHAT TO DO ABOUT DRY EYES

Postmenopausal women are especially susceptible to dry-eye syndrome. According to Michael S. Berlin, MD, Director of the Glaucoma Institute of Beverly Hills at Cedars-Sinai Medical Center, that's because a reduction in oestrogen production can go hand-in-hand with a reduction in tear production. If your eyes sting, burn or feel scratchy, it may help to humidify your home and work environments – and also to wear sunglasses outdoors. You can also buy artificial tears – Hypromellose – which can be used safely to 'top' up your own tear level. Rohit Mehta of the Nutri-Centre* also recommends Specialist Herbal Supplies' Eye Wash Mixture, an eye bath featuring eyebright, raspberry leaf, bayberry, golden seal and buckwheat leaf, which can be used any time eyes are dry or tired.

Don't be tempted to turn to over-the-counter eye drops to combat any redness, however. While these are OK for special occasions, eyes can become dependent on them very quickly. In a study at Baylor College of Medicine in Houston, scientists found that patients with unexplained conjunctivitis – redness, swelling and tearing – had been overusing eye drops, which are meant to be used for three consecutive days at most. (If eyes still hurt after that, see a doctor.) Patients had used the drops daily for between three and 20 years. Once the patients stopped the drops, the condition cleared up, usually within a month.

Some people believe that glasses make our eyes lazy – and what we really need isn't a new pair of Armani frames, but an eye workout...

throw away your specs

THE BATES METHOD

There's no question that glasses are a godsend for millions with less-than-perfect sight. But they may encourage wearers' eyes to become lazy. The less frequently you give your eyes a workout – even by just going without your glasses whenever you safely can – the *less* they may achieve without the aid of lenses.

The good news is that this downward spiral can possibly be stopped – even reversed – with the Bates Method, a technique which keeps eyes strong and healthy. About a century ago, Dr William H. Bates cupped his eyes in the palms of his hands to help himself relax at the end of an exhausting day. Just a few minutes later, he found his eyes no longer ached and he felt infinitely zippier. From this simple start, he devised a regime which combines relaxation exercises with stimulation exercises. Techniques include regular blinking, swaying the body with the eyes closed ('sunning'), twice-daily splashing of the eyes with cold water several times, focusing exercises, 'shifting' – or rapidly moving your gaze around – and palming. All is revealed in his bestselling *Better Eyesight without Glasses** and we explain a couple of simple exercises here.

Bates exercises can be practised simply at home, but are best first taught by a recommended teacher (*see Directory*). One famous Bates Method devotee was the author Aldous Huxley, whose sight condemned him to milk-bottle glasses at 45. Within a couple of months of starting Bates, he was able to read without glasses.

The following relaxation exercises will give you some idea of what the Bates Method can offer you; they also work as terrific de-stressors, even for those with 20/20 vision. Do them without glasses or contacts. Breathe calmly and deeply and don't strain or try to over-achieve.

(NB Eye problems can accompany various illnesses, such as diabetes or glaucoma; experts suggest that you should be screened for these before undertaking any vision improvement programme.)

Palming A method for resting your eyes in what Bates called 'perfect blackness', free of visual demands. Rub your hands briskly together for about 20 seconds until you feel heat and tingling. Then cup your hands and place your palms over your closed eyes without actually touching them or applying any pressure. Rest your fingers lightly on your forehead and concentrate on your breathing. Without straining or opening your eyes, see the blackness before you.

Blinking Many people with refractive sight problems don't blink enough. Deliberate blinking – which also helps fight dry eyes – is simple: make dozens of delicate butterfly blinks for 10–20 seconds, several times a day, gently turning your head from left to right, and back again. Frequent blinking momentarily rests the eyes, stretches the eye muscles, massages the eyeballs and exercises the pupils by continuously dilating and contracting.

what the bates method did for me...

AGE: 45
PROFESSION: MANUFACTURER'S AGENT

'At 39, my sight started to deteriorate. I realised I was seeing things in a blur and went along to be fitted for glasses. The optician diagnosed an astigmatism (I had had a squint as a child) and myopia. He prescribed glasses and I very quickly couldn't see without them. In 1996 an article about the Bates Method inspired me to find a local teacher. I started with five minutes' practice daily and built up to ten. As well as palming, blinking and sunning, I was given exercises such as looking for a different colour for each day so you see with your brain as well as your eyes. You pick out all the red around you: letter boxes, hats, flowers, etc. It was my 'goal' to be able to read the writing on a Cointreau bottle label about four feet away on the kitchen table. About nine days in, after palming, I saw the word 'Cointreau' perfectly clearly for one micro-second. After six or seven sessions, I took my glasses off and have never needed them again. I do my practice for 20 minutes twice a day, before and after work. The Bates Method has changed my life. Nobody tells you that there are alternatives to glasses. For me, this is nothing less than a miracle...'

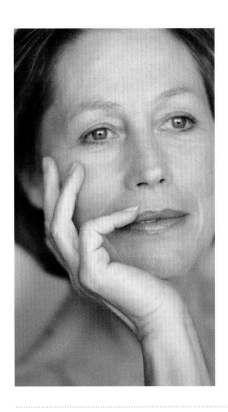

THROUGH THE PINHOLE

Another option to turn eyes into regular little Arnold Schwarzeneggers is pinhole or Trayner glasses* (available from many health-food shops) which you wear, instead of your usual prescription, for just 15 minutes daily during everyday activities such as using the computer, reading or watching TV. Hundreds of tiny pinholes force the eyes' ciliary muscles both to relax and to exercise, building up flexibility and strength and reminding eyes how to focus on their own without tight muscular control – helping to avoid headaches and visual stress. It takes a week to get used to them. Manufacturers say they may also reduce the heart rate – a well-known stress indicator – by up to 4 per cent during ten-minute test periods.

what pinhole glasses did for me…

AGE: 55

PROFESSION: REAL ESTATE AGENT

'I have worn glasses for distance most of my life. In my late forties, I started to have problems reading and focusing. I didn't want to wear bifocals so I decided to look for other ways of treating my sight problems. I found Trayner Pinhole Glasses at a health exhibition and the people on the stand explained they are helpful for all kinds of health problems. I started wearing these lightweight glasses for 20 minutes a day, plus an hour before I went to bed, watching TV or reading. You're aware of the holes for about five minutes but then your eyes adjust and they simply fade away so you see normally. When I first started wearing them, I still had to take my reading glasses around with me in case the lighting was bad or the print small. After three months, I noticed a significant improvement in both long- and near-sight. My eyes were so much better I barely wore my glasses at all. At an eye check four years later, my optician told me my astigmatism had gone and my vision was back to 20/20. I said, 'It must be the pinhole glasses'; he said, 'That's ridiculous.' But I know the glasses work; I just think the optical world is threatened by alternative sight improvement techniques.

'When I first got a computer, I suffered burning, redness and irritation. So now I keep a pair of Trayner glasses beside the computer for the odd symptom of eyestrain and I can work for two or three hours without any problems. My one message would be: stick with it. Even if you don't experience any improvements at first, persist because they can really change your life.'

SUPPLEMENTARY STORY

We know that antioxidants are powerful helpers for our eyesight. Jo Fairley has her own theories about the link between diet and vision.

how jo threw away her glasses…

'Ever since childhood, I have had an astigmatism - one eye doesn't focus on exactly the same point as the other. I wore specs off and on through childhood and for almost 20 years as an adult. About three years ago, I noticed that things became blurred when I wore my glasses - basically all the time. The reason, a somewhat bemused optician told me, was that my eyes had actually improved considerably - odd because, generally, an astigmatism is for life. He told me firmly that the improvement could not be diet related but I have my own theory. I eat a very healthy fruit, veg and whole grains diet but I also noticed that the improvement coincided with beginning to take blue–green algae, which is extremely high in beta-carotene, the 'eyesight vitamin'. If I run out of the algae and forget to stock up, it becomes harder to read number-plates or the digital numbers on the video recorder. Now I have virtually stopped wearing my glasses, my eyes have become steadily stronger; I can sit in front of a VDU for long stretches without strain. Yet when I wore glasses, taking them off for a few minutes and trying to read or look at the screen made my eyes hurt.

'My advice would be that unless you're· in actual physical danger through not wearing them – for instance, driving – then it's worth giving specs a rest whenever you can.'

getting rid of milia

Milia are tiny oil-filled cysts just under the upper layer of the skin, usually found near the eyes or on the cheeks, most often on oily or acne-prone skins. But they can develop around the eye area whatever your skin type. 'When you wear glasses, sweat builds up in the area where your frames rest,' explains Wilma F. Bergfeld MD of the Cleveland Clinic Foundation. 'The excess oil gets under your skin and forms milia.' Prevent this by wiping the area under your glass frames with a soft cloth and occasionally clean your glasses with an astringent, cleanser or soap. If the milia don't disappear, don't attempt to pick or remove them yourself. Visit a doctor or dermatologist who will probably 'nick' the top with a sterile scalpel or electric needle. Skin peels can also be effective.

choosing glamorous spec frames

Despite advances in contact lens manufacture – and leaps in laser surgery – more than half of all people with sight problems choose to wear specs. Then of course there's sunglasses – the positively glamorous side of specs – where we can all indulge the Jackie O in our souls, and at the same time protect our eyes against damaging UV light, which may cause inflammation of the cornea, cataracts and degeneration of the macula – the most important part of the retina for vision. Even on a moderately cloudy day, up to 80 per cent of UV light can still reach the eye.

Specs can be a great accessory – enhancing good points, minimising less attractive ones, and balancing face shapes. Trouble is that until the recent past, guidelines on how to choose a new pair have been limited to vision criteria only – perish the thought that you might consider how they look. As spec wearers ourselves – Jo for an astigmatism (in the past) and presbyopia (Sarah) – we have taken a keen interest in putting these guidelines into practice.

The choice of sizes and shapes nowadays is enormous. Materials are mainly plastic or, today's fave, metal: usually titanium and stainless steel. Not only do these look elegant, metal is durable and should last for two to three years, by which time most people want a new pair anyway. Or *pairs*: many women choose to have two or more sets, discreet for day, more flamboyant for evenings. But beware of rimless specs: although they suit most faces, they are more fragile because the lenses are unsupported.

Today's frames are smaller as well as lighter. But unless you're remorselessly trendy – and very young-looking – very small frames tend to be unflattering for older faces. Aim for medium- or larger-size frames which camouflage the eye area and its bags and wrinkles. Large-framed sunglasses effectively prevent UV light getting to the vulnerable skin of the eye area.

It's worth finding an optician who will give you a personal consultation. Also, take time to look around and see that you're getting the best deal price-wise.

The guidelines for choosing the most flattering frames are straight-forward. Gather up several pairs, and consult with assistants at the stores before making your final decision:

- Avoid frames the same shape as your face; if you don't know your face shape, find out with the simple technique on *p.96*.

Oval face Can wear just about any size and shape frame: for fun, try angular or rounded 'aviator' shapes or small, round wire frames.

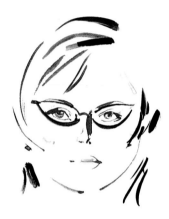

Round face Go for shapes that will slim down your features, e.g. cat's eye, above, rectangular or square.

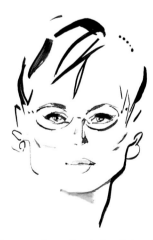

Square face Look for light, thin frames in an oval shape.

Long face Opt for wide frames, not too small, to counteract the length and narrowness of your face. Steer clear of small, square styles.

- Make sure your eye is in the centre of each frame.

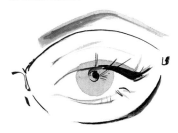

- Close-set eyes will appear more wide apart with lightweight, thin, small frames and a narrow bridge.

- The top bar should follow or echo the line of your eyebrows.

- Owners of one and a half, or even double chins, should look for (non-extreme) cat's eye or oval frames which are higher at the temple and so distract from the chin.

- Try toning the frame colour to your hair: silver, gold, grey, tortoiseshell, etc. If you want to go superfunky, try combinations such as turquoise or red with salt and pepper hair; olive, bronze or antique gold with fair or red hair; shiny black with olive or dark skintones.

- Ensure frame sits comfortably on your nose; small – but not major – adjustments can be made.

- Shorten long noses with a lower bridge; for short noses, choose a higher bridge in a light colour.

- If you suffer from headaches under strip lighting, you may want to try having your reading glasses tinted to cut the brightness.

SUNGLASSES

- Always choose sunglasses which give 100 per cent UVA and UVB absorption; this is especially important as you get older because it helps protect against radiation reaching the lens and possibly causing inflammation of the cornea or cataracts.

- For very hot climates, also look for infra-red protection to keep your eyes cool and comfortable.

- Buy plastic (e.g. acrylic or polycarbonate) lenses if possible, which don't break as easily as glass and are less permeable to UV rays. If you do buy glass, opt for toughened or laminated.

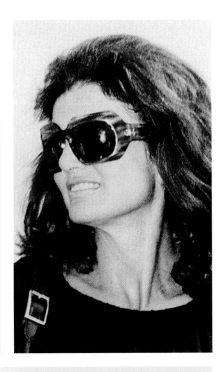

know the jargon:

Photochromic lenses change tint with light intensity so are good for driving or whenever the amount of light may vary, e.g. with time of day or where you are.

Polarised lenses reduce glare from light that bounces off flat surfaces, e.g. roads, water or snow.

Fixed tint lenses (made from plastic) are good for very light-sensitive people or those who have had cataracts.

DO YOU NEED SUNGLASSES EVEN WHEN IT'S CLOUDY?

Yes, yes and yes! For the same reason you should wear sunscreen even when it's overcast: there is still plenty of harmful UV light getting through. Good sunglasses are much, much more than a fashion accessory: they help to keep your eyes healthy. According to Dr Hugh R. Taylor of Johns Hopkins University, USA: 'When it comes to eyes, the more protection you have against UV radiation the better, especially against UVB radiation.' Wraparound or large-frame glasses are best, as they block more light, not only giving you protection against vision damage but also helping to stop wrinkles forming around the eye zone and keeping eyes cool and comfortable.

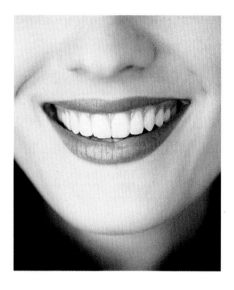

toothtalk

A wide smile with gleaming teeth is one of the most attractive assets for anyone. But teeth often get relegated to 'poor relation' status, possibly because they may seem less important than smooth skin or glossy hair. But taking care of your teeth, gums and mouth and finding a good dentist is essential.

Meticulous daily dental care is vital always, but particularly as we get older. The big thing to avoid is the build-up of plaque, the layer (mainly composed of bacteria) on the surface of teeth which leads to disease of both teeth and gums, and to dental caries (tooth decay). You can prevent plaque by brushing and flossing teeth regularly and thoroughly, and having regular check-ups with the dentist and hygienist. The same care can prevent gum disease, caused by bacterial infection, which increases in frequency as we age, causing receding gums and sometimes even loss of teeth.

Although hormones have never been definitively proved to be linked to gum disease, some dentists notice that the state of women's mouths alters cyclically, which suggests at least some hormonal connection. So it may be worth considering scheduling dental check-ups mid-cycle if possible and also taking extra care of teeth, gums and mouth around menopause.

London-based dentist, David Klaff, President of the British Academy of Aesthetic Dentists, helped us compile these Top Tooth Tips for keeping your pearly whites gleaming with health.

TOP TOOTH TIPS

▷ Consult your dentist to set up an examination and hygiene programme about every three to six months routinely, depending on your individual needs.

▷ Change your toothbrush every month; ask your dentist about the most suitable design for you and the best brushing technique. Rotary electric brushes currently seem to show excellent results for controlling plaque, removing food debris and stimulating the gums (please remember to change the head every month.)

▷ Clean your teeth when you get out of bed in the morning to remove debris.

▷ Floss your teeth regularly at night.

▷ Consider also using a water-jet/water-pick at night (available via your dentist or at a pharmacy) to flush out debris.

▷ Eat well: nutritional deficiency may cause gum disease by reducing resistance.

▷ Eliminate unnecessary acidity in the mouth, caused by sugar, citrus fruit and stress; it increases the risk of tooth decay and gum disease by allowing bacteria to flourish.

▷ Drink lots of water – particularly if you like eating citrus fruit or drinking orange or grapefruit juice (while citrus fruits probably contribute to acidity in the mouth, as above, you shouldn't miss out on the vitamin C benefits).

▷ Take positive steps to relax and combat stress: many dentists believe that stress also causes an acid environment in the mouth.

▷ Opt for gentle, non-stinging mouth sprays. (Look for plant-based natural sprays, like Janina Programme Opale Spray Cleanser, *see Directory*)

▷ Don't smoke: as well as causing yellowing teeth and bad breath, smoking prevents healing and contributes to disease by restricting blood supply.

beating bad breath

Bad breath, or halitosis, is a confidence downer of the first order. Dr Mervyn Druian**, who runs the London Breath Centre and is a spokesman for the British Dental Association, says bad breath is not just a one-off social discomfort, it can cause marital break-ups and even spell the end of promising careers.

Fortunately, however, it's relatively simple to treat. There are plenty of at-home measures you can follow, but if the problem persists, do consult your dentist. Very, very rarely bad breath could indicate a disease condition, such as diabetes, liver or kidney disease or a cancer. So don't ever let it go on for weeks or months.

Why it happens

Some 90 per cent of stale-smelling breath is due to the millions of bacteria living – and dying – in your mouth. The dead bugs form the whiffy sulphurous gases. Bleeding gums cause an unattractive combination of dead and dying blood cells to add to the bugs. The bug population also shoots up when there's infection or inflammation. Saliva, your mouth's waste-disposal operator (also a very efficient antiseptic), just can't cope, so the dead cells hang around creating problems.

Bacteria also get trapped in the dark folds at the back of the tongue where oxygen (which knocks out the sulphur compounds) can't reach easily.

Other causes of bad breath include: broken or cracked fillings which can trap food particles, sinusitis or rhinitis which can cause a bug-laden drip from the back of your nose into your mouth during the night, smoking (a major cause of very unpleasant breath), poor digestion plus any activity that dries up saliva and allows decaying bugs to make a takeover bid for your mouth. So beware of dieting, only eating one meal a day, not drinking enough water or drinking too much caffeine, and medications including anti-allergy drugs, diuretics, tranquillisers, blood pressure lowering drugs and any drugs containing sulphur. Basically, anything that makes you feel as if a gerbil has slumbered in your mouth overnight may make it smell that way too.

Hormonal cycles from puberty to menopause affect breath as well, creating more sulphurous compounds for a couple of days before menstruation, around ovulation and during menopause (because of a slightly drier mouth and an increased likelihood of bleeding gums due to stress).

Consulting your dentist and following the guidelines below should keep the problem at bay.

Is it you?

Check your breath in one of the following ways:

- Lick the soft part of your wrist, using the farthest back part of your tongue, wait a few seconds then sniff.
- Rub a piece of tissue or gauze at the back of the tongue, then smell it.
- Draw a piece of dental floss back and forward several times between your top back teeth, then give that the sniff test.
- Dentists may also use a device called a halimeter.

If the result gives you a nasty moment, don't despair, there are a range of simple remedies.

What to do

The Top Tooth Tips on the previous page will go a long way to solving any long-term problem but for an instant fix, try the following:

- Brush carefully on the outside and inside of your teeth and gums then sluice with a specific antiseptic rinse: try RetarDENT toothpaste, and RetarDEX rinse (made by Rowpar Pharmaceuticals); or Janina Ultrawhite Toothpaste and oral spray (brilliant for travelling).
  NB avoid rinses with alcohol; they may provide an instant fix but the alcohol will then dry the mouth making bad breath more likely.
- Floss thoroughly.
- Use a special tongue cleaner which you can buy at a pharmacy or use an upside-down spoon, rubbed back and forth across the tongue at the back of the mouth.
- Chew on a sugarless dental chewing gum.
- Stop smoking.

What's the alternative?
Herbal Helpers

- Try an infusion of myrrh; or make your own peppermint, rosemary, fenugreek or sage infusions with 1 dessertspoon of fresh or dried herbs infused in a cup of boiling water and strained.
- Chew on cinnamon or licorice root, star anise, cloves, parsley, apple or carrot.
- Plant-based 'green drinks' may also help: try a tablespoon of liquidised alfalfa or wheat-grass juice twice daily, added to water or fruit juice.
- Try homoeopathic remedies such as Kali. phos. to remove a bitter taste on waking; for a metallic taste, try Merc. sol. in the 6X potency, twice a day for ten days.

If you're entirely happy with your teeth, you obviously don't need even to think about cosmetic dentistry. If you're not, consider the following:

*Are you self-confident about smiling, or do you ever put your hand over your mouth when you beam? *Do you look at friends and envy their smiles? *When you smile at yourself in the mirror, do you see any defects in your teeth such as white or brown stains, overlapping or protruding teeth? *Are your gums rosy-pink and clean-edged – or red, swollen and/or receded?

If you answer '*yes*' to any or all of these, it's worth consulting a dentist experienced in this type of work. Unfortunately, although the results may make you feel infinitely better, they come with a hefty price tag. So do please take time and trouble finding a good dentist, who will make sure that the work on your teeth is not only aesthetically pleasing but also corrects any problems and protects teeth against future damage.

WHAT YOUR DENTIST CAN DO FOR YOU

Scaling and polishing
Make a regular three- or six-monthly appointment with the dental hygienist to remove plaque and surface stains, and give teeth a brightening polish. Ultrasonic scalers are generally available; the latest technology is the air-abrader – an 'airgun' which fires high-speed abrasive powder at the teeth, giving excellent results in stain removal.

Bleaching
Whitening teeth professionally with either carbomide peroxide or hydrogen peroxide is currently illegal in the UK – despite its use on hair, skin and nails – because of an alleged carcinogenic link. However dentists in America, Asia and mainland Europe are all bleaching teeth legally. The British Dental Association is trying to get the legislation changed and one manufacturer of dental-bleaching equipment is negotiating with the Government.

Although British dentists are unable to offer bleaching, many will consent to do it if the patient asks and if their teeth are sound and mouth healthy. Bleaching can improve the hue and brightness of teeth by 60–70 per cent. However stains caused by tetracycline treatment in early youth are less likely to respond satisfactorily, and bleaching won't touch the big white patches on teeth cause by demineralisation; the only way to remove those is with micro-abrasion (polishing with a mild, safe form of hydrochloric acid). Where there are existing white fillings, the bleach may penetrate down the sides of the fillings and cause sensitivity. Fillings may need to be replaced after bleaching.

Laser technology is the latest painless, effective – but costly – tooth whitener in America and the UK and looks set to become the choice of the future.

Crowns
The traditional way of repairing a broken or unsightly tooth. The tooth is ground down to a peg and a replica fitted over the top. Top dentists are now working in porcelains so hard that internal metal supports, previously needed as a reinforcement, are no longer necessary. So crowns look better, last longer and never have a black line around the margin. With healthy gums, a porcelain crown will last 20 years.

Bonding
Sticking tooth-coloured material to an existing tooth is an alternative to crowning. The tooth is etched using a weak acid which creates a rough surface on the tooth to which composite or porcelain in-lays (which fit entirely within the confines of the prepared tooth) or on-lays (which fit over the prepared tooth and cover all or most of the biting surface) are attached (*see Veneers, below*), depending on the problem. Bonding is far easier than other means of fixing. It's particularly helpful for filling gaps between widely-spaced front teeth. Expect to need replacements every five years or so.

Veneers
A popular solution for badly discoloured or misshapen teeth – a very thin layer of porcelain, rather like a false fingernail, is bonded to the tooth. Increasingly, veneers are so superthin that they can be applied without removing any of the tooth. Disadvantages are that veneers can chip and, in rare cases, they may fall off, usually because of poor technique. Since teeth darken with age, veneers will need to be done at intervals to match other teeth.

Implants
Titanium screw implants have revolutionised the replacement of lost

teeth; until recently their use was limited to places in the mouth where there was sufficient bone to screw in the implants. Now, however, advanced surgical techniques mean that surgeons can graft the patient's own bone from another part of the body into the mouth as a 'bed' for the implant.

Amalgams

Removing amalgam fillings and substituting composite (plastic and ceramic) or porcelain fillings will give you an all-white yawn instead of a mouth like an ironmonger's. For larger fillings, where shrinkage is a big problem, the dentist takes an impression and the filling is made in the laboratory and pre-shrunk before use. These fillings are also stronger and can be excellently colour-matched but the are more expensive.

Healthwise, there has been on-going controversy on the topic of mercury in amalgam fillings. Mercury is a powerful neurotoxin which has been shown to escape from fillings and to lodge in tissues. That's enough for an increasing number of dentists to stop using it. However, some dentists – and the dental governing bodies in America and Great Britain among other countries – stalwartly maintain that it is perfectly safe and there is no link between ill health (apart from temporary and minor problems) and mercury fillings. But we know of many women who are delighted to have had their mercury fillings removed. At the very least, their mouths taste fresher; at the most, all sorts of chronic symptoms such as headaches, joint aches, skin conditions, fatigue and non-specific ill-health improve. David Klaff adds that amalgam fillings are also responsible for causing cracks and fractures in teeth. However the current range of tooth-coloured fillings, although becoming more durable, cannot yet match the 15-year-plus lifespan of the amalgam filling, and require a more sophisticated and dexterous hand to fit them well. NB Mercury vapour may be released as the fillings are removed, so mercury amalgam fillings must be replaced by a dentist who is experienced and takes all due precautions.

Orthodontics

Using fixed braces, a trained orthodontist can correct the alignment of teeth, adjust the relationship of teeth and jaw to give a better bit, improve the shape of a sticking-out or receding jaw and correct congenital anomalies such as cleft lip and palate. In extreme cases, the upper and lower jaw are so out of alignment that surgery is also necessary. Adult orthodontic work, mainly private, is becoming more common and makes up about 40 per cent of most dentists' practices. The latest ceramic technology means that fixed braces can be tooth-coloured rather than silver. Treatment may take 18 months to two years.

what veneers did for me…

AGE: 40, PROFESSION: ADVERTISING SALES EXECUTIVE

'My teeth had always looked disproportionately small because I'd ground them in my sleep until they were almost straight across. They'd yellowed a lot, too. Veneers offered an affordable way of getting them fixed. At my initial consultation with the cosmetic dentist, computer imagery superimposed an image of eight new teeth onto a picture of me, allowing me to see how I could look.

'The first thing they did was take a putty "cast" of my teeth. Then they smoothed my teeth down under local anaesthetic and filed away some of what was there before I was fitted with a temporary plate. That was cemented into place so that I didn't have to live with stumps while the veneers were being prepared. I was back walking around after about three hours, feeling a bit achey but otherwise fine. The plate felt strange, like a set of false teeth, and what was left of my teeth felt very sensitive to hot and cold.

'My second visit – to have the veneers permanently cemented into place – took about two hours. The main discomfort, aside from more local anaesthetics, is having to keep your teeth totally dry so the cement will stick – of course the moment someone tells you that you can't have a drink of water, you're desperately thirsty. They had to tug the plate off first and the new teeth had to be scraped and smoothed a bit; my mouth felt a bit gritty while that was going on, like having fillings smoothed. Because of my tooth-grinding I'd altered my bite, so it meant there were extra alterations to ensure the lip fitted over the teeth properly at a third visit, after any swelling from the anaesthetic had subsided. I had a very disconcerting lisp, but that went after the third visit.

'They did feel enormous at first, but now they just feel like they've always been there. Friends have said: "I knew something was different, but I couldn't work it out." That's exactly the subtle reaction you want. But now I really realise how tooth-grinding destroys your looks – and I regret it like mad! All those years when I could have had smile-worthy teeth…'

rejuvenating surgery

YOU'RE SO VEIN...

We have a love-hate relationship with our veins. We love them when they're invisible, pumping blood healthily from A to B , but often become extremely self-conscious about them when they start to show. Today, you can zap them, collapse them – even have some veins completely removed. If you're vain about the appearance of yours, here are the latest options...

SPIDER VEINS ON THE FACE AND LEGS...
(aka telangiectasia, dermal flares or broken veins)

THE CAUSES: In fact, the veins aren't 'broken' at all – they simply become more obvious as skin thins with the years. Some women are genetically predisposed to them, especially the pale and fine-skinned. Aggravating factors include hormonal changes due to pregnancy/menopause, the Pill, HRT, injury, sunburn and alcohol.

'Spider veins are very common in women from 20 up,' says our 'vein expert', Mr John Scurr**. 'It's almost impossible to find a woman who hasn't got them – but some are more self-conscious about them than others.'

Spider veins can also be painful; the pain is often cyclical and related to periods.

THE FIXES *Electrolysis:* Using a similar needle technique to hair removal, an electrical current is passed into the skin to cauterise the vein; the blood is then absorbed into the body. 'This treatment is available through beauty salons, but you need to be very sure that the beautician knows what she's doing and has the back-up to deal with potential problems, such as infection,' advises Mr Scurr.

Micro-sclerotherapy: 'This uses an ultra-fine needle to inject a "sclerosing" solution – a detergent substance – into the vein.' (In the US, saline – a salt solution – is commonly used.) The solution irritates the vein lining, causing the sides to stick together so that the top, just under the skin, is no longer filled with blood and visible.

Sclerotherapy leaves no scab or obvious mark. Sometimes results are instant, but in other patients there may be up to a three-month wait for veins to clear. In some cases, blood slowly leaks back into the veins so they become apparent again. The length of the session – and the number – will depend on the extent of the problem.

Laser treatment: Lasers can be used for removal of spider veins on the legs or face. It is vital that they are used properly, by a qualified surgeon, and, even then, Mr Scurr is cautious; laser treatment can leave some scarring, as it burns the skin and can create blistering. Mr Scurr prefers PhotoDerm pulsed light therapy – one of the 'new generation' laser-type technologies – which uses a high-intensity light filtered to a very narrow wavelength to heat and destroy the blood vessels. (Different surgeons have different laser preferences, however.) PhotoDerm works best where there is greatest contrast, i.e. red veins against pale skin. The light, delivered in pulsating flashes, feels like a rubber band snapping at the skin. Afterwards you may look as though you have a slight sunburn in treated areas; if you're unlucky, you might peel. But as the redness fades, so do the underlying flares. Repeated treatments may be necessary. 'To get the best results, avoid exposure to the sun for three months before treatment.'

'But,' Mr Scurr adds, 'spider veins are like weeds in the garden. If you're predisposed towards them, you're likely to get another crop, at some stage in the future...'

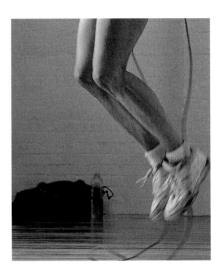

VARICOSE VEINS ON THE LEGS

THE CAUSES: These are dilated superficial veins; they can range from a minor bulge through to a prominent bunch-of-grapes effect. They occur when veins in the legs aren't able to return blood efficiently to the heart. Our veins are equipped with a series of one-way valves that direct blood flow towards the heart. When the valves work poorly, blood stagnates in the veins, causing them to become swollen and twisted. 'Anyone who stands around a lot is also vulnerable, as are pregnant women,' says Mr Scurr. Over the years, there is a loss of tone in the valves and veins, leading to a higher incidence of varicose veins. Sufferers may complain of aching, tingling, tired legs, irritation, cramp or pain on standing. There are potential dangers in ignoring obvious varicose veins, he adds. 'Over time, the skin around the ankle may start to discolour. The skin there also thickens and may actually break down, causing an ulcer; these are difficult to heal and – not to put too fine a point on it – nasty, smelly and unpleasant.'

THE FIXES: Before treatment, you'll be given a clinical examination and an assessment (which may include an ultrasound scan, to measure blood flow). *Support hose:* In some women, surgical support stockings or tights may keep minor varicose veins under control, but these are hot and sweaty to wear in summer. (Sadly, Lycra fashion tights aren't powerful enough to do the job of surgical support hose – though Mr Scurr feels they may have a helpful role as a preventive measure.) *Drug treatment:* 'New drugs, which constrict the muscle, actually have an effect similar to elastic stockings,' says Mr Scurr. In the UK, the most commonly used drug is called paroven; in France, Daflon is extremely popular. They work by improving tone in the vein wall, giving a constricting effect – but only for as long as you are taking the drug; side-effects, he insists, are minimal. *Surgery:* When it comes to more drastic options, 'the earlier treatment is embarked on, the better the results'. For more advanced veins, surgery may be the best solution. After a light general anaesthetic, initial incisions are made in the groin, to cut off the blood supply to the legs during surgery; in some cases, there will be incisions made behind the knees. Then the varicose veins are hooked out through the incisions. Mr. Scurr prefers to wrap the legs temporarily in bandages, then replace them with compression stockings after 12 hours (so the patient can shower). For the first few days, the stockings are worn day and night, then removed at night; they can be taken off for a shower but bathing or swimming is not advised. In all, you will need to wear them for about ten days. Infection, meanwhile, is extremely rare,

but if any wounds become red and angry, the doctor should be informed, and, probably, antibiotics prescribed.

SELF-HELP
• Regular exercise is excellent prevention. Walking is ideal; walking barefoot on the beach or wading in the sea provides increased stimulation.
• Avoid sitting for long periods of time, because the pressure of a chair against the back of your legs impedes circulation. If you work at a sedentary job, get up and walk around every hour for a few minutes.
• While sitting in a chair, lift your legs straight out in front of you. Point and flex your feet several times to stimulate calf muscles and assist your circulation.

THE ALTERNATIVES
Although overnight results are impossible with alternative therapy, leading naturopath Jan de Vries believes that a combination of diet, exercise and prescribed homoeopathic remedies (i.e. Hyperisan, Urticalcin and Aesculus hipp., or horse chestnut) can be effective. He advises patients to avoid alcohol, nicotine and salt. For some varicose vein patients, Jan de Vries also prescribes twice-yearly courses of vitamin E. 'I would always try an alternative before surgery.' Dr Joseph Pizzorno suggests a diet rich in dietary fibre with liberal amounts of cherries, blackberries, bilberries and other dark berries, which contain high levels of bioflavonoids, together with garlic, onions, ginger and cayenne. If you don't mind taking a long-term approach to the problem, it may may be worth consulting a naturopath for an individual prescription of herbs and supplements.

ESSENTIAL STEPS IN CHOOSING A SURGEON

Just because this is often called 'cosmetic' surgery, don't forget that all surgery – to any part of your face, scalp or body – is an invasive procedure which carries risks, some potentially life-threatening. It is also very expensive – little cosmetic surgery is available on health services or on medical insurance – but just because surgeons charge a lot doesn't mean they are good. It is vital that you take time and care choosing the person who you're putting in charge of your looks – and your life. Most important of all, according to the surgeons we talked to, is to have a good relationship with your surgeon and to be thorough in your questioning – but not aggressive.

We recommend that before you finally decide on surgery, you try the other non-surgical lifestyle options we write about in this book.

STEP 1: SHORT LIST

There are three main ways of finding one or more surgeons to consider.

a. Ask your family doctor; be aware, however, that many won't know *either* the best person to go to *or* the most appropriate procedures.

b. Ask friends for recommendations.

c. Ask your doctor to get a list of consultant plastic surgeons with an interest and expertise in cosmetic (also called aesthetic) surgery.

We do not recommend you approach the clinics who advertise in the back of glossy magazines. However good they sound – and many may be entirely competent – this is often where the problems occur, with unqualified staff and/or poor facilities.

STEP 2: CONSULTATION

a. Make an appointment to see one or more surgeons for an initial consultation. There will almost certainly be a fee, which is usually refundable if you decide to go ahead with that surgeon. However, paying for a consultation is always a wise investment.

b. See firstly whether you get on with the surgeon. It's crucial you like and trust the person. Talk to them about all the different options: a good rule of thumb is that if you feel you are the object of a selling/marketing operation at this point, the surgeon is probably more interested in his fee than in you, the potential patient.

c. Ask for detailed information on the procedures you are contemplating (many surgeons provide their own fact sheets), possible complications, pain relief and recovery times. Some patients like to see before and after pictures – these are fine as a point of comparison but remember you will never be shown the worst results. Remember that no wise surgeon can or should guarantee a specific result.

d. Also ask about whether the anaesthesia will be a general anaesthetic, deep sedation or local anaesthetic. This will affect how groggy you feel after surgery and how long you need to spend in hospital.

e. Check out the surgeon's qualifications and training: ask him/her what professional bodies he/she is a member of and ring them to confirm.

f. Make sure your surgeon is comprehensively insured.

g. Ask whether he/she has had any legal cases brought against them and what happened.

h. Check out the surgical team and the hospital or clinic: does the surgeon work regularly with a particular team of qualified anaesthetists and experienced nurses?

i. Before you leave the consultation, make sure you have a clear understanding of the possible procedures, risks and recovery times; ask for these details in writing plus the precise costs and the number of follow-up visits (most reputable surgeons include follow-ups for the following six to 12 months, or as long as they consider necessary in individual cases).

STEP 3: THINKING TIME

Don't feel you have to make a decision immediately. Sleep on it, talk about it, consider the other non-surgical possibilities. If you decide to go ahead, you will be asked to sign a consent form. Read it thoroughly before signing. However be aware that the consent form is designed to protect the surgeon, and the medical system, rather than the patient. Signing the consent form implies that the risks and possible complications involved in the procedure(s) have been explained to you – and that you understand them. If something is not clear, do not sign until you have asked more questions and received satisfactory answers.

See Directory for where to get lists of qualified surgeons in the UK.

medical matters:

techniques

In the last few years, the range of rejuvenating techniques has greatly increased. Although facelifts and other cosmetic surgery procedures are still as much in demand as ever, many women are choosing to start younger with less invasive techniques, such as laser re-surfacing and chemical peels, to brighten tired skin and reduce fine lines and wrinkles. Remember that in most cases, as with surgery, you must be prepared to look worse – sometimes much worse – before you look better.

SKIN PEELING, DERMABRASION AND LASER RE-SURFACING

These techniques have revolutionised the treatment of facial blemishes: fine lines, poor skin texture, dark circles, acne scars, brown spots, moles, birthmarks and port wine stains. They must be performed by experts, usually by a cosmetic surgeon or dermatologist, in a reputable medical clinic – never in a beauty salon. They should improve skintone and texture but will not 'lift' sags or bags, tighten loose skin or remove deep scars.

Because they are all based on revealing new skin which is very sensitive to UV light, you must be prepared to keep out of the sun and zealously protect your face with high factor sun preps (SPF25–30 or total block) and a floppy hat.

CHEMICAL SKIN PEELS

These can deep-clean and soften skin, they may also remove lines, e.g. vertical furrows round the mouth. They come in three basic strengths, depending on the depth to which the chemical agent applied penetrates. Strength is governed not only by the type of peel but also by the concentration of active ingredient(s), the number of coats applied and also what pre-treatment was used. Skin is

often pre-treated with Retin-A, itself a peeling agent, or with alpha-hydroxyacids (AHAs). The milder the chemical, the safer the procedure – and the less effective at removing lines. And vice versa: as peels increase in strength, so do the risks of scarring (all peels carry a risk of scarring), irregular pigmentation, loss of pigmentation. Peels of different strengths may be used on the same patient, e.g. a medium peel on the face, with a light peel on the neck.

Light or Superficial Peels

These work on the horny layer and upper epidermis to promote exfoliation; they're ideal for freshening the skin and are often called 'skin-freshening peels'; they are usually backed up with home use of tretinoin (Retin-A) or AHAs.
What's used: high-concentration (20–25 per cent) glycolic or lactic acid; low-concentration (10–25per cent) trichloracetic acid (TCA); Jessner's solution, a predictable and safe combination of salicylic acid, resorcinol and lactic acid peel.
Recovery time: Sometimes called 'lunch-hour' peels, these usually cause only a few hours' slight flushing and some flaking for a couple of days.

Risks: Scar formation.
A closely spaced series of light peels can also be carried out by some cosmetic dermatologists to rejuvenate skin without the recovery period needed for a medium to deep peel.
What's used: high concentration (50–70 per cent) TCA; Jessner's solution plus TCA in low (15–25 per cent) concentration, or high concentration (70 per cent) glycolic acid. Light peels will soften or eradicate fine to moderate wrinkling, crêpiness and some forms of pock scars, reduce or shrink pore size, improve skin colour and smoothness.Each peel will probably induce an evening of uneven colour.

Medium (or Moderate) Peels

Medium and deep peels are sometimes called skin-rejuvenation peels. A medium peel will penetrate through the horny layer and upper epidermis to the upper dermis. One or two peels will improve skin colour markedly, eradicate deeper lines, wrinkles and furrows by causing surface blistering and peeling; the peel stimulates the production of new collagen and elastin fibres and may also soften shallower acne scars, eliminate thicker age spots, even mottled colouring and eradicate some early pre-cancerous growths.

What's used: higher (35–50 per cent) concentration TC; full-strength (88 per cent) phenol; or two-step peels with first Jessner's solution, or glycolic acid, followed by 35 per cent TCA.

Recovery time: Swelling, blistering, oozing and crusting may last for seven to fourteen days; strong painkillers may be necessary.

Risks: Excessive lightening or darkening of the skin; scar formation.

Deep Peels

These go further still, to the mid to lower dermis, and deal with deeper wrinkling and scarring problems.

What's used: phenol (the Baker-Gordon formula or Baker's peel is a special modification of phenol solution).

Recovery time: Swelling, blistering, oozing and crusting may last for 14 days or more; skin may be red for eight to twelve weeks afterwards.

Risks: Permanent slight loss of pigmentation (said to be almost inevitable); pigmentation irregularities (so darker-skinned women must be warned of possibly permanent changes in pigmentation); excessive lightening or darkening of the skin; elevated scars. The effects of phenol absorption into bloodstream can include severe liver, kidney and heart-rhythm problems in people with pre-existing conditions.

DERMABRASION

This technique uses different instruments – e.g. a small drill-type instrument with a pear-shaped head studded with diamond dust, or a wire-wheel brush – to 'sand' away upper layers of skin to remove scars and create a smoother surface.

Recovery time: The skin reddens, swells, becomes itchy, dry and possibly painful for several days or even weeks before the scabs fall off and the new soft 'baby' skin grows through.

Risks: Causes enlarged pores, discoloration and bleeding in the treated area, so may leave a 'tidemark' at the edges. The main risk, as with all similar techniques, is in going too deep into the skin, so creating a lasting scar, rather than removing problems. Temporary reactions may include tiny whiteheads (milia).

LASERS

In expert hands, laser treatment is said to be more predictable and safer than dermabrasion and chemical peels. Rapid shallow pulses of laser light burn away the top layer of skin, reducing wrinkles, smoothing and tightening skin, removing age marks and mottling, and helping with acne scarring. But be cautious: lasers are still new 'toys' for surgeons and represent sizeable financial investment. There are no long-term studies as yet, and lasers can inflict serious damage, literally burning the skin. For skin rejuvenation by resurfacing, the most popular (and extensively tested) type is the CO_2 (carbon dioxide); the two leading brands are Silk Touch and Ultra-Pulse. The newer Erbium: Yag laser is useful for very superficial treatment, e.g. on crows' feet, though shallow application of CO_2 lasers may be equally, or more, effective. Q-switched Ruby or Nd: YAG are mostly used for brown spots and moles.

Recovery time: Skin will be noticeably pink for at least six weeks (about three weeks with the Erbium:Yag).

Risks: Permanent pigment change; post-operative bleeding; burns; lasting scars.

what laser resurfacing did for me…

AGE: 59
PROFESSION: AROMATHERAPIST,
'I don't mind being 58 but not looking 58 – and raddled. A top laser surgeon wrote "smoking" and "sun damage" on my notes and said I was a good candidate for treatment. An information sheet told me about the possible downsides, including white patchiness on the skin (like vitiligo), and redness for 14 days (which actually lasted a month). I had a "twilight" anaesthetic, which just put me under. My face was covered in a thick layer of antiseptic cream and my eyes shielded. The surgeon spent nearly an hour going backwards and forwards over my skin – rather like a child colouring in a picture. I was terrifically woozy afterwards and my face had been covered in gauze, over an antiseptic pack. I was given painkillers and very expensive tablets in case I developed herpes, but I felt no pain at all. The next morning, my face was bright red and swollen! I had to put on a special pure moisturising cream every hour or so, except while sleeping. That prevented any scabbing, but over the next few days, my skin went very papery and brown. The cream kept it from coming off like a snake's. My face would sometimes heat up, like a hot flush – but I breathed deeply and it went right away. By the second week, I could work again. After two weeks, with foundation, my skin looked beautiful: fresh and clear without any lines around the eyes. My sun spots went and the skin round my lips is much better. I feel absolutely brilliant.'

'FILLERS' AND LIP RE-SHAPERS

Many women with a thin mouth (due to nature or ageing) long for plumper, 'bee-stung' lips. There are several temporary or permanent measures.

TEMPORARY RE-SHAPERS

Collagen injections

Disadvantages include short-term results, about two to six months, and at least one, preferably two, patch tests four weeks beforehand because of possible allergy (3 per cent risk) to the purified bovine collagen.

Hyaloform and Hyalangel Injections (see p.148 for one woman's experience.)

These options, based on hyaluronic acid, are increasingly taking over from collagen; they last about the same time, but cause many fewer allergy problems (0.03 per cent).

Autologous fat

Your own (autologous) fat, often taken from the stomach, is processed and injected with multiple needles into numbed lips (where it doesn't last so well), naso-labial lines, hollow cheeks or acne scars; the supply is inexhaustible and safe, and the results may last up to two years or more. (Hands can also be treated this way.)

PERMANENT FILLERS

More permanent options include injecting micro-droplets of silicone into the lip, but many surgeons reject this method because the silicone can cause skin ulceration, and in some countries it is actually illegal.

Permanent surgical re-shaping

Skin is removed from an over-long upper lip, or skin plus tissue from too-thick ones.
Recovery time: Two to seven days.
Risks: The usual risks of anaesthesia and surgery.

Gore-Tex

Over-thin lips can be enhanced by Gore-Tex (the biologically compatible membrane which is used in cold-weather clothes and equipment including skiwear), shaped and threaded into the lip, or by inserting a dermis (skin) graft.
Recovery time: Two to seven days
Risks: Lip induration (abnormal hardening) with Gore-Tex; rejection.

SoftForm (see right.)

The latest 'filler' is SoftForm, a purified and more pliable variant of Gore-Tex, used for lips thinning with age, and/or naso-labial lines (the grooves running from nose to mouth); it's fed in and out of the area to be filled through a cannula (or needle), via two tiny cuts. A permanent treatment (although removable), it's very popular with people who get fed up with collagen which may last from two to six months. It looks and feels very natural, and is actually 'adopted' by the skin's fibroblasts.
Recovery time: Bruising, swelling and sensitivity may last a day up to about a week, depending on exactly what is filled.
Risks: Infection (reduced by use of antibiotics); poor result – place of implant must be accurate and depends on the skill of the surgeon.

what SoftForm did for me…

AGE: 56
PROFESSION: ACTRESS

'At 56, I had started to notice fine lines on the upper lip; a surgeon recommended Softform, a fairly new procedure – and heart-stoppingly expensive. But it was permanent – so no upkeep, also it had been used for years in vein and artery surgery, with no record so far of hardening, shifting or rejection by the body. During the procedure, which lasted my lunch hour, my face was covered up with a scarf-like cloth, with a hole cut for my mouth. I had a local anaesthetic, first with a gel on the inside of the lips, then a massive injection to numb the whole area. Basically you don't feel a damned thing. Six incisions were made along the upper lip. Then the SoftForm thread was threaded through using an ultra-fine needle, almost as thin as a hair. You could feel things going on – yet absolutely no pain. The incisions were closed with tiny stitches; skin glue is also used. Immediately afterwards, my lips were a bit swollen – but I went straight back to work without anybody noticing. Within two hours, the anaesthetic had worn off and it was a little tender and sore where the stitches had been but basically pain-free. The swelling was worst at the end of the second day; by the third day, it had started to go down. I'm incredibly pleased with the results and I'm now going to have the grooves running from nose to mouth filled with SoftForm. I can see a real improvement though friends simply said how well I looked. So I haven't enlightened them…'

BROW SMOOTHERS

Only lucky souls escape a lined or furrowed brow. If a fringe fails to disguise the problem, surgical techniques are an option. As well as the endoscopic brow lift (*see opposite*), there are several other less invasive procedures.

Botox

Injections of a plant bacterium called Botulinum toxin (Botox) have been used for years for blepharospasm (eyelid twitching) and squints and appear to be completely safe. Botox is ideal for vertical frown-lines, unlike collagen. You lose the habit of frowning and, with the release of pressure, the lines start fading almost immediately. The initial effect lasts about three months and some surgeons claim the effects become long-lasting after several injections and a year or two of immobilisation.

Recovery time: Nil.

Risks: Safe in experienced hands but toxic if wrong dose is given; a small percentage of patients (about 5 per cent) develop immunity to Botox, usually after repeated doses; if the injection is misplaced, the patient may not respond or may develop a (temporary) droopy eyelid. (Placement can be checked by using an EMG machine which records when the needle is right in the muscle.)

Arteplast (Artecol)

This combination of 40 per cent collagen and 60 per cent PPMA (polymermethyl-methacrylate), a dental cement, is said by some surgeons to be effective on superficial facial lines, including the forehead, and is also used for cheek implants.

Recovery time: Nil.

Risks: Permanent and uncorrectable irregularity of the treated area; allergy (prolonged swelling and redness).

what Botox did for me...

AGE: 40,
PROFESSION: JOURNALIST

'I am a squinter. I'm always losing my glasses or peering at things – and as a result, at 40, I've developed two frown-lines running vertically between my brows. A friend suggested Botox – and pointed me in the direction of a very experienced doctor.

'An anaesthetic cream was applied to my forehead; the only thing used to numb it. Then he gave me two injections, one into each frown-line. The needle doesn't move – and you can't feel it; the paralysing toxin is simply injected into the muscle and it's frozen from that moment on. I have a very low pain threshold, but there was absolutely no "ouch" factor. It felt a bit weird afterwards, and my brow was numb – rather like what happens to your lip when you go to the dentist. But I wasn't conscious at all of the fact that I couldn't now frown; my forehead didn't feel paralysed, just very natural.

'I was told that it would last around three months – and it did, just about. During that time, my forehead looked smoother and I suppose I looked a little younger – or maybe less cross! – but I can't say that it made a dramatic difference. Even my husband didn't notice. So, I'm not going to have it done again. The upkeep seems a lot of bother. And I'd rather invest the money in a couple of spare pairs of spectacles.'

HAIR TRANSPLANTS

If medical treatment for thinning hair (*see p.108*) falls short of your expectations after giving it a good try with a reputable trichologist, you may want to explore the surgical route. Micrograft hair transplants, using a laser, are usually performed on the front and temples to give more coverage. A few hairs at a time are taken from the rear of the scalp and implanted into the thinning areas. The results may be good, even excellent, but in less than experienced hands can be disappointing. It can take many months to show any result.

Recovery time: Seven days.

Risks: Infection, poor result.

what Hyalangel lip enhancement did for me...

AGE: 43
PROFESSION: TV WRITER

'An expert at lip enhancement advised me the most suitable substance to make my lips fuller was Hyalangel. I had two local anaesthetic injections, one in each side of the mouth, but it was still incredibly uncomfortable. He repeatedly injected my top lip, moving the fine needle a few millimetres each time. My lip area was a little red and swollen afterwards, but completely like my own. I decided my lips weren't quite full enough and had more injections. After about three months, the lips deflated and went back to normal quite quickly. The upkeep is time-consuming and expensive. But having fuller lips is certainly addictive.'

FACELIFTS

At one time, a facelift involved such prolonged bruising, swelling and visible scarring that patients had to disappear for months afterwards. Today's high-tech medicine means much shorter in-patient stays and, in general, shorter recovery times. The rule of thumb is that the more extensive and the deeper the level of surgery, the more impressive and longer-lasting are the results – but also the longer the recovery time.

Endoscopic Facelift and Brow Lift

Endoscopic or keyhole surgery for faces is a recent arrival. The surgeon inserts the endoscope (a surgical telescope) through tiny cuts in the top of the head which heal rapidly, leaving no visible scars. A minute camera on the endoscope allows the surgeon to operate inside the face and brow by watching progress on a large television screen.

The 'endoface', which is performed relatively rarely (usually by cranio-facial surgeons), is most suitable for patients under 50 with mild to moderate sagging and heaviness of the cheeks and jowls. Facial tissues and muscles are re-positioned through five small cuts behind the hairline and one inside each lower eyelash line. Post-operative swelling should subside by 14 days, in the worst case, six weeks. The 'endoface' should give a younger-looking upper face and jawline, plus improved skin texture but is not as effective as 'open' (as opposed to endoscopic) facelifts in patients with severe sagging, particularly of the neck.

The 'endobrow', which can be combined with any type of facelift, involves just three small cuts on the scalp, unlike the traditional brow lift which necessitates an Alice-band cut from ear to ear. It can be done in a day and corrects furrows, lines and heavy brows. Unlike a conventional brow lift, it does not significantly raise the hairline so is suitable for patients with a high forehead. It is an ideal procedure to lift a heavy brow (especially for men because the scars don't show).
Recovery time: Swift. One patient was ballroom dancing four days afterwards. Temporary changes in sensation over the forehead and scalp may last three to six months.
Risks: Damage to sensory nerve with numbness in forehead and scalp; damage to motor (movement) nerve to forehead.

Mask (or Sub-periostal) Lift

This is suitable for the same group of patients as the 'endoface'. The soft tissues of the face are detached from the bone and re-positioned. Some of the facial bone structure can also be altered. Two small cuts are made inside the mouth; the other cut runs from ear to ear.
Recovery time: Results are usually dramatic, although there is considerable swelling and most patients need six to eight weeks' recovery time.
Risks: The Alice-band cut is likely to feel numb for two to three months after surgery and there is a risk of temporary injury to the facial nerve, particularly with surgeons less experienced in this technique.

Skin Lift with SMAS Lift

The most commonly performed lift is the skin lift where the surgeon cuts around the ear, pulls up the skin, tightens the musculoaponeurotic fascia (the deeper layer of fibrous tissue and the sling muscle which embraces the jawline), and removes the excess skin. The results will last up to three years, at most.

Most surgeons combine the skin lift with a SMAS lift: the skin is lifted from the SMAS (subcutaneous aponeurotic system – the layer where the muscles are attached to the skin), through a cut which runs around the ears and down into the hairline. The SMAS and the muscle are repositioned and excess skin removed, to correct heavy cheeks, jowls and sagging neck in patients of any age. It can give quite dramatic results in older patients and usually lasts ten years providing patients keep a constant weight.
Recovery time: Patients are leading a normal life within two weeks.
Risks: Permanent damage is extremely rare; short-term problems include haemorrhage, haematoma, skin necrosis, temporary facial nerve damage (very rare).

Extended SMAS Lift

The extended SMAS, which needs a very experienced facial surgeon, goes further down to smooth out heavy lines between nose and mouth more effectively than with any other SMAS lift.
Recovery time: Usually about three weeks.
Risks: Same as skin lift; there is a much greater risk of injury to the facial nerve in inexperienced hands.

Eyelid Surgery (Upper and/or Lower Blepharoplasty)

This removes the fatty tissue, extra skin and wrinkles which build up around the eyes. Scars, positioned in the upper eyelid groove just above the

crease or under the lower eyelashes, should be virtually invisible. The only painful bit is removing the stitches. Operating from inside the eyelid (trans-conjunctival surgery) avoids stitches but is only suitable for young patients with minimal skin to remove.
Recovery time: Seven to ten days.
Risks: Pulling down of lower eyelid if excessive skin removed, excessive scar tissue formations, haematoma, dry eye syndrome (grittiness), watery eyes.

Cheek Implants

These are traditionally made of silicone but the cheek may also be built up with collagen or the patient's own (autologous) fat. The most recent advance is hydroxyapitite, a synthetic with a similar composition to bone, which is mixed with the patient's blood to make a paste which can be moulded and applied directly to the bone. Recommended for cheeks or other bone-deficient sites, but not for chins where there is too much motion.
Recovery time: Seven days.
Risks: Asymmetry, infection.

Ear Correction (Otoplasty)

Surgery to pin back protruding ears, an inherited condition, can be performed as early as five years old. Incisions are made in the groove behind the ears so that the scars are hidden from view. (NB Babies may be able to have protruding ears corrected with a soft pliable rod which re-trains the ear.)
Recovery time: Seven days.
Risks: Incomplete correction, haemorrhage, infection, skin necrosis.

Nose Re-shaping (Rhinoplasty)

Surgery can either beautify or correct injuries – in which case it may come under the NHS or private medical insurance. Bumps can be removed, a broad nose slimmed down or the tip altered. Underlying excess bone and cartilage are usually removed from inside the nose, leaving no scars.

Noses can also be built up with cartilage or bone. Silicone is not advised because it tends to become infected.
Recovery time: Mouth breathing is necessary for several days after surgery which can be uncomfortable. 90 per cent of swelling and bruising should go down in two to three weeks, although nose shape may go on changing for up to six months.
Risks: Haemorrhage, unfavourable result, asymmetry.

Chin Augmentation (Mentoplasty)

Permanent re-shaping of receding chins is sometimes performed at the same time as nose re-shaping to get a better profile. The implant is traditionally silicone although new materials, including HTR, polymers are starting to be used. The incision is usually made inside the mouth or under the chin. People with long jaws can also have bone removed to improve the shape of the jawline.
Recovery time: One week for implants, two weeks if bone removed.
Risks: Infection, damage to mental nerve (which controls sensation in chin and lower lip) by anaesthetising chin.

Chin augmentation can also be performed in a procedure called genioplasty. This involves cutting into the bone of the chin below the roots of the teeth, re-positioning the bone and fixing it with a plate.
Recovery time: Two weeks.
Risks: Much less risk of infection than with mentoplasty; same risk of damage to mental nerve.

Breast Reduction and Breast Uplift (Mastopexy)

Over-large, pendulous breasts can be surgically reduced and uplifted. Breasts are marked with a special pen before the operation with the patient standing. Under general anaesthetic, the nipple is detached from the skin but left attached to the breast tissue, an incision made vertically down and then under the breast, skin and breast tissue is removed, the nipple replaced and the wounds sewn up.

Scarring will fade but is permanent. More recent techniques avoid a scar under the breast but leave a wrinkled vertical scar which takes a few months to become even.

Pregnancy must be avoided for one year to avoid stretching the scars so it's not recommended for would-be mums.
Recovery time: Two to three weeks.
Risks: Haemorrhage, infection, skin and, very rarely, nipple necrosis, asymmetry.

Breast Augmentation

Demand for this once common operation dropped off sharply after the scare that silicone implants filled with silicone gel may lead to an increased risk of cancer or of auto-immune disease, particularly if accidentally ruptured. Although subsequent research appeared to show that these risks are no greater than normal, some patients developed other chronic problems (e.g. aches, pains and skin irritation) which may prove to be due to the implants. At the moment, no one knows. However, implants may form hard lumpy scar tissue which is an undisputed problem. Improved implants with a textured surface reduce this risk.

Patients now have a choice: saline-filled implants (which don't look or feel very natural and may leak); silicone gel-filled implants (which give the best shape and feel); or triluscent implants filled with soya bean oil (which have the advantage of being radio translucent so that they allow better imaging in mammography) – these fall halfway between saline-filled and silicone gel-filled implants in feel and shape.

Recovery time: Two weeks.

Risks: Haemorrhage, infection (very rare), capsules contract and harden, asymmetry.

Liposuction

The removal of fat by suction means that many areas of the body can be re-contoured, including face and neck (particularly double chins and back neck humps), breasts, arms, waist, abdomen, buttocks, inner and outer thighs and knees. It is suitable for removing stubborn localised areas of fat – it is not an alternative to exercise and sensible eating.

Recovery time: Seven days, although bruising takes up to four weeks to fade.

Risks: It's more complex than it seems and can cause nasty problems if not done by an expert (one woman ended up in intensive care after poor surgery and there have been deaths reported). If too much fat is removed, the skin will ripple or sag irreversibly. Poor liposuction can cause grooves and ruts which are difficult to put right. And if you put on weight again, it settles somewhere else which can lead to odd shape changes.

Liposculpture

This is another name for liposuction but sometimes involves injecting fat into depressed areas to recontour the body. It also includes superficial liposuction which involves removing fat just below the surface of the skin with a very fine cannula (syringe). Results can be excellent but you must have an expert surgeon.

Liposculpture can also be done on the face and jawline, with good results.

Recovery time: As for liposuction.

Risks: As for liposuction.

Ultrasonic Liposuction

With the patient sedated and under local anaesthetic, tiny incisions are made in the skin at the affected area and the ultrasound probe slid into the tissue. Surgeons using this technique claim that by employing a specific frequency of ultrasound, the fat can be dissolved and suctioned off, more fat can be removed and the skin is said to shrink better. However, other surgeons dispute the benefits and say the risks are higher.

Recovery time: Same as liposuction.

Risks: Same as liposuction, plus skin necrosis which can be a serious complication, so this should only be done by experts.

Abdominal Reduction (Abdominoplasty)

This 'tummy tuck' operation takes out the excess skin and fat which often affect women after pregnancy and which defies exercise. Tummy muscles can be tightened at the same time. Liposuction is often carried out simultaneously for best results.

Recovery time: Three weeks.

Risks: Infection, haemorrhage, asymmetry, poor-quality scars, skin necrosis.

Varicose Veins

See You're So Vein, p.142.

stephen glass's tips for cosmetic surgery patients

Many women take a 'Ssssh, don't tell a soul approach' after having cosmetic surgery. Make-up artist Stephen Glass*, who has many clients asking for advice after facelifts, recommends:

• 'If you wear glasses, have a tint put in them before the operation: it will disguise bruising or puffy eyes.'

• 'Manual Lymphatic Drainage massage is the only thing to drain the face and disguise puffiness. But bruising can be effectively covered with a product like Estée Lauder Maximum Cover which stays put – and matte – all day...'
(*See p.74 for guidelines on how to apply cover-up make-up.*)

• 'Use stronger toned lipstick to take the focus away from the eyes.'

• 'Stick to make-up colours that will play down any redness. Pink, burgundy, even brown is a bad idea – instead, choose greys, or greens or slate blues.'

• 'Get a new haircut or a make-up make-over. Then you have an instant explanation when anyone says, "You look great – what have you done?".'

• 'Women often take longer to heal than the doctor says – so give yourself plenty of time and don't make plans you may have to cancel.'

diary of a facelift

Ellen, now 51, is a successful international businesswoman, currently living in London. She wrote her diary for us over the last six years.

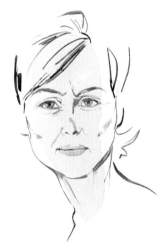

March 1992 Read an account in Vogue of woman's suffering following a facelift. Vow never to be so vain.

December 1993 Dinner with friends; husband — 12 years younger than I am — says, 'Didn't Emma look beautiful? She must be about your age, but there's not a line on her face.' Ponder.

February 1994 Met old friend who has had laser treatment on upper lip to reduce lines, and looks five years younger.

April 1994 My 47th birthday. Realise that since 45, face has begun to sag. Focus on deep frown-line.

September 1994 Particularly harsh bright morning — look in mirror and decide I need advice. Ask beautiful Emma what I can do. She suggests top London plastic surgeon called Barry Jones.

October 1994 BJ says three procedures would make great difference. Brow lift would smooth away frown-line,

removal of excess skin round eyes would get rid of hooded look, and then — rather frighteningly — he draws line with finger round my ears where the incision would be if had lower part of my face 'lifted'. Leave clutching information on all three.

November 1994 Mention brow lift to husband.

December 1994 Go to business function with husband where everyone but me in their mid-thirties. Become convinced that after 50, gap between our ages will become more apparent. Mention possibility of having eyes done.

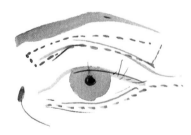

January 1995 Ring BJ's office to say will have all three operations. Mention facelift to husband who rejects it out of hand. Is gradually won round.

Friday, January 20th, 1995 – D-Day Jump in taxi at 6.30 a.m. Arrive at Wellington Hospital in London, fill in forms, meet anaesthetist and theatre nurse. BJ draws lines on face where frown and sag. At eight o'clock sharp, in elasticated stockings (to prevent deep vein thrombosis), am wheeled into theatre. Op takes five hours. Wake up on glucose drip, worried

as can't see very well. Nurse says eyes still 'seeping' slightly (due to ointment to stop eyes drying and getting sore).

January 21st, 1995 – After interminable night of sickness, wake at last without feeling nauseous. Look in mirror. Horrible sight! Hair glued to head, eyes bruised and puffy with white sticky tape round them; face slightly swollen.

Leave this afternoon. Go to bed early with head up on five pillows to help reduce the swelling. Discover I have a circle of staples in my hair and whichever way I turn I cannot get comfortable. Can't read because side of my face is swollen so glasses hurt nose and ears.

January 22nd, 1995 Bruises are moving — in the right direction. Eyes are definitely getting less puffy. Beginning to see shape of nose again. But still have two black eyes surrounded by white sticky tape, bruising on both sides of neck and hard swelling under chin.

Try to work but feel too tired. Very strange using telephone as ears completely numb. And glasses still too heavy for bruised nose and ears. Husband reads me Rudyard Kipling short stories. Eyes sore during the night, so put on witch-hazel-soaked sterile eye pads.

January 23rd, 1995 Swelling round eyes down but still look like victim of domestic violence. Nurse takes tape off eyes and pulls stitches out — surprisingly un-painful.

January 25th, 1995 Contort body and wash hair. Have less surface bruising but skin looks jaundiced. Forehead smooth and rejuvenated. Am thrilled. Swelling around mouth almost gone and lips beginning to regain shape.

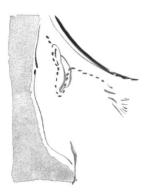

January 26th, 1995
Rest of stitching goes, so do awful staples. Taught how to massage face, eyes and chin. Eyes now have dark under-circles of bruising but can see their new shape — and am delighted.

January 27th, 1995
Still enough bruising to keep me inside, but physically almost completely well again. Swelling under chin uncomfortable, numb ears strange, and short sharp pain if raise eyebrows. Neck looks rather bullish with swelling both sides. Nights still a problem as scalp tender.

February 3rd, 1995
Two weeks since the op. Still very slight bruising under left eye. Began week working normally, but by Wed evening was incredibly tired. Nurse removes two stitches from each ear — they should have begun to dissolve but hadn't for some reason, and were irritating. Get first really good night's sleep since operation.

February 12th, 1995 Bad week. Fainted at theatre. Spend today sleeping and resolve to have snooze every afternoon next week.

February 17th, 1995 Much better physically. Incisions at bottom of scalp healed almost completely. Top of scalp and ears still numb. Neck swollen. Begin having facial massages which leave swollen cheeks and throat feeling softer. BJ said it takes six months to get full effects of surgery so am fairly relaxed.

February 20th, 1995 Face now definitely looking younger, and people start asking guarded questions. 'You look great, what's happened?' Have hair restyled to give them a reason for the transformation.

March 3rd, 1995 Swelling on cheekbones going down, although neck still slightly tender. Ears and edges of cheeks now only half-numb. Went to hospital for well-woman check-up and doctor talked about my getting pregnant! Proof I've lost years off my face.

April 14th, 1995 My 48th birthday. Can honestly say look as I did in my mid-thirties — eyes wide open, cheeks don't sag, neck looks better than for 15 years and frown line a slight crease in the skin.

March 1998 Husband now frightfully pleased and I look in the mirror every morning and say, 'Thank you, Barry Jones'. The bandage-like feeling has still not completely left but I look ten years younger, and I couldn't be happier about it all.

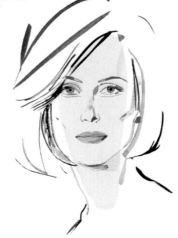

EXPERT ADVICE

Barry Jones, leading London aesthetic plastic surgeon, says:

TWO WEEKS BEFORE SURGERY
It's vital to avoid any drugs which may cause bleeding and so increase bruising; these include aspirin, and aspirin-containing compounds, non-steroidal anti-inflammatory drugs such as brufen and ibuprofen, vitamin E and compounds containing vitamin E (that includes evening primrose oil and fish oils), garlic and garlic capsules. All of these should be stopped at least two weeks before the surgery and not recommenced for at least two weeks afterwards.

AFTER CARE
It's very important to rest for the first three days and to sleep with four or five extra pillows so that the head is always above the chest to reduce blood pressure in the face and therefore encourage swelling to dissipate. It's essential to avoid any strenuous physical activity for the first two weeks after surgery. Eyepads soaked in witch-hazel and cooled in the refrigerator are soothing to the eyes for the first 48 hours or so.

It's helpful to shower and wash the hair on alternate days; this is an easy way to keep the wounds and suture lines clean. Normal daily activities can be re-introduced gently after two weeks and most patients will be fit to return to work by two to three weeks, depending on exactly what has been done.

Patients should avoid strenuous physical exercise, such as running or aerobics, for four to six weeks. Also bleach-based hair colourants which contain potentially irritating synthetic chemicals should be avoided for six weeks after; try gentler vegetable colourants after three weeks.

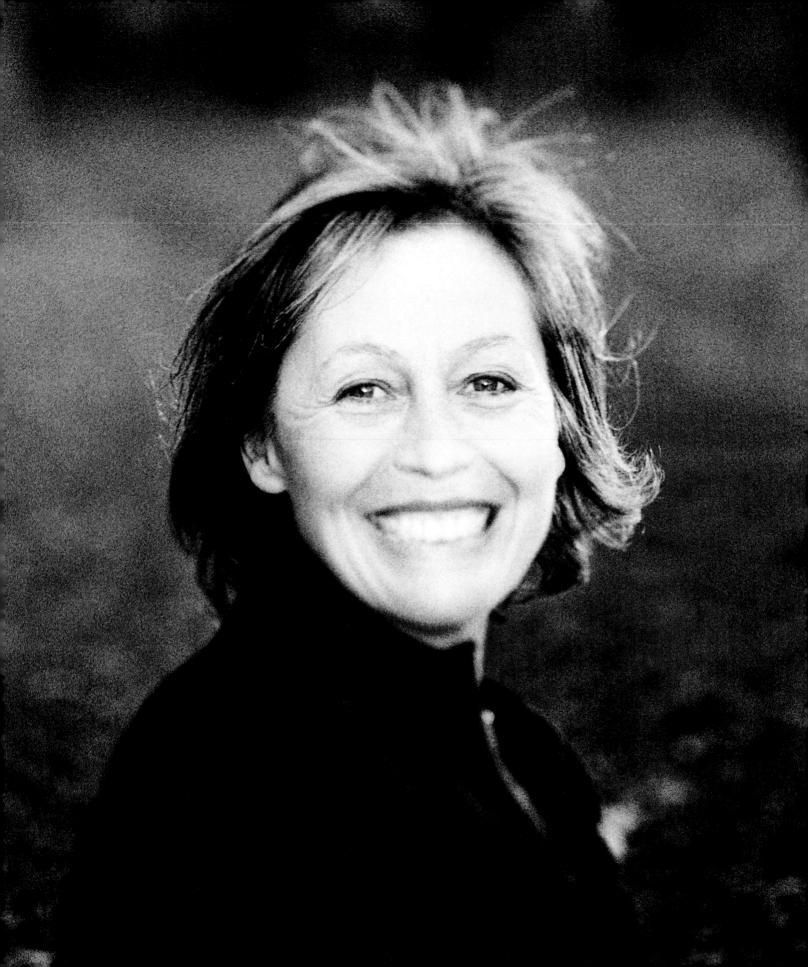

At this age, there is an art to feeling fabulous. To waking up every morning refreshed and full of life. To having the energy to do everything we need to do (and some spare for what we want to do).

When we were children, it came naturally. And it still can – now that

how to **feel** fabulous part 2

more is understood than ever before about superfoods, easy-but-energising exercise, health-protecting supplements – and the role hormones play in our well-being. So we talked to the experts – worldwide. Uncovered the latest thinking on ways to live life to the full. And spoke to real, glowing women about their secrets for feeling fab forever – so that we could share them with you...

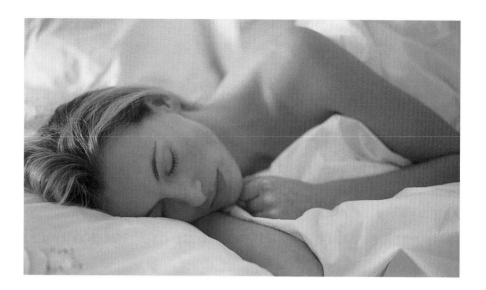

desperately
seeking **slumber**

More women complain of sleeping problems than men. For many of us, sleep has become the sex of the 1990s – and, according to experts, most of us aren't getting enough...

At any age and every stage, the better we sleep, the better we feel – and the better we live. But unfortunately, not all mornings begin brightly, especially around menopause. One problem is that the hot flushes associated with dwindling oestrogen levels tend to jolt women awake throughout the night, because oestrogen has a direct effect on sleep. And in mid-life, we tend to have weighty responsibilities and worries which compound sleeplessness: unruly children, ageing parents, work worries.

Many menopausal women, having previously relied on sleeping like babes, suddenly find they are waking at 2, 3 or 4 a.m. – their bed more like a battlefield than a cosy nest.

In general, sleep complaints increase significantly with age; some researchers believe that this is due to the reduction in levels of many hormones as we get older. Researchers like Dr Karen Moe in Washington are, meanwhile, worried at the huge number of prescriptions for sedative-hypnotic drugs which people turn to for relief. The carry-over effect of these can, she says, exacerbate all sorts of problems from sleep apnoea (snoring so extreme that it disrupts breathing) to the way your brain works – and may also contribute to falls and subsequent fractures.

After a bad night – let alone a succession of them – your body feels achey and drained. You're irritable,

foggy and edgy, because you haven't had the rest you needed. And you're not alone. Between five and ten million people in the UK have problems sleeping, and around half a million are estimated to suffer serious sleep disorders. In the US, meanwhile, 70 million people have trouble sleeping.

Today, most of us have so many commitments and chores to perform that sleep gets shuffled down the priority list. According to Stanley Coren, Professor of Psychology at the University of British Columbia and author of *Sleep Thieves**, 'We cheat our bodies of sleep every night because the pressures of modern life insist that we take less than evolution programmed us to get. Before electric light, people went to sleep before the sun went down and slept for an average of nine and a half hours – two hours more than now.' The knock-on effect of this shortage, he believes, 'is we are becoming clumsy, stupid, unhappy – and dead'.

Sleep deprivation undermines the immune system. When human guinea pigs were kept awake for four hours beyond their usual bedtime, blood tests taken next day showed a marked dip in key defences against infections and cancer. Not getting enough sleep may even make us fat. Ignoring our rest needs makes us prone to overeating, seeking quick boosts from sweets and snacks because our energy reserves weren't topped up by adequate sleep.

But how can each of us tell what our individual optimum sleep quota is? If you can work efficiently and stay alert all day after a few hours' rest, consider yourself lucky – your nightly respites are satisfactory. If that's not enough, daytime tiredness is likely to be the biggest symptom. 'The acid test for insufficient sleep is whether you have trouble staying awake during the day,' suggests Professor Jim Horne, who runs the sleep laboratory at Loughborough University. If you find that you are tired all the time, try sleeping more – and tune in to what that does to your alertness. Set an earlier bedtime for a week and sleep longer. (If you don't experience improvements on the new regime, however, consult your doctor; there may be another physical cause.) Those who say they exist on four hours' sleep may only need that much, biologically. But if you're an eight-hour sleeper and you're only getting four, you will soon be running on empty.

how much sleep is enough?

Experts often tell us that we need less sleep as we age. But when we asked Dr Joseph Pizzorno for his top anti-ageing secrets, eight hours' sleep was at the top of the list. 'Adequate sleep is absolutely necessary for long-term health and regeneration,' he explains. 'While many different processes occur during sleep, perhaps the most important for rejuvenation are, firstly, the scavenging effects of free radicals in the brain, and, secondly, increased production of growth hormone.'

Free radicals – responsible for a lot of the damage elsewhere in our bodies (including to our skins) – can build up in the brain. 'Sleep functions as an antioxidant for the brain, because free radicals are removed during this time,' says Dr Pizzorno. If you sleep for less than eight hours, however, the 'clean-up' task may not be completed. 'Most people can tolerate a few days without sleep and fully recover. But chronic sleep deprivation appears to accelerate ageing of the brain – so your brain will start to function less well.'

And as if that wasn't enough of an incentive to get the full eight hours, consider this: growth hormone – mostly produced during sleep – has been called the 'anti-ageing' hormone, for its ability to stimulate tissue and liver regeneration, muscle building, the breakdown of fat stores, blood sugar normalisation, 'and a host of other beneficial actions,' reports Dr Pizzorno. 'Basically, it helps convert fat to muscle...'

It's certainly true that as people age, they tend to sleep less. 'The average person of 50 years or older sleeps almost two hours less than they did as a teenager,' observes Dr Pizzorno. 'But this diminished opportunity to secrete human growth hormone and scavenge free radicals in the brain probably plays a significant role in the degeneration of ageing.' He believes we should all try for the magic eight hours.

And to anyone who can't imagine they can get everything done that they need to do *and* manage eight hours' shut-eye, we'd say this: getting the extra sleep seems to make it easier to whizz through tasks. Whereas not getting enough can make for entire 'lost' days when life can be compared, at best, to swimming through treacle...

PAY OFF YOUR SLEEP DEBTS

If you find that you 'get behind' with your sleep then as soon as you can, pay off your 'sleep debts', as Professor Coren calls them. Losing one hour's sleep a night means we end up with a sleep debt of seven hours by the end of the week. 'This is the equivalent of losing a full night's sleep – and you start to show the symptoms of someone who's done just that.' Which might include itching or burning eyes, blurred vision, headaches and/or feeling chilled, as well as waves of sleepiness or fatigue, irritability or weepiness; short-term memory is also affected. The way to get back on track is napping and sleeping in on the weekend, when you have the opportunity. To avoid the knock-on effects of a nap keeping you awake at night, take it before 3 p.m.

SLEEP-EASY STRATEGIES

Popping sleeping pills is always an option but managing stress, eating well and taking regular exercise will ultimately induce a far better quality of sleep. 'About 90 per cent of all insomniacs can be cured through self-care,' says Peter Hauri, Director of the Mayo Clinic's Insomnia Programme, USA. So try these sleep-inducing tactics...

◆ Start preparing at lunchtime – if you keep stress levels under control during the day, you're less likely to be frazzled come bedtime. Take a ten-minute break, around lunchtime, for some deep breathing or yoga.

◆ Avoid caffeine (in coffee and tea, chocolate, cola, guarana-based products and some pain-relievers) in the afternoon and evening; it takes nearly ten hours to leave your system. NB Decaffeinated doesn't necessarily mean caffeine-free.

◆ Regular daily exercise encourages deep sleep but do aerobic exercise early in the day, or you may be too revved up to nod off. (An early evening walk is a great way to wind down, we find.)

If I'm exhausted, I clear my mind by imagining a blank, white canvas. When you're tired, problems escalate, so I go to bed as early as I can.
AMANDA BURTON

◆ Avoid alcohol and cigarettes before bedtime. Alcohol may help you nod off but as it breaks down in the system, it disrupts sleep later on, so you wake up and find it difficult to get back to sleep. Nicotine acts as a stimulant.

◆ For perfect slumber, the sleep 'hygienists' are agreed that we should establish a regular daily pattern of going-to-bed and getting-up times.

◆ Finish your main evening meal at least two hours before bedtime: digestion – and the blood sugar surge from food – can keep you awake.

◆ Have a warm, milky drink an hour before bedtime: it helps reduce anxiety and promote sleep.

◆ Have a warm pre-bedtime bath: it raises body temperature and the natural sleep-preparation mechanism is triggered as the body cools again.

◆ Ban TV and newspapers from the bedroom, and don't use it as an extension of the office, a place to eat, pay bills or talk on the telephone. Bad sleep rapidly becomes a vicious cycle; someone who's having problems sleeping will read or watch TV or look at work papers – which in turn stimulates them and can prevent sleep, or trigger poor-quality sleep. Experts believe that images of bad news or violence on TV can interfere with good sleep on an unconscious level.

◆ Keep the bedroom warm but not stuffy; try to have fresh air circulating.

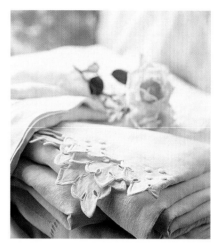

◆ If there is a street light outside your window, or you wake early in the summer, invest in heavier curtains – or wear a sleeping mask in bed.

I think sleep keeps you young. I like 10 or 12 hours but I usually manage eight. I have trained myself to sleep in planes, trains, even cars.
CAROLINE HERRERA

◆ Noise is one of the greatest pollutants. Uncontrollable noise when you're trying to sleep can disturb your sleep and result in physical tension next day. If you can't change it, make sure you have a battery of aids from ear plugs to personal stereos; play soothing sounds or 'white noise', which blots out other noise.

◆ Write a To Do Tomorrow list before bedtime – and keep it by the bed. Then if you wake up thinking of another task jot it down – and get back to sleep.

◆ Don't forget to get your oats! A bowl of porridge or muesli in place of supper is nutritious, good for the nervous system and an anti-depressant.

sleeping beauty

What if you could spend eight hours every night at a spa? Most of us would leap at the chance. Well, not for nothing is it called 'beauty sleep' – because the sleeping hours deliver the perfect opportunity for skin to repair and regenerate itself. According to Jack Mausner, PhD, Chanel's Senior Vice President of Research and Development: 'Sleep time is the optimum time to repair. The skin is in a faster state of regeneration.' And according to clinical studies carried out by Estée Lauder, certain healing compounds (anti-inflammatories, antioxidants) are actually absorbed better at night.

Some skin experts, however – including Eva Fraser and Eve Lom – go so far as to suggest that skin should be left naked at night. (Although we've tried that, and given up, because for us it's just plain tight and uncomfortable; personally, we are big fans of facial oils for night treatments – *see page 49 for suggestions* – and serums, which seem to give our dry skins the extra nourishment we feel they need.) But whether you apply a special night cream – or use your favourite daytime moisturiser – is really a matter of personal preference, but if you like the richer, nourishing texture of a night cream (or a facial oil), go for it – confident that the shinier, more slippery texture won't interfere with make-up application. Night-time is certainly the right time for using heavier treatments on scalp, hands and lips that you wouldn't get away with in the day, too – even sleeping in cotton gloves and socks if a product demands it. After all, nobody has to be a beauty in the pitch dark...

TRIED & TESTED
── NIGHT CREAMS ──

These were the products – designed to be used overnight and capitalise on the skin's capacity for repair – which did best among our testers. You'll find reviews for some of them in our Tried & Tested Miracle Cream section (*see pp.16–17*), but we've also included other creams that some of our testers reported as being 'overnight sensations'...

Clarins Extra Firming Night Cream
8.57 MARKS OUT OF 10 (££££) – *see p.17 for more about this cream.*

Estée Lauder Advanced Night Repair Protect Recovery Complex
8.4 MARKS OUT OF 10 (££££) – *see p.16.*

Avon Retinol Night Cream
7.87 MARKS OUT OF 10 (££)
This cream uses what Avon describe as a 'microsponge' technology to deliver pure vitamin A into the skin. According to Avon's own consumer tests, fine lines and wrinkles were visibly diminished in two weeks, and in four weeks, complexions appeared brighter and more even-toned. However, less than half our testers said they would actually invest in this cream.
UPSIDE: 'a really excellent product – I noticed a big difference in softness, brightness – my skin glowed' ◆ 'skin definitely looked and felt smoother; neck, especially, looks years younger. This is a must-have for every woman whose skin has passed the first smooth bloom of youth' ◆ 'a girlfriend asked what I was using as she noticed my skin looked firmer.'
DOWNSIDE: 'there was a slight tingling and pinkness' ◆ 'did not like smell or greasy texture; very chemical smell.'

Lancaster Oxygen Repair for the Night
7.14 MARKS OUT OF 10 (££££+)
This cream uses Lancaster's patented oxygen carrier system to deliver pure oxygen molecules to the skin, together with a list of ingredients (think 'complex of magnetic particles A.M.C.S.-K.', 'spherolin K', etc.) which seem guaranteed to baffle anyone without a degree in astrophysics. What you probably do want to know is that it's lightweight and non-greasy. Meanwhile, less than half the testers said they would buy it.
UPSIDE: 'my skin definitely looks younger – I've never used a product that had so much effect so quickly and so obviously; however, having used it for six weeks my skin reached a "plateau" in improvement and I couldn't detect any further difference' ◆ 'no side-effects or irritation and I have sensitive skin' ◆ 'fine lines less noticeable especially on forehead, eyes and mouth area' ◆ 'overall a real pampering product' ◆ 'most of my fine lines have been reduced to a minimum and large wrinkles have softened immensely'.
DOWNSIDE: 'I liked the texture of this cream but was disappointed that I didn't really look any different after using it'.

Prescriptives Nightclock
7.11 MARKS OUT OF 10 (££££)
This emulsion features a yeast extract (labelled 'Tissue Respiratory Factor' by Prescriptives), time-released moisturising ingredients, green tea and vitamin E, together with 'enzyme inhibitors' that help counteract the enzymes that break down collagen and elastin in the skin. It's recommended for skins over thirty. Two-thirds of the testers said they would buy this product.
UPSIDE: 'improved face and neck noticeably; looked younger and fine lines reduced, especially round eyes and forehead' ◆ 'my skin was very "strokeable" – soft and smooth – in the morning' ◆ 'I really like the cream; it's evened out my skintone; my oily panel seems much less so and my skin generally plumper; there was a definite improvement in fine lines and my husband says my skin looks better' ◆ 'I was told by a new friend I didn't look old enough to have a 19-year-old and a 23-year-old and I think it must be the cream' ◆ 'after two weeks, my skin looked fresher and less tired; gives fast results which people notice'.
DOWNSIDE: 'came out in red blotches all over my face after the third application, so I stopped using it.'

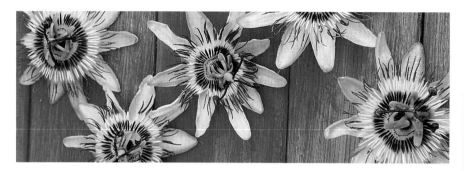

NATURAL SLEEP REMEDIES

Millions of prescriptions for sleeping pills are handed out every year and though they will work – mostly – they traditionally do so by depressing brain function, resulting in a quality of sleep that's less restorative.

The body soon develops a tolerance to sleeping pills, so people may soon need to raise their usual dose in order to get the same effect. Many sleeping pills are highly addictive and, in some cases, may actually lead to increased anxiety and stressful feelings during the waking hours; sudden withdrawal also leads to problems. In the last few years, some sleeping pills have had to be hastily taken off the market by manufacturers as unacceptable side-effects emerged when millions of human guinea pigs put them to the long-term test in real life…

If you've tried our 'better sleep guide-lines' (see p.158) and still find sleep elusive, it is worth trying the complementary route.

Acupuncture
Insomnia can be treated by a qualified acupuncturist. Or try sending yourself to sleep using acupressure: use your thumb to stimulate the acupuncture point in the centre of your abdomen, one hand's width below the navel.

Aromatherapy
To a warm bath add five drops each of chamomile, lavender, rose, geranium, neroli, sandalwood or lime-flower oil, blended into 5ml (1 teaspoon) of 'base oil', such as almond or jojoba.

Herbs
Herbal sleeping remedies are perfectly safe, says Andrew Chevallier of the National Institute of Medical Herbalists. 'There should be no significant side-effects and you won't have a hangover.' NB Buy organic herbs whenever possible. Many dried herbs have literally been drenched in chemicals. Look for ready-to-use products or infuse your own herbal teas.
• German Chamomile *(Matricaria recutita)*
• Lime flowers *(Tilia)*
• Valerian *(Valeriana officinalis)*
• Hops *(Humulus lupulus)*
• Lavender *(Lavandula)*
• Skullcap *(Scutellaria lateriflora)*
• Passion flower *(Passiflora incarnata)*

Homoeopathy
Try one tablet of Ars. alb. 30C or Belladonna 30C – or consult a homoeopath.

Hypnotherapy
Consult a qualified practitioner, buy a self-hypnosis tape or learn to DIY.

Relaxation Tapes
Most music shops (and some natural-food stores) offer a selection of relaxing 'New Age' music that can help you unwind. Or listen to plainsong, or your favourite calming music.

Supplementing Sleep
Some somnologists recommend a night-cap of minerals including calcium and magnesium to combat nervousness, muscle tension and aching joints.

And if all else fails, opposite are the top instant face wakers, to make you *look* as if you've had eight hours.

sleep affirmations

We find saying these are wonderfully effective at helping us chill out – particularly when we are worried about not getting enough sleep. Vary as you wish.
● Lie on your back and un-tense your body from head to toe – just run through your body from scalp to toes in your mind, letting all the tensions of the day evaporate.
● Breathe slowly and gently – try visualising your breath as a wave on the beach, rippling gently up, pausing, then flowing out again.
● Say to yourself: 'Today is over and tomorrow is not yet here; now I'm going to have a restful/delicious/restorative sleep and wake up gleaming.'
● Try noticing and appreciating nice sensations like the coolness of the pillow and sheets, softness of the duvet, supporting firmness of the mattress – or the feel of your partner's skin.

TRIED & TESTED
INSTANT FACE WAKERS

Clarins Double Serum 38
8.25 MARKS OUT OF 10 (££££)
This light, fluid gel – like the La Prairie serum, which also scored well – works in two ways: it's designed to give an instant boost (which is what our testers were originally asked to comment on) and act as an intensive anti-ageing treatment. It features 38 ingredients (hence the name). All but one of our testers said they would buy this product.
UPSIDE: 'skin instantly felt like silk and the texture was much improved' ◆ 'skin on cheeks felt very smooth and lines around eyes less deep' ◆ 'face uplifted and seemed more "refined"' ◆ 'make-up went on incredibly smoothly and stayed put all day: ◆ 'it evened out my skintone and fine lines appeared less noticeable' ◆ 'a tiny drop went a long way' ◆ 'skin looked immediately plumper and glowing' ◆ 'relaxing fragrance'.
DOWNSIDE: 'skin felt immediately firmer, but not nourished.'

Lancaster Oxygen Mask
8.11 MARKS OUT OF 10 (£££)
This ten-minute mask is designed to be used every few days or whenever dry, dull skin needs a lift. It can either be left on the skin or applied more generously, then tissued or rinsed off. More than three-quarters of our testers said they would buy this product.
UPSIDE: 'this lives up to its claims, tested after a night out. The result was excellent: a much, firmer, smoother, brighter complexion' ◆ 'I didn't look nearly as exhausted; my face was not so much uplifted as evened out! Top marks for refreshing and relaxing' ◆ 'my skin immediately looked healthier; my face was plumped up like a cushion' ◆ 'people remarked I was looking well'.
DOWNSIDE: 'no feeling 'tighter'; I was disappointed in that' ◆ 'face felt cleaner but otherwise no different from normal.'

Clarins Beauty Flash Balm
8 MARKS OUT OF 10 (££)
This was the original 'face-waker' and is a by-word with beauty editors as a quick pick-me-up, applied for 10–15 minutes in a thick layer. Its primary effect is to tighten the skin, helping to make fine lines and wrinkles less noticeable. It can also be used as an intensive beauty treatment two or three times a week. Three-quarters of our panellists said they would buy this product.
UPSIDE: 'I could see the difference immediately; the tone was improved, my skin felt tighter and my make-up seemed to glide on; skin looked revitalised, firmer and younger' ◆ 'it gave a boost to my confidence as well as my skin' ◆ 'the most exciting cream I've ever had' ◆ 'after three months of using this product occasionally, I find it matches the claims made for it; it makes me feel pampered and I honestly can't find fault with it' ◆ 'I used it on the back of my upper arms and legs and found it was excellent for ridding the skin of slight blemishes – so I'd buy it for that.'
DOWNSIDE: 'needed a moisturiser as well' ◆ 'results only lasted 30 minutes after which skin felt too taut' ◆ 'when applying make-up afterwards, it flaked as I blended it in'.

Yves Rocher ADN Mask
7.75 MARKS OUT OF 10 (£)
This cream is designed as a boost for devitalised skin, to be used once a week – in the morning, then tissued off before putting on make-up. Three-quarters of our testers said they would buy this.
UPSIDE: 'I loved this product! It gave my face an instant lift and make-up stays on longer after using it' ◆ 'best mask I have ever used; it's a great boost for skin in winter and in the morning gives an instant lift and glow' ◆ 'worked well as a desperate "first aid" measure when I was looking very tired and worn and I even received a few compliments'.
DOWNSIDE: 'no visible difference and after I removed my make-up my skin was all blotchy' ◆ 'didn't quite live up to claims; result lasted only three to four hours'.

Clarins Skin Firming Concentrate
7.5 MARKS OUT OF 10 (£££)
A light, fluid gel, this can be used either as a one-off treatment or on a daily basis over moisturiser. It has a dual moisturising and astringent action, which explains the toning effect. It's targeted at women with loss of facial tone, but also as a preventative treatment after 25-plus – and two-thirds of our testers said they'd buy it.
UPSIDE: 'gave a pleasant invigorating feeling, skin felt firmer and smoother and it gave the skin a glow best seen without make-up' ◆ 'this is a winner – it gave the impression of plumping out fine lines round my mouth as well as an overall smoother look and radiance' ◆ 'skin looked firmer and had a better colour for a couple of days' ◆ 'removed those early morning creases that appear after heavy sleep' ◆ 'I've taken to using it to give my face a mini-lift if I'm going out in the evening'.
DOWNSIDE: 'skin felt rather dry after use – I had to use far more moisturiser than usual' ◆ 'feel I need something heavier in the moisturising department; it wasn't good enough, at my age' ◆ 'make-up seemed to drag and blotch.'

La Prairie Cellular Face Complex with Caviar Extract
7.5 MARKS OUT OF 10 (£££££+)
Incorporating real caviar, this luxury product is said by La Prairie to provide immediate firmness, radiance, freshness and evenness of complexion – and also to prolong youthful appearance on a longer-term basis. Two-thirds of the testers said they would invest in this.
UPSIDE: 'my make-up glided on – and people commented on my skin. I really felt it did improve my complexion' ◆ 'my skin felt like velvet and my neck in particular benefited – the best cream I have used' ◆ 'brilliant product for the neck area; my skin was flaky and thirsty due to central heating, but this cured the problem and now I use it most days' ◆ 'even my husband commented it gave my face a youthful glow' ◆ 'it took about 20 minutes for the skin to be uplifted – though it never felt tight. The skin was soft, smooth and the tone vastly improved, while the crêpiness on my neck completely disappeared. My foundation seemed to stay on longer and the results lasted 24 hours'.
DOWNSIDE: 'no obvious improvements.'

NB The lowest scoring product in this category was awarded just 4.75 marks.

Forget aiming to look like Kate Moss or going for Jane Fonda's burn (and getting scorched). The new thinking on fitness is: take it easier. For the ultimate daily workout, scientists are now agreed that nothing beats regular, moderate exercise: a mix of cardiovascular, stretch and gentle weight-training. Think too of standing straighter, breathing better and acquiring grace. Sure, if you feel energetic, go for a run, play a game of tennis – or whatever you enjoy. But there's no need for exercise to leave you huffing and puffing, achey and flushed as a beetroot. (Which, if you're not used to it, can even be downright dangerous.) And the good news is: if you want to feel fabulously fit forever, it's never too late to start…

the breath of life

In the beginning, we breathed. Rhythmically, deeply. Inhaling through our noses and filling our bodies and brains with oxygen. Exhaling through our mouths and breathing out all the waste carbon dioxide. Then life and all its stresses knocked the natural breathing pattern sideways, leaving us alternately gasping and holding our breath…

When we're anxious or nervous, we tend to breathe shallowly. Usually when we breathe we take in about the equivalent of a tumblerful of air – just one-third of our lungs' capacity. If you could spread out the lining of your lungs, there would be 100 square metres (40 square yards) of it. In your lungs are 600–700 million air sacs, all waiting to be filled. Once the air gets to them, they circulate the oxygen round your bloodstream. In turn, your blood sends back the waste carbon dioxide to be exhaled. Breathe inadequately – just at the top of your lungs – as most of us do, and a lot of the waste never gets expelled. (And you may puff as if you've been running for a train, although all you've been doing is walking to the phone.)

Getting back to breathing properly is an almost instantaneous route to feeling better, in every way. What's more, like that other great health and beauty staple – water – it's completely free and under your control.

Try it now, wherever you are. Breathe slowly in through your nose, let the breath go down to your belly, put your hand there and inflate it like a balloon. Feel the breath go up to your head, clearing your brain. Now gently breathe out through your mouth. Try it again – and don't force it or your shoulders will go up, neck stiffen and jawline tense. Breathe as lightly and softly as a puff of breeze on a calm day.

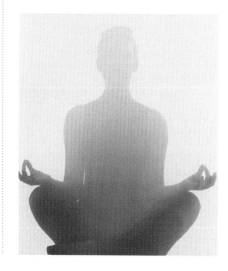

Do this all the time, everywhere, particularly when you feel anxious, and you'll notice how much better you feel instantly – more alert, relaxed, in touch. You may not realise that breathing is also calming your heart rate, helping to normalise your blood pressure and decrease your risk of heart disease.

Alternate nostril breathing – a mainstay of some types of yoga – has been shown to help brain clarity and concentration. It may seem confusing at first but you'll get the hang of it very quickly; then it's second nature and you don't even have to think.

◆ Keeping your mouth closed, push all the spent air in your body out through your nose.
◆ With your right thumb pressed firmly against the right side of your nose to keep it closed, take a deep breath through your left nostril.
◆ Now push your right forefinger against your left nostril, lift your thumb and breathe out through your right nostril.
◆ Pause for a second then repeat the other way around.
◆ Repeat this pattern several times and marvel at how well you feel.

You can use your breathing to express anger or frustration as well. In moments of fury, sit or stand with a straight back, take a long deep breath, hold it for about 15 seconds, shaking your hands and arms, then push it out vigorously – with a big roaring moan if there's no one else around.

Last thing at night, as you lie in bed gazing at the ceiling, try closing your eyes, letting your mind roam and breathing your way to sleep. In through your nose to the count of four, hold for one, then out to a count of six, or eight, or…

STRAIGHT TALK

The inside story on how to lose five pounds – and get taller – in five seconds. Plus a lot more…

To some of us, posture seems about as old-fashioned as pressing dried flowers, relevant only to Edwardian ladies. But, second to breathing – with which it's intimately connected – improving your posture is probably the cheapest, quickest and simplest method of improving your appearance and the way your body systems work. If tension builds up in the muscles and connective tissue, the balance of your whole body is disrupted, leading to a sagging tum, aching muscles and joints, and poor circulation, plus indigestion, headaches and even cellulite (because the body's detox systems are not flowing freely). Long-term wear and tear may lead to osteoarthritis.

> *Good posture –*
> *and real jewellery –*
> *are the only things that*
> *can improve on nature*
> *once a woman gets*
> *to a certain age.*

HELEN GURLEY BROWN

'Beauty and health are posture-deep,' says manipulative physiotherapist Warwick McNeill of Physioworks in London, an innovative practice which specialises in detecting and correcting the underlying postural problems that cause intractable chronic aches and pains.

Most of all, good posture means being effortlessly relaxed and at ease with your body – never tense or rigid.

quick fix:

Just try this posture-perfecting exercise for starters…

◆ Stand with your feet one hip-width apart, toes facing forwards, knees 'soft'.

◆ Make sure your weight is on the centre of your feet; roll forward onto your toes, then back on your heels to understand the wrong positions, then find the mid position.

◆ Breathe slowly and rhythmically, in through your nose and out through your mouth.

◆ Tighten buttock muscles, but don't stick your bottom out – again find the mid position between sticking out and tucked in.

◆ Draw in your tummy muscles – imagine you're sending your navel towards your spine.

◆ Remember to go on breathing – there's a tendency to hold your breath when you're tightening your muscles.

◆ Think tall – imagine a thread drawing the crown of your head to the ceiling, look straight ahead, letting your chin and jaw relax; let your shoulder-blades drop.

◆ Some yoga teachers suggest that pupils simply remember how they felt when they heard good news – then stand and walk like that, with chest lifted, shoulders back and head held high.

◆ Still breathing gently, prowl gracefully round the room like a cat. Try it with bare feet, on a lawn or sand if possible. Your feet should be facing forwards, or at five minutes to one on the clock face, second big toe leading, heel touching the ground first. Let your hips roll and your arms swing gently.

◆ Keep breathing – and think feline…

planning ahead

True postural fitness depends on long-term tactics. The key support system for the spine is the transversus abdominus muscle which wraps round your middle like a Victorian corset. If that is floppy, the spine suffers. Studies have shown that the muscle is far weaker in people with bad backs. Some gym workouts can actually make matters worse by emphasising limb strength: as the muscles in your arms and legs get stronger and shorter, a floppy middle tends to get even weaker.

Strengthening the 'corset' physically with simple exercises helps enormously, so – perhaps surprisingly – can visualising the muscle 'corset' in your mind's eye as you move about throughout the day. Visualise – and strengthen. Visualise – and strengthen…

Physically, you need to aim for exercise which incorporates limb and trunk strengthening so that you control the middle of your body. Postural fitness is best done slowly and gently. Yoga, t'ai chi, Pilates, Feldenkrais and ballet plus hands-on therapies such as Alexander Technique, hellerwork, rolfing and muscle-based physiotherapy (called physical therapy in America) are particularly suitable for anyone wanting to improve their posture.

physioworks perfect posture plan

Long-term strategy: find your corset and get your back in fine fettle

1 Finding your corset

Locate your 'corset' muscles by kneeling on all fours and gently pulling in the wide belt of muscle over your tummy button and below – not the area above.

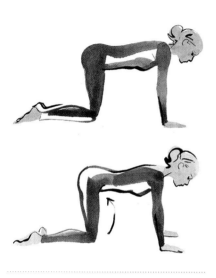

2 Single leg lift

Lie on your back with your knees bent, feet facing ahead. Place a hand on each hip-bone. Pulling in your 'corset', gently lift one knee towards you, raising the foot from the floor. Hold for a couple of seconds with your thigh as near vertical as possible then lower it gently. You will feel your pelvis roll very slightly from side to side – the object of the exercise is to use your corset to keep your pelvis as still as possible. Repeat on alternate sides for one to two minutes, twice daily.

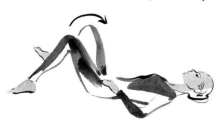

3 Single leg over

Starting in exactly the same way, keep your left knee pointing to the ceiling and let your right knee drop out to the side, right foot planted on the floor. Slowly return it to upright. Use your corset all the time to control the pelvic roll. Repeat as above.

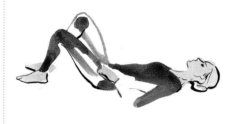

4 Shoulders right

Standing upright, find the correct position for your shoulders by having someone lay their hand on your lower trapezius muscle. Now draw it in very gently – imagine the hand pulling back your shoulder-blades – not your whole shoulder. (This is a subtle – not a big – movement.) Your shoulders should be square, rather than slouching and/or sloping like a ski run. Take care that your shoulders don't shrug up or your arms move backwards; keep your lower ribs still and don't let them lift up.

5 Behind basics

In a standing position, find the muscle in your bottom (the gluteus medius posterior) by imagining you are placing your hands over the back pockets of a pair of jeans. Now face a mirror and pull in those muscles. Let your legs turn out slightly from the hips and feel the arch of your feet lift.

6 Knee bends

This perfect basic exercise teaches your brain to have control over the alignment of trunk, knees and feet.

◆ Stand facing a mirror with your bare feet parallel, hip-width apart.
◆ Pull your navel in towards your spine without bending your back.
◆ Tense your bottom muscles, pointing the kneecaps straight ahead.
◆ Gently draw your shoulder-blades back to square your shoulders – don't let your lower ribs rise.
◆ Pull your chin in and back gently, lengthening your neck.
◆ Now bend your knees slightly; only go as far as you can while keeping your body in the same position and your knees directly over the middle toes.
◆ Repeat 20 times.

WATCHPOINT: Don't stick your bottom out.

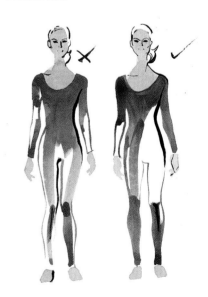

7 Nods for necks

Stand with your back to a wall, your heels about 5cm (2 inches) away (or sit on a stool); touch the wall with the back of your head, then start nodding your head gently. This will lengthen the back of your neck and you will feel your head slide up the wall.

8 Sitting pretty

Help align your lower spine when sitting by rocking forward on the bones of your bottom so you sit on the front side of the bones...

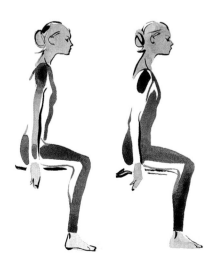

10 Wrongs and rights

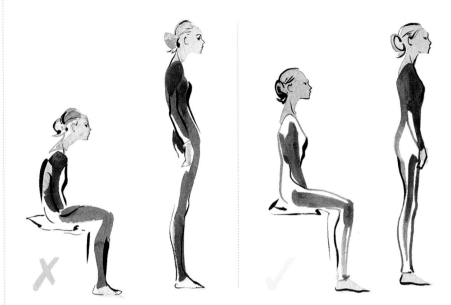

Sarah's first Alexander Technique teacher set her homework which involved looking at the way other people sat and stood. The problems are plain to see. The key thing to avoid when sitting is slouching and the goal at all times is to have ears and thighs in line, plus instep when you're standing. Not only will you look miles better but you'll avoid aches and pains and allow your organs to work optimally.

Remember to keep the rest of your body relaxed, knees a hip-width apart, feet firmly planted on the floor. (Sitting habitually with your knees together turns off natural postural muscles and encourages bad posture.) Support your lower back with a fat cushion or a lumbar roll. Practise sitting well by putting your chair in front of a mirror. Support your lower back and sit as above. Now gently draw your shoulders back into the correct position, without lifting your chest or sticking out your lower ribs. (It's easiest to monitor what your body is doing if you do it in a minimum of undies.)

9 Sit to stand

When you get up from a seat, the trick is to move from your hips and follow the crown of your head. Most people get out of a chair with their chin leading, straining the neck and spine. Instead, try putting your hands on your lower back, then bend at the hips, looking down at your toes so that your weight is well forwards. Then rise, keeping your lower back in its natural curve. Practise this ten times a day – or whenever you get up from a seat.

TIP: When sitting, change your position every 20 minutes.

our **fabulously easy** fitness programme

Yoga-based routines, walking, dancing round the kitchen – or anywhere else – plus a DIY sleek and tone workout based on body-conditioning Pilates are our nominations for the greatest all-round gentle exercise. (Add in swimming if you're a mermaid.) Think in terms of spending about half an hour every day, if possible – but at least five days a week – on these types of exercise. Get a mix – and, above all, do what you enjoy. Because the bottom line is that there's nothing more attractive and elegant than a woman who moves gracefully and with controlled vitality. Whether she's thirtysomething – or eightysomething…

Exercise naturally induces many of the anti-ageing mechanisms that scientists try to bring about by much more complex means, from hormone supplements and calorie restriction to gene therapy. It builds muscles, burns fat, makes heart and lungs work more efficiently, lowers the density of damaging sugars in the blood and is a major factor in protecting you against osteoporosis – brittle bone disease – which causes 200,000 fractures a year in the UK, a horrifying 40 per cent of which prove fatal. Weight-bearing exercise makes bones stronger and more dense – try anything where your weight is directly pressing on the ground – walking, jogging, dancing, skiing, etc. (Cycling, although great exercise, isn't weight-bearing.) Resistance exercises, such as lifting weights and swimming, will keep bones and muscles healthy.

Remember: gentle exercise should be just that. If you have aches and pains, any medical condition, or you haven't exercised for a while, consult your doctor before starting any exercise programme. If you feel a twinge during exercise, stop pushing yourself and return to something gentle.

INSTANT ENERGISERS

■ With your forefingers and thumbs on each ear, rub ear rims and lobes
■ Pull and wiggle the fingers of each hand in turn
■ Shake your hands vigorously, up and down, side to side
■ Pull, rub and wiggle the second big toe of each foot

ARE YOU GETTING ENOUGH?

Here's the bottom line, from the Health Education Authority: half an hour of moderate-level physical activity, at least five days of the week – and preferably every day. Sarah Williams, spokeswoman for the HEA, explains: 'Moderate activity is anything that makes you feel warm and breathe a little more heavily. That could embrace brisk walking to cycling, swimming – even vigorous housework or washing the car. People should try to find ways of fitting physical activity into their routine so that it doesn't become a chore – and vary the activity. If you're out of shape, split it into two 15-minute chunks – then increase to half an hour at a time. It's amazing how quickly fitness improves.'

get **going!**

When exercising is the last thing you feel like, Champneys – the UK's leading health spa – suggests ways of getting off the couch and out of the door…

◆ Use aromatherapy oils such as grapefruit, geranium and frankincense to give you a boost.
◆ If you have an exercise bike or other exercise equipment at home, put it in front of the TV and promise yourself that you won't watch your favourite programme unless you are working out at the same time.
◆ Find an 'exercise buddy'; you will motivate each other.
◆ Have a massage every week, if you can; it will help your circulation and make you feel less sluggish in winter. Trade DIY massages with your partner or 'massage buddy'.
◆ If you feel unmotivated, tired or get the munchies during winter and can't face the great outdoors, try full-spectrum light therapy. Over-production of melatonin, the sleep hormone which is turned on by lack of light, will cause the same symptoms that make animals want to hibernate in winter. Bright light counterbalances these symptoms. *(See p.235 for more details on winter depression or SAD.)* If you possibly can, remove your glasses or lenses and go out as often as possible on bright days.
◆ Eat a carbohydrate-rich diet to keep energy levels up *(see pp.188–190).*

exercise for happy hearts

Before menopause, the hormone oestrogen seems to help protect us from heart disease. But as oestrogen levels fall, so our risk goes up. Heart disease kills one in five women, and it's the second biggest cause of premature death among women after cancer. What is certain is that taking exercise – in tandem with stopping smoking, eating wisely and reducing excess stress – is one of our best bodyguards...

For post-menopausal women, evidence is emerging that even a little exercise can go a long way. In a seven-year study of the link between physical activity and survival time in more than 40,000 women in Minneapolis, the Minnesota School of Public Health found that those who took moderate activity – such as bowling, gardening or a long walk – as little as once a week were 24 per cent less likely to die over the course of the study than those who weren't physically active at all.

But more is undoubtedly better. The fittest people live the longest and because the heart is a muscle it will get stronger and be more efficient if it's asked to work harder. You do this through 'aerobic' exercise. This means working relatively hard and steadily for a sustained period which makes your heart pump harder in order to provide the other muscles with supplies of fresh oxygenated blood.

Exercise helps you achieve two things: a more efficient pump which leads to a larger heart muscle; and a lower resting heart beat, or pulse (which also translates as a healthier heart). It happens like this. As your heart gets bigger, it can pump more blood per beat so it doesn't need to beat so often. So, as your heart gets fitter, the heart rate gets lower – at work, rest and play – and returns more quickly to a resting rate after exercise.

Getting your heart fit is simple if you follow our suggested exercise programme.

If you do five 30-minute sessions a week, you're there. Alternatively, mix and match with other aerobic activities from the list on the right.

If you are completely unused to exercise, start with eight minutes every other day for the first week, then add on three minutes per session each week.

Don't forget also to add on the three to five minutes' warm-up and cool-down time either end.

heart news

The American National Institute of Health recently recommended that people with moderately raised blood pressure and no risk factor for heart attacks (such as positive family history) should exercise regularly for a year and lose 4.5kg (10lb) in weight before resorting to pharmaceutical drugs. They should also stop smoking immediately, reduce salt intake, drink a maximum of two small glasses of red wine daily and, above all, relax.

AEROBIC ACTIVITIES

For everyone:
Dancing/walking/dynamic yoga
Re-bounding on a mini-trampoline
Swimming/aquarobics
Cycling
Jogging/running
Mountain hiking
Ball games (tennis, badminton, volleyball, basketball)
Martial arts (kick-boxing, karate, judo)

For more advanced exercisers:
Skipping
Rollerblading
Skiing, both downhill and cross country
Windsurfing, skin/scuba diving

Exercising once or twice a week reduces the risk of heart attack by 36 per cent, compared with no exercise; three or four times weekly by 38 per cent; five times or more per week by 46 per cent.

The fittest people live the longest, but the good news is that exercise brings about the biggest jump in life expectancy even for people who go from nothing to being moderately active. According to William Evans, Director of the Knoll Physiological Research Center at Pennsylvania State University: 'If you're a sedentary person, any regular exercise of moderate intensity – even if it's mowing the lawn, house cleaning or climbing the stairs – will allow you to live longer.'

walking back to happiness

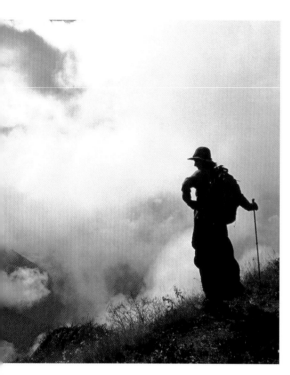

The problem with most of us is that we know we should exercise – but we don't, because it's boring, complicated, inconvenient (or a combination of all three). That's where walking wins, every time: it's free, it's easy, most of us are naturally good at it – and it's simple to fit into everyday life. (And walking from A to B is a double-whammy: free transport and a free fat-burner.) So step right up for the perfect walking workout...

Our biggest health and fitness secret is that we walk, walk, walk, walk, walk – at every opportunity. Across the park, to meetings. In the evenings, with friends, as a social activity – or instead of taking the car to a restaurant.

We walk at weekends, in parks and in wide open spaces. And we've found that if we have to do without our walks, our stress levels soar and we feel decidedly unsparkling...

Today, research has confirmed that nature's greatest fitness and looks booster is walking, at a normal-to-brisk pace. Unlike jogging or running, walking doesn't jolt and jar the skeletal structure every time your foot hits the ground. Yet it can raise your heart rate to around 50–70 per cent of its maximum – similar to aerobics, cycling and swimming – which boosts your heart health.

Ideally, you need to walk for 20–30 minutes (or more), five times or more a week. (If you start to walk to get from A to B, instead of always driving, it's surprisingly easy to fit that into even the busiest lifestyle.) Yet according to the Pedestrian Policy Group, the average distance walked per person has actually plummeted by more than 20 per cent in the past twenty years – with disastrous consequences for our fitness, putting us at risk of heart disease, premature arthritis and osteoporosis through lack of exercise. The solution is simple: lace up those trainers (or those comfy brogues), and put one foot in front of the other...

Walking strengthens hips, thighs, stomach and bottom muscles (plus arms and shoulders if you swing your arms as you walk). It speeds up the metabolic rate so that calories are burned faster even when the walk's over.

What's more, walking also appears to boost our immunity. According to a study carried out by Dr David Nieman, PhD, a Professor of Exercise Science at the Appalachian State University in Boone, North Carolina, 'Walking seems to prime the body's immune system, preparing it to fight disease before we even feel the first sniffle.' Among the women in Nieman's study, those who walked briskly for 45 minutes a day, five days a week, were sick with colds or flu for only five days during the 15-week study period – timed to coincide with the peak cold season – as opposed to ten days among the sedentary women.

I don't believe you need any more than bending, stretching and walking – not very different from how we exercised back in the cavewoman era. Keeping dogs disciplines me to exercise when they do. I always make sure I have a young dog among them – to maintain the pace!

KATIE BOYLE

stomp and stretch warm-up march

Always warm up and cool down before and after exercising. This energising march also gives you a speedy workout if you're short of time.

● **March briskly** on the spot for two minutes. Still stomping, add in some stretches.

● **Shoulder shrugs:** lift your shoulders up to your ears and down; with your elbows bent, circle your shoulders slowly backwards and then forwards.

● **Arm swings:** swing arms vigorously to front and back.

● **Knee lifts:** lift your knees high so that your thighs are parallel to the ground.

● **Alternate knee lifts:** still lifting your knees, alternate your arms and legs: touch your left knee with your right arm and vice versa.

● **Chest presses:** bring your arms together across your chest so that the elbows, wrists and fists touch.

● **Hamstring curls:** with arms swinging loosely, bring your heels up to your buttocks.

● **Upper back squeezes:** squeeze your shoulder-blades together as you march.

● **Walk on the spot** for one minute, arms swinging, until you gradually come to a stop.

walkfit secrets

Fitness experts Chrissie Painell and Anne O'Dowd RSA developed the excellent walking audio-cassette Walkfit* which tells you how to make walking your optimum workout; it's perfect to play on a Walkman as you start to get into the habit of striding out. We asked them for their top tips to help develop good walking and breathing techniques...

1 Walk tall. Lift up from the chest, keep your shoulders relaxed back and down. This will help you to breathe more deeply.

2 Breathe in through your nose and out through your mouth.

3 Keep your elbows bent at 90°. (Imagine you are holding an egg in each hand.) This will help ensure that upper body movement comes from your shoulders.

4 Your heel should land first. Then roll through to the balls of the feet and toes. Push off with the back leg as you bring your other leg forward.

5 Try to glide along. When your stride is too long, you break the forward motion and slow yourself down. If your hair is flopping up and down wildly, you may be over-striding.

6 Keep your abdominal muscles pulled firmly in to support your back.

7 Try to avoid swinging your hips.

8 Avoid dehydration. And avoid eating a large meal before your walk. Drink water before, during and after your workout, ideally sipping from your water bottle every 10–15 minutes.

9 Plan a well-lit route.

10 Remember: warm up and cool down for three to five minutes, walking more slowly at the beginning and the end of your workout.

STEPPIN' OUT – MUSIC TO WALK TO

From the Walkfit team, their top ten of music suggestions to get you in the mood for walking...

1 **Simply the Best** by Tina Turner (to warm up)

2 **Do Ya Think I'm Sexy?** by Rod Stewart (to warm up)

3 **Closer than Close** by Rosie Gaines

4 **Remember Me** by The Blueboy

5 **What Becomes of the Broken Hearted?** by Robson & Jerome

6 **Cosmic Girl** by Jamiroquai

7 **One and One** by Robert Miles

8 **Follow the Rules** by Livin' Joy

9 **Hallelujah Chorus** from Handel's *Messiah* (to get you to the top of the hill or mountain!)

10 **Everything** by Mary J. Blige (to cool down)

How can you tell if you're walking at the optimum pace? You need to have your heart rate raised – but don't overdo it. The easiest test is the 'talk' test: you should be able to pass the odd sentence as you walk, but if you can have a lengthy, effortless gossip, you're not working hard enough.

Eat within 60–90 minutes of exercising to reboost energy levels.

walking advertisements

Walking advertisements – literally – include Michelle Pfeiffer ('walking burns fat and gives me energy for the day'), Hillary Rodham Clinton, Suzanne Somers (who calls it 'a mind-cleanser'), Sophia Loren, Catherine Deneuve and former tennis star Chris Evert, who has traded her tennis racket for a pair of walking shoes.

shoe savvy

The beauty of walking lies in its total simplicity: expensive gear and flashy Spandex are superfluous. But if you're planning to go walkabout regularly, do invest in a pair of supportive shoes. We are great fans of the Ecco range from Denmark*, which combine style with amazing comfort; their shoes are often smart enough for meetings – but supportive enough for an eight-mile hike. Many are lace-ups, which stop the foot 'rolling' as you walk.

Alternatively, look for a pair of walking trainers in a sports shoe store. If you can't find a pair specifically for walking, ask for 'cross-trainers', which are designed to be suitable for a range of sports, including walking. Ask for advice in a sports shoe shop, if you need guidance. Most of us have one foot bigger than the other, so always fit for your bigger foot (and, if necessary, wear an extra sock on the other foot), rather than squeeze your toes into a shoe size too small. (Adequate toe space is vital.) Heels shouldn't grip too tightly: leave enough space to fit a pencil between your heel and the back of the shoe, to avoid blistering. Half a size larger than usual may make the difference between exquisite pleasure and total torture. The soles should be flexible, so that you get a full range of movement through the foot. When you're trying on shoes, always wear the socks you'll usually be walking in. (You might want to keep at least two pairs of walking shoes of slightly different sizes, one for winter and one for summer; you should also replace pairs approximately every six months, if you walk regularly, as the heels get worn down.) And remember: for long, wet walks, two pairs of socks – or changing into a fresh pair mid-way – can prevent agonising blisters caused by damp-sock rub.

more shoe talk

All the shoes you choose to wear – at any time – are key to body alignment. High heels throw your weight forward to your forefeet. Compensating for the disruption can involve your entire musculo-skeletal system: watch out for head, shoulder and back aches, not to speak of throbbing feet and injured calf muscles. The best advice is to wear low heels with plenty of room for your toes – crease marks on your feet mean toes are cramped.

Because your bones become more rigid as you age, high heels become even more of a problem from the age of 40 onwards. Wearing them very occasionally is okay – not at all is best, and certainly not for a standing-around sort of party or for dancing – or walking...

And if you are determined to get on your high heels, don't wear backless shoes or mules and do protect corns with special tubing.

SEVEN GREAT REASONS FOR WALKING...

◆ Walking contributes to stabilising blood sugar levels, helping to avoid swings in mood and energy.

◆ Walking can lift your mood because, like all exercise, it releases endorphins, your brain's own mood-elevating compounds.

◆ Walking is weight-bearing exercise so it helps fight osteoporosis.

◆ Research shows that people who combine exercise – like walking – with healthy eating are more likely to keep off weight than those who only diet. Not only that, it can actually peel off pounds. According to Dr Craig Sharp, Professor of Sports Medicine at Brunel University, 'At a fairly moderate walking pace, you will burn up about five calories a minute, walking 20 minutes a day burns 100 calories a day – about 3 kilograms or 8 pounds a year.'

◆ A regular walking programme builds endurance in the large muscle groups that stabilise and support the spine, helping to prevent (and even cure) back pain.

◆ It's great for the heart. Walking strengthens the heart, making it pump blood more efficiently through the body – and raising the level of HDL ('good') cholesterol, which helps cleanse the surplus fat from blood vessels and so reduces deaths from heart disease.

◆ Walking can even help your reaction time, says Wanda Spirduso, EdD, a Professor of Kinesiology and Health Education at the University of Austin, Texas: 'Exercisers' muscles work better,' explains Dr Spirduso. 'But so do their minds...'

BRAIN BAGS

If you carry a shoulder (or hand) bag, swap it from side to side. Don't use your shoulder as a hook, try to hitch a bag round the back. Preferably use a rucksack like the one Jo is striding out with below – very chic and savvy!

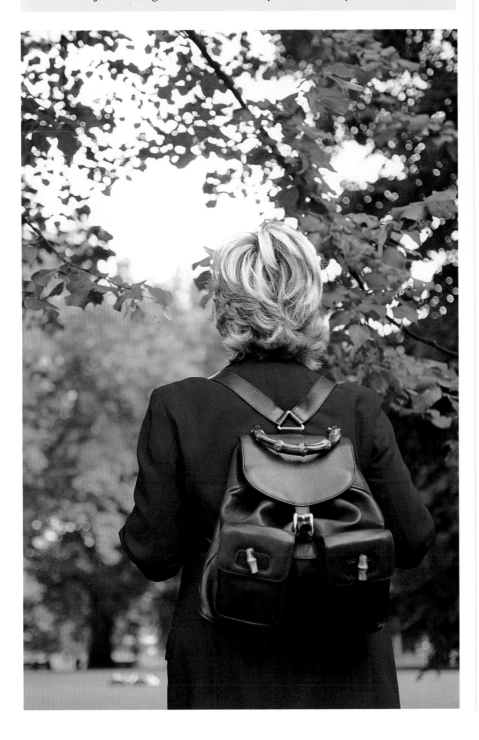

take strides not Prozac

When you're feeling blue, walking can put you back in the pink. The Exercise Laboratory at the University of California claims that 'a vigorous walk can be more effective than 400mg of tranquilliser'. And since walking is suitable for everyone – from the overweight and the elderly, not to mention pregnant women, there really is no excuse not to lace up – and step out...

no sweat

Everyone sweats, and when it's hot or we're nervous, we sweat even more. Research shows, however, that one in five is embarrassed by perspiration and nearly two-thirds of women report wetness after using their regular deodorant.

There is a range of simple measures which may help to stop wetness and prevent body odour:

◆ frequent regular washing, plus thorough drying
◆ shaving armpit hair
◆ loose clothing made of natural fibres, e.g. cotton or silk
◆ shoes rather than boots
◆ combined deodorant and antiperspirant products, such as Mitchum for Problem Perspiration
◆ stronger products such as Driclor, which contains aluminium chloride; this is used at night then washed off in the morning before applying a normal product.

reach for the sun

The Salute to the Sun is considered the perfect way to greet the day, stretching the body into wakefulness by unkinking muscles and banishing creakiness. It also helps de-mist foggy minds. Yoga sessions usually start with this gentle Salute to the Sun, to warm the muscles. You need to do it barefoot and make sure that you're on a non-slip surface – and don't try to reach for the sun immediately on getting out of bed; do some warm-up exercises (or go for a walk) first...

1

Stand straight with your feet hip-width apart. Toes should be spread and the weight evenly distributed between heels and toes; knees should be straight but not locked. Hold in your tummy. (You will feel your back straighten.) Breathe in slowly and deeply. As you breathe out again, bring your hands up and place your palms together at chest level, keeping your forearms straight but not stiff.

11

Breathe out and stretch your arms either side of your body until they come to a resting position, putting you back ready for Position 1.

Repeat the whole sequence from start to finish, this time leading with your left leg in Position 4. Build up until you can go through the entire cycle five or six times, to warm and loosen up the body. Keep the entire movement fluid and as smooth as possible, your breathing steady.

NOTE: *If you have neck or shoulder problems, go through Positions 1–5, then skip right to position 8. This will still be enough to get your energies flowing... Once you have reached for the sun, your muscles are warm – and you are ready for some individual yoga postures.*

10

Breathe in as you slowly and gently uncurl your body, with your head coming up last. When you're upright reach your arms forward and stretch them up over your head, eyes looking straight ahead, breathing naturally.

9

You are now going back to Position 3, so breathe out, bringing your left foot forwards parallel with your right foot, several inches apart. Hands are by your side on or towards the floor (whichever is comfortable for you), forehead facing your knees, which are bent.

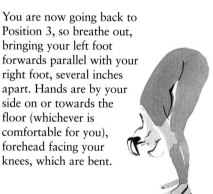

2

Breathe in and stretch your arms over your head; hold your tummy in to prevent your back over-arching. Your arms should be in line with your ears, elbows and knees straight, palms a few inches apart, fingertips reaching upwards. Look straight ahead, but don't let your chin poke forwards.

WATCHPOINT: Don't let your shoulders rise; feel your shoulder-blades sinking down even as you reach for the sky...

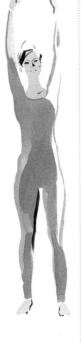

3

Bend your knees slightly. While keeping your arms and body stretched, breathe out slowly and bend forwards, keeping your head tucked in towards your knees. Bring your hands to the floor, next to your feet. (Don't worry if you can't reach that far; let them dangle, then take another deep breath – as you exhale, your hands will drop. As you become increasingly flexible, you may be able to straighten your knees and even touch your forehead to them.)

7

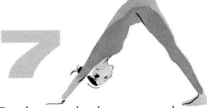

Breathe out and tuck your toes under. Without allowing hands or feet to move, raise yourself on your forearms as far as you can. Leaning on your knees, push your bottom up so you're back in the box position and then push your hips up. Tuck your head in, so that you're looking through your legs. (This is called the mountain position because of the shape the body makes.)

WATCHPOINT: You can only do this with your toes gripping the floor. Remember to keep breathing, and try not to tense your shoulders.

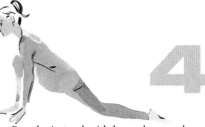

4

Breathe in, and with knees bent and palms flat on the floor next to your feet, stretch your right leg as far back as possible. (Fingers are spread and pointing forwards.) Drop your right knee to the floor. Your front left knee should be directly above your ankle. Eyes up, look straight ahead. Breathe out slowly.

5

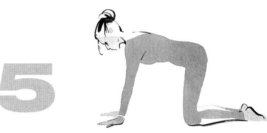

Inhaling, bring your left knee back so that it's next to your right knee, creating a box shape with your body. Hold your tummy in and ensure that your shoulders are directly over your hands. (Now you'll be looking at the floor.) Keep breathing deeply and naturally. (NB If you are at all stiff or have neck or shoulder problems, we suggest you stop here. See note opposite and skip to step 8.)

6

Breathing in, slide your hands forward a few inches. Keeping your knees and feet on the floor, bottom raised, maintain your weight on your arms and lower your trunk very gently to the floor. Now lower your forearms to the floor. Lift your head slightly; keep your shoulders back and down and make sure you don't strain or over-arch your back and neck. Only come up as far as possible – this may be a very small distance.

8

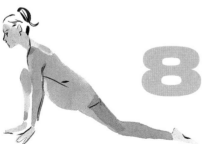

Breathe in; bring your right foot forwards between your hands, letting your back foot uncurl and your body slide backwards so that once again you are in Position 4. Make sure your front knee is aligned with your ankle and uncurl your back toes.

yoga wisdom

In the quest for grace, strength and flexibility, yoga has topped the charts for thousands of years. Yoga fans see it not as a form of exercise but as a way of life, thanks to the amazing physical and mental benefits it delivers, bringing mind and body into balance.

Yoga postures (aka asanas) exercise every part of the body, stretching and toning all the joints, muscles, spine and skeleton, as well as massaging the internal organs to make them work efficiently. Yoga is something that you can literally enjoy forever. We know women in their seventies and eighties who took up yoga in mid-life – or even later – and as a result have stayed amazingly limber, with extraordinary elegance. What's more, you don't need expensive equipment or snazzy clothing – simply a few minutes of peace and quiet. And because of the emphasis on deep breathing, with movements that help the body's natural energy to flow, yoga exercises can quickly re-energise you when you're flagging…

YOGA BREATHING

In yoga, it's important to breathe from the diaphragm, rather than from the chest – breathe in and out through the nose, not the mouth. Babies breathe naturally from the diaphragm – think of their little tummies, rising and falling – but adults tend to breathe from the chest and the more stressed-out we are, the shallower our breath becomes.

To learn diaphragm breathing, stand straight with your feet together, shoulders down, hands resting on your hips. Then inhale deeply and push your stomach out from the diaphragm; it will inflate like a balloon. When you breathe out, your tummy will contract again.

the tree

This is wonderful for improving balance – and surprisingly challenging at first. Stand up straight with your feet together. Shift your weight to your right foot; bend the left knee and place that foot against the opposite thigh/knee as high as you can get it. The knee should point outwards, with the sole of your left foot flat against the leg. Bring your hands together in the prayer position in front of your chest; keeping the palms together, slowly extend your arms above your head, elbows slightly bent. Focus on a point in front of you, breathing rhythmically and gently. Hold in position for 15 seconds to start with (building up to 30 seconds as your balance improves). Repeat, with the opposite leg.

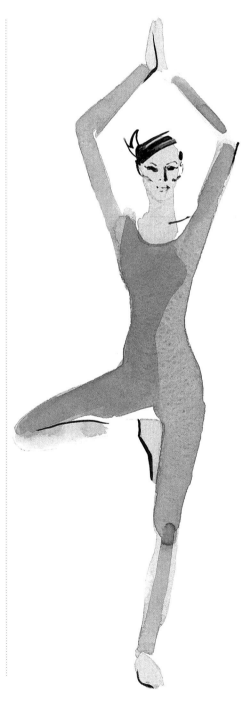

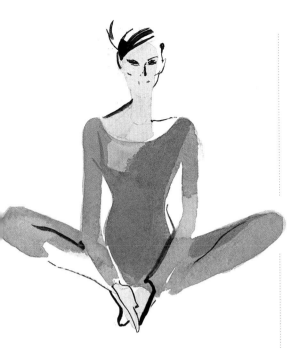

spinal twist

This boosts mobility and loosens up the spine, so it's good for muscle problems in the hips and back. Sit on the floor with both legs straight in front of you. Bend the left leg at the knee and place it over the right leg, with the foot flat on the floor outside the right knee. Put your left hand flat on the floor just behind your body. Then gently twist your torso and place your right hand on the floor, beside the left knee. Follow that line so that you are looking over your left shoulder, keeping your shoulders parallel to the floor. Very gently push your right elbow into the left knee. Hold for 30 seconds, then switch sides. Repeat.

As always, be gentle and don't push yourself further than is comfortable. Practised regularly, the spinal twist will soon boost your flexibility more than you can imagine.

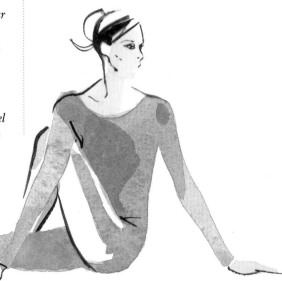

the butterfly

This improves hip flexibility and stretches the groin area. Sitting on the ground with your back straight, bring the soles of your feet together. Take hold of your feet with both hands and draw them in towards the groin, being ultra-careful not to over-stretch. Keeping your back straight, hold the position for 30 seconds and gently release. Then repeat.

relaxation pose

This is the classic way to finish a yoga workout, relaxing the body and stilling the mind. Lie on your back with your arms by your side, palms facing upwards, legs slightly apart and eyes closed. Try to make your body as symmetrical as possible. Breathe deeply into your abdomen and then up into your chest so that your breath feels like a rolling wave. With each breath, allow gravity to help your body sink deeper into the floor. Be aware of all the parts of your body that are in contact with the floor. Bring your awareness to any tension in your body and let them gently relax. (This is a powerful time to repeat any affirmations to yourself.) Stay in the relaxation pose for at least three minutes or until you feel totally relaxed and ready to face life with a renewed charge of positive energy.

YOGA ESSENTIALS

◆ Exercise slowly.

◆ Don't stretch the body to the point where it's uncomfortable.

◆ Make sure the room is warm – or that you're wearing a cosy jumper.

◆ Try to turn off the telephone or exercise in a place where you won't be disturbed.

◆ Wear comfortable clothing and take off any jewellery that might get in the way.

◆ On wooden or tile floors, always perform yoga exercises with bare feet, so that you don't slip.

◆ If you don't have a special exercise mat, you may want to use a thick towel to cushion yourself against the hard floor.

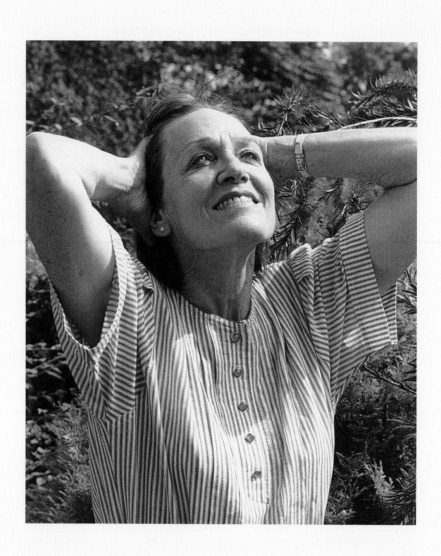

Suzanne Adamson

We are inspired by Suzanne because, in her sixties, this reflexologist and yoga teacher – who helps women from new mums to pensioners discover the joy of relaxation and exercise – is as lithe and limber as a teenager. And because – having reinvented herself when her children were grown – this South African author of *The Reflexology Partnership** is proof to all women that life really can begin at mid-life…

'I took up yoga in 1974 – not in a big way, but to keep myself in balance after my husband died; I'd just left Kenya, where I'd been training racehorses and growing coffee, to build a new life in Scotland as a health visitor, with three small children. Yoga practice helped maintain balance while adapting to a totally new way of life – the perfect combination of physical exercise with mental relaxation.

'I'd always taken good health for granted, until a bout of viral hepatitis and encephalitis soon after my husband died. Feeling healthy again was such a joy and relief that the importance of valuing and nurturing one's health became indelibly imprinted in my mind. I began to get interested in complementary medicine. Working as a health visitor, I encountered so many lonely old ladies, in a poor state of health, taking fistfuls of medication – and I thought: "There's got to be a better way of doing things…"

'My children were growing up and going to college and had their friends. I realised I'd got them to the stage where they could look after themselves and it was time for a fresh start. In the end, I flew the nest! And came to London…

'I started going to talks on complementary medicine. Reflexology, in particular, fascinated me. The idea that by massaging points on the foot you could have such a dramatic effect elsewhere in the body was a revelation. So I began to study reflexology, massage and bio-magnetics, and to train as a yoga teacher. In my work as a yoga teacher, I realised how amazing yoga was for the elderly and for people with physical disablement, once you get them to start and out of that state of hunched-up-ness – it really is never too late. So many of my older pupils have told me how their thyroid problems were better, their asthma improved, or their blood pressure had stabilised.

'Yoga is now part of my daily life. I recently went for a bone-density test, to check out whether I was at risk for osteoporosis, and the technician said that in her experience people who do yoga are the only ones she sees whose bone density is the same in both ankles.

'I always do 15 minutes of breathing practice, first thing in the morning; physically, my body is a happy body and more comfortable to live in when I'm doing an hour and a half of yoga every day. But when I'm fantastically busy I'll have to decide whether to do my yoga or have an extra hour's sleep – and sleep usually wins, because my body really needs seven hours.

'I became a vegetarian ten years ago. People say that being vegetarian doesn't do a lot for your bones, but I feel fantastic on the food I eat: a great variety of vegetables, lots of brown rice, seeds like sunflower and pumpkin, almonds and other nuts and tofu in lots of different forms. I eat some cheese and the occasional egg. As a treat, every now and then I indulge myself with a little chocolate – and love it. I only drink very occasionally – if I'm out and it's someone's birthday.

'I don't know if it's the yoga, the food I eat, or just good luck, but I had no problems with menopause; I was so busy I didn't really have time to notice what was going on. I think if you are walking around and being active, keeping life in balance, there is no need to take anything for menopause at all. And the only supplements I take are Hawaiian Pacific spirulina, for extra protein, and Sunrider's Beauty Pearl*, which is bio-available calcium.

'Ageing well is all a question of balance, I feel. There is so much stress in the world but the vital thing is to try to tackle it before it gets to you, physically or mentally. But for me, there is a tremendous sense of freedom being in my sixties – as if I've been given an open ticket to life. (Getting my free bus pass was very symbolic!) I just make sure to nurture my sense of wellness – so I can enjoy the moment and get on with the adventure of life. Without being distracted by an uncomfortable body…'

sleek and tone pilates style

The body-conditioning technique known as Pilates – which several of the team working on feel fabulous forever **swear by – is a system of slow, sleeking and toning exercises that can be used to spot-target specific areas of the body – from bad backs to saddlebag thighs via weak pelvic floor muscles (these slacken after childbirth and naturally with ageing – sometimes leading to stress incontinence and/or reduced sexual pleasure). This ability to overcome physical problems non-invasively and/or improve angst areas makes Pilates one of the most effective all-round forms of exercise – and great for anti-ageing.**

Pilates (named after its founder, Joseph Pilates) is now increasingly being taught in workout studios or by personal trainers around the world. Explains Anne-Marie Petash*, a leading London Pilates instructor, 'The focus of attention is on the three main control centres of the torso: the deep inner and outer abdominal muscles, and the pelvic floor muscles.' This results in a stronger spine, improved posture, reduced back pain (even in long-term sufferers), and an amazingly sleeked silhouette; even the notoriously hard-to-tone tummy area can be impressively tightened.

The following spot-targeted exercises, explained by Anne-Marie, tighten up the whole pelvic area. The result: a tighter tummy, more control – and better sex. Beat that!

A

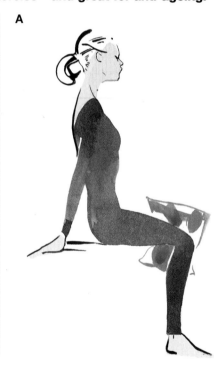

B

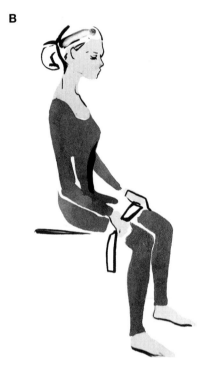

PELVIC FLOOR EXERCISE 1 (Illustration A)

◆ Sit on a straight-backed chair and place a firm cushion between your knees.

◆ Keep your feet hip-width apart. Lengthen your spine by placing your hands either side of you, and very slightly behind you, on the chair.

◆ Draw your sitting bones together – which will raise your bottom slightly in the chair – and squeeze your inner thighs together. Squeeze on the cushion for seven slow breaths. Inhale through the nose and, as you exhale, pull the abdominal muscles in towards your spine.

◆ Do three sets of this exercise. For the second set, move the cushion halfway up your thighs. For the third set, place it right at the top of your thighs.

PELVIC FLOOR EXERCISE 2 (Illustration B)

◆ Same position as above, without the cushion, so your inside knees are around 7.5cm (3 inches) apart to start with. Place a strap or a belt around your thighs just above the knee. Keeping a firm, tight grip on the strap, push your legs outwards. Draw the sitting bones together and hold this position for a set of seven breaths, pushing against the belt for resistance, without releasing at any time during these breaths. Then release the strap and do two more sets of seven breaths each, moving the feet and knees very slightly further apart each time on each set.

WATCHPOINT: Don't tense up your neck and shoulders, and keep lengthening the spine.

the good sex (and everything else) workout

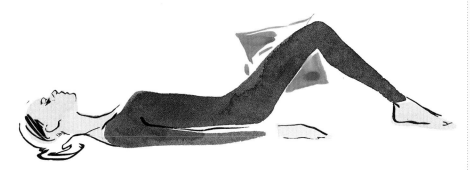

PELVIC TILT

Lie on your back with your knees bent and your feet parallel, hip-width apart and facing forwards on the floor. Place a firm cushion between your inner thighs. Stretch your arms forward on the floor, palms down. Start with your spine in a relaxed position. (The small of your back will be slightly off the floor.) Slowly inhale in this position and then exhale, gently squeezing the inner thighs. Pull your navel down towards your spine and curl your tailbone slightly off the floor. You will now feel the small of your back pressing into the floor. Exhale and curl your spine down to a relaxed position. You are now back where you started; slowly repeat ten times.

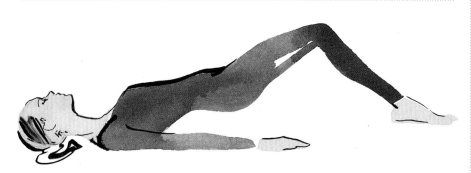

PELVIC LIFT

Start in the same position as for the pelvic tilt. Go through the same movements and breathing as for the pelvic tilt, but this time peel your spine off the floor to the level of your shoulder-blades. Hold the position and inhale. Make sure your feet stay firmly flat on the floor and don't roll in either direction.

As you exhale, bring the spine back down to the floor, vertebra by vertebra, returning to your neutral position. Keep tipping the pelvis upwards on the way down. Repeat ten times. (NB If you feel any pressure on your back, place your feet on a low, wide stool.)

WATCHPOINT: Keep your jaw and neck 'soft'; don't allow them to tense up, or your chin to jut out.

I'm not a health fanatic; I eat a reasonable diet and just add in extra vitamin C if I remember. But for the last 15 years I've been doing Pilates – a system of long, slow stretching exercises – at Alan Herdman's studio in London's West End. I'm convinced it's the key to suppleness and good health. You slowly develop a very strong, sleek musculature, which not only helps keep the figure but prevents back pain, because the stomach muscles become so strong.

You're very closely supervised so you have to do every exercise perfectly, ensuring the maximum results in just an hour and a half once or twice a week. On a cold winter's morning I always think, shall I go? But I always feel so fantastic afterwards that it's worth it. Lately I've also taken up fast-walking, a couple of times a week, because my doctor said I wasn't getting enough aerobic exercise. Together they mean total fitness.

HONOR BLACKMAN

the baked bean workout

Stay full of beans forever and discover the strengthening and toning power of weight training...

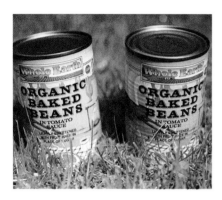

Women lose about a third of their muscle mass between the ages of 35 and 80, but inactivity, not ageing, is the major cause for the slow slide into creakiness when steps seem steeper, groceries become heavier. According to Research Into Ageing, even healthy people lose strength at some 1–2 per cent per year, and some may decline even faster. Strong muscles are of course essential to support your bones.

The good news is that weight and resistence training can reverse muscle decline. Two groups of women were observed for a study at the Jean Mayer USDA Human Nutrition Research Center on Ageing at Tufts University, Boston: one group remained in couch potato mode, while the other group came in twice a week to lift weights. One year later, the inactive group was even less active than before; their muscles and bones had aged. But according to the study's co-ordinator, Miriam E. Nelson, PhD, 'The women who lifted weights changed, too – but in a miraculous way: after one year of strength training, their bodies were 15 to 20 years more youthful.' And it really is

never too late to turn back the clock: a recent study showed that women aged 75 to 93, who exercised gently for a total of three hours a week, improved the strength of their thigh muscles by around 25 per cent in only 12 weeks. This is equal to a rejuvenation of strength of some 16 to 20 years. And in yet another study, it was found that muscles remain capable of improving with use even in the tenth decade of life.

You certainly don't need expensive equipment for weight training. If there are a couple of cans of baked beans in your larder, you've the recipe for a simple upper-body workout to regain strength – and improve posture. We asked fitness pro Gloria Thomas (who's coached at top London gym, The Harbour Club) for this baked bean workout. It's suitable for every woman because it can be done sitting or standing. Start slowly, but 'Do each exercise until your muscles become tired,' says Gloria. 'If you ultimately find you are doing endless repetitions, switch to a slightly larger can of beans!'

WATCHPOINT:
Don't forget to breathe!

SHOULDERS
Sit in an upright position. Your abdominal muscles should be pulled in, your shoulders back and down. Your head and neck should be relaxed. With a can of baked beans in each hand, bring your hands to shoulder level, with your palms facing forwards and arms straight. Inhale and take the

can of baked beans up above your head to a count of two, then slowly lower to the starting position.

BICEPS
Keep the same sitting position as before with your upper arms by your side and your palms facing each other, holding the cans. Keeping your elbows close to the body in a fixed position, bend your arms, palms upward, and curl up towards shoulders for two counts; lower to a count of four.

TRICEPS
Do this exercise one arm at a time, or both at the same time if you're used to exercising. Once again, keeping the same position as above, grasp a can of baked beans between the thumb and forefingers of each hand. Take your arms behind your head so that your elbows are just above either ear. Straighten your arms upwards until your baked bean can is overhead. Take care not to lock your elbows. Slowly return to starting position.

BACK
This is great for strengthening the muscles of the back and for posture. In the same sitting position as above, hold a can of beans in each hand and take your arms out in front of you at shoulder level. Now take your arms around to the side, pulling your shoulder-blades together, for two counts. Your hands should end up in line with your shoulders, making you into a T shape. Slowly go back to your original position.

SWIM TO HEALTH

Some biologists believe mankind came from water. That, they say, is why we need to drink so much water, why we do so well on fishy food and why infants up to six months old have the same diving reflex as aquatic mammals like dolphins: drop a baby into water and it will submerge, stop breathing, slow down its heart rate, then re-emerge, turn its head to the side, breathe and dive again. (Dolphins' flippers, incidentally, have exactly the same bones that we have in our arms and hands.)

Whatever our evolutionary background, there is no doubt that swimming is wonderful exercise. Water's innate buoyancy makes it the perfect environment for workouts for all ages – whether it's for re-hab from injuries or keeping fit. Water exercise can improve the way your body works overall; in particular it imp roves digestion and sleep patterns, reduces 'bad' cholesterol and of course makes regular swimmers sleek and toned. It is also a resistance exercise, so helps protect you against osteoporosis. You needn't even know how to swim. Water workouts in a swimming pool or the sea can be ultra-simple...

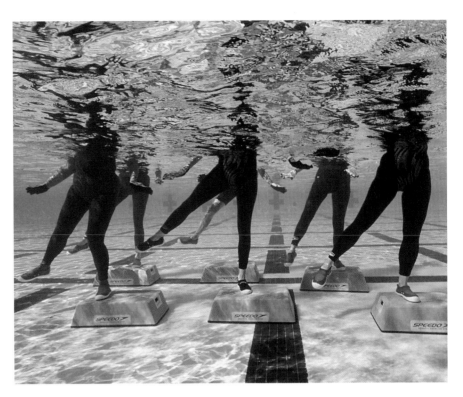

◆ Walk in water

Walk in chest-height water from one side to another, then walk backwards; keep your arms swinging.

◆ Crab walk

Now walk sideways, like a crab, across the pool, your body at right angles to the side. Keep your feet pointing straight ahead and bring them together after each step; don't turn when you reach the other side, simply lead with the other foot. Repeat both walks several times; work up to a run if possible.

◆ Trunk twist

Stand in shoulder-deep water, legs a shoulder-width apart, knees slightly bent. Extend arms straight out to sides, parallel to surface, palms facing forwards; swing body round to the right and the left.

◆ Front-back leg raise

Stand in chest-deep water at right angles to pool wall, holding onto bar. Raise your outer leg straight up in front of you. Lower leg and continue the movement to the back, keeping your knee and back straight. Turn round and repeat on other side.

◆ Side leg raise

Stand in chest-deep water at right angles to pool wall, holding onto bar. Lift outer leg directly to side, keeping toes forward. Repeat on other side.

◆ Arm pull

Stand in shoulder-deep water, legs a shoulder-width apart. Bend knees slightly. Extend arms directly in front of you, palms down and hands cupped. Keeping your elbows straight, pull your arms down past your body and behind. Then turn your hands around so your palms are facing down and push arms back to starting position.

WARNING: Swimming is a wonderful exercise but, if you have a bad neck and/or back, beware of breast stroke. According to physician and back expert Dr Richard Petty, it can exacerbate the condition unless you keep your face in the water. Some sufferers report that back crawl gives the most benefit.

cellulite: the bottom line

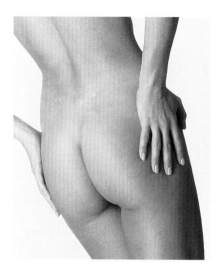

Action plan for dimpled derrières...
About 95 per cent of women say they have some degree of cellulite, the orange-peel skin on thighs and bottom, which ranges from dimples to the full-blown mattress look. Exactly how this trapped fat forms is uncertain, but the root cause is female hormones – men don't get cellulite. It's not insoluble, but it won't disappear overnight. Allow at least four to six weeks on the programme below to see changes. (But just think how long it took to appear!) We are doubtful that cellulite ever disappears 100 per cent, but most women will see a big improvement.

DIY CELLULITE SOLUTIONS

◆ Clean up your diet: exclude fatty sugary treats and fat/salt combinations.
◆ Feast on high-fibre fruit and veg.
◆ Eat plenty of complex carbo-hydrates to keep your blood sugar balanced *(see p.190)*.
◆ Eat lots of fresh, nutritious, preferably organic food; processed foods have lost many nutrients.
◆ Avoid artificial additives, e.g. pesticides, colourings, sweeteners, etc.
◆ Take supplements with vitamins C and E. Cellulite researcher Dr Karen Burke, from New York, recommends 1–6g of vitamin C daily and 400 iu of natural vitamin E in capsule form.
◆ Eat little and often; never skip meals – it forces your body to store fat.
◆ Never yo-yo diet, it encourages your body to lose weight above your waist and store it below.
◆ Investigate food allergies or intolerance *(see p.198)*.
◆ Drink at least 2 litres (3½ pints) of still, pure, room-temperature water daily to flush your system.
◆ Reduce alcohol as much as possible; opt for organic wine.
◆ Try stretching exercise, e.g. yoga and dance, which stretch and tone rather than body-build; swimming is a great all-rounder, plus a brisk daily walk.
◆ Brush your skin – one of the cheapest and most effective ways of budging cellulite.
◆ Don't take diuretics: they ultimately cause more water retention. Slimming pills also cause fatigue and irritability.
◆ If cellulite won't budge and you are taking prescribed hormones, investigate alternatives.
◆ Try massage – but beware of big claims; massage that is too violent may damage the lymph system and cause more problems. Experts recommend manual lymphatic drainage massage *(MLD, see p.61)* or gentle self-massage with anti-cellulite oil.
◆ Most specific cellulite products improve skin appearance and feel, but any 'shrinking' may be short-lived.

PROFESSIONAL CELLULITE SOLUTIONS

IONITHERMIE
A salon treatment combining plant and mineral preparation with a gentle electric current; good for tone and texture and may be useful in combination with a basic home treatment programme.

MESOTHERAPY
An expensive medical therapy where minute quantities of pharmacological drugs are injected into the cellulite deposits to boost circulation, stimulate drainage and digest hard-lump tissues around cells. Should be combined with a basic home treatment programme.

CELLULOLIPOLYSIS
Invasive medical technique where electrodes encased in long needles are inserted into the cellulite. In a small unpublished study by a leading British cosmetic surgeon, only half of the patients said they saw any improvement.

SURGERY
No surgical intervention, e.g. liposuction, liposculpture or ultrasonic liposuction, has been shown to remove cellulite – and may damage circulation and the lymph system.

BEWARE! Clinics promising miracle cellulite cures spring up like mushrooms everywhere. Regimes are expensive, clients may be asked to pay up front and results seldom seem to match promises.

TRIED & TESTED

ANTI-AGEING BODY CREAMS

In our experience, women seem reluctant to invest in body creams – the 'poor relation' to face-saving miracle creams. However, our testers were extremely impressed with some of the top products in this category – which you may like to try to help improve dryness, goose-bumps – and even stretch marks...

Fenjal Body Milk
8.8 MARKS OUT OF 10 (£)
A new product from an old favourite range, this light but rich body milk contains active ingredients including vitamin E and vitamin B5. All of our testers said they would buy this excellent value lotion.
UPSIDE: 'definitely left skin silkier, smoother, plumper and brighter; not even a tingle on my sensitive skin' ◆ 'compared very well with costlier treatments; this is excellent and achieved noticeable results very quickly' ◆ 'rough areas like elbows, knees and soles of feet were transformed' ◆ 'my body – apart from neck and back of hands – looks 20 years younger!'
DOWNSIDE: 'bottle too big for travelling.'

Guerlain Issima Body Serum
8.75 MARKS OUT OF 10 (£££££)
This heavenly scented, luxuriously textured emulsion has an anti-free radical action and is designed to give long-lasting moisturisation, and to firm and tone. Four-fifths of testers who tried it would buy it.
UPSIDE: 'has given my skin a very pleasant smell and a softer, younger feeling; particularly good on elbows, knees, arms, legs and thighs. Lovely to use' ◆ 'the ultimate in luxury – I felt like Cleopatra!' ◆ 'sank into the skin really easily and left it lastingly hydrated' ◆ 'skin on upper arms appeared tighter' ◆ 'after using this serum my skin felt reborn; it will be on my Christmas list from now on'.
DOWNSIDE: 'not quite moisturising enough for mature skin' ◆ 'very good when used regularly, but shins were very dry and scaly again after one missed application'.

Decleor Système Corps
8.5 MARKS OUT OF 10 (£££)
Suitable for all skintypes but particularly designed for dry, dehydrated or 'lifeless' skin, this light, creamy milk is rich in natural plant ingredients. All but one of the testers said they would buy this product.
UPSIDE: 'it has improved areas where I had goosebump-type texture; lumpiness on inner thighs and arms has improved' ◆ 'I liked the fact I could dress immediately without worrying about it getting onto underwear' ◆ 'emulsion had a lovely feeling which stayed all day, like wearing silk undies' ◆ 'beautiful fragrance – no need to wear any perfume' ◆ 'marked smoothness on neck and elbow areas almost immediately'.
DOWNSIDE: 'pump dispenser difficult to use; did not improve dry elbows at all' ◆ 'immediate blotching on neck and throat but acclimatised after a few days' use'.

Vitace Body Lotion
8.4 MARKS OUT OF 10 (£££)
The name of this range gives away the key ingredients in this body lotion: antioxidamt vitamins A, C and E. All of the testers said they would buy this product.
UPSIDE: 'marvellous on legs, particularly after waxing; completely removed dry patches' ◆ 'liked the easy-to-use and lightweight packaging' ◆ 'immediately after use, skin was velvety and I did not feel at all greasy' ◆ 'pigmentation marks on my sun-damaged décolletage have improved' ◆ 'a real improvement in hardened skin on knees and with age spots on legs'.
DOWNSIDE: 'didn't like the smell at all'.

Estée Lauder Re-Nutriv Extra-Rich Firming Body Moisturiser
8.3 MARKS OUT OF 10 (££££)
This light, non-greasy cream promises to firm and tone slackened skin, prevent roughness – and Lauder actually make the claim that 'natural extracts will diminish the appearance of stretch marks caused by dramatic weight gain or loss.' Though it got some raves, only six out of ten testers said they'd buy it – most of them deterred by the high price, and a few by the smell.
UPSIDE: 'having recently had a baby, my stomach and thighs have benefited as it has helped tighten skin' ◆ 'skin on arms and lower neck improved drastically; I have never used such a pleasant product before which actually improved skin' ◆ 'my skin feels young, soft and silky again'.
DOWNSIDE: 'my usual cocoa butter moisturiser is equally as good and only a fraction of the price' ◆ 'a strange, buttery smell – not pleasant for a luxury lotion'.

Lancaster Oxygen Body Lotion
8.3 MARKS OUT OF 10 (£££)
A lightweight, gel emulsion, this uses a patented technology said to deliver oxygen to the skin. It contains fruit acids for skin-brightening, plus plant extracts. Despite very high scores from some testers, only just over half said they would buy it, largely due to price and/or packaging.
UPSIDE: 'loved the sheen it gave and saw a particular improvement in upper arms, décolletage and legs' ◆ 'very moisturising indeed; the effects last for a couple of days and flakiness on legs had gone in three days' ◆ 'goes a long way' ◆ 'quickly absorbed – unlike some body lotions'.
DOWNSIDE: 'no noticeable difference from any other body lotion and left my skin smelling rather unpleasant' ◆ 'only criticism is it's quite thick so you get through it quickly!'

Dr Hauschka Body Milk
8 MARKS OUT OF 10 (££)
Just over half the testers said they would buy this entirely natural product, made to a recipe based on herbs and oils such as peanut oil, olive oil, jojoba oil and extracts of sage, carrot and blackthorn.
UPSIDE: 'I had a skin reaction during the trial period but the skin cream was so soothing that I was able to avoid my usual steroids' ◆ 'skin was soft and smooth, with a fresh smell'; 'it helped very greatly in dry areas; I suffer flaky, sore skin on my legs in winter but using this has meant I haven't had it at all' ◆ 'I have had athlete's foot and nothing helped; using this cream has treated the skin, which was quite raw in places' ◆ 'both invigorating and soothing'.
DOWNSIDE: 'the texture was a little thin' ◆ 'it is very runny and if you were using it all over you would quickly use it up' ◆ 'slightly medicinal smell'.

NB The lowest scoring product in this category scored just 4.62 marks.

guidelines for golden girls' wardrobes

While exercise enhances body image and makes your wobbly bits less wobbly, the right choice of clothes can also work figure-slimming, confidenceboosting miracles. So 'Wardrobe Doctor' Amanda Platt* – a London-based freelance personal shopper and wardrobe consultant – offers this wisdom on stylish dressing for those of us of a certain age...

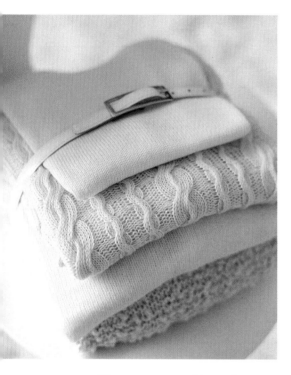

◆ 'Treat age as something to be cherished, rather than something to fight. If you're at ease with who you are, you'll look better in everything.'

◆ 'After a certain age you really can't get away with cheaper clothes. Buy fewer, better-cut clothes, because they'll give you extra help. Your big outlays should all be in neutral colours. After 25, cut is everything. Save up for things that don't date.'

◆ 'If you wear a baggy jacket you'll just look big all over. But if you invest in a jacket that is tailored and cut in at the "kidneys" – that area at the back, just above the waist – it will improve your shape, whatever shape you have.

◆ 'Small shoulder-pads can give a crisper line to T-shirts and knitwear, and balance a larger bust. (Not necessary for the broad-shouldered.)'

◆ 'Sleeves and skirts should get a little longer as we get older. Elbow-length sleeves – or below – are safest, to avoid the sight of underarms wobbling in the wind...'

◆ 'Frills and flounces are the kiss of death. Think crisp tailoring and clean lines – and keep it simple.'

◆ 'If you have any beautiful body part, dress to show it off – whether it's a neck, wrist, ankle, or waist. It distracts the eye from less-than-perfect parts...'

◆ 'Invest in good underwear, fitted by an expert. It's worth its weight in gold for the extra support and/or cinching-in that it delivers.'

◆ 'Get fitted regularly for a new bra. Bulging over your straps or cups makes you look as if you've put on weight.'

◆ 'Keep clothes dark from the waist down; dark tights, dark shoes, dark skirt creates a streamlined look. Then you can wear colour next to your face, to frame it.'

◆ 'Flat shoes are the most practical but they can make some women's ankles look bigger. I always have 1cm ($^1/_2$ inch) extra added onto the heel at a shoemaker's – that little bit of lift can make all the difference in the world...'

◆ 'Save jeans for gardening. Switch to slacks and tailored pants; they are also more comfortable.'

WHAT ALL WELL-DRESSED WARDROBES SHOULD CONTAIN...

◆ A good quality steam iron

◆ A professional steamer (or steam your clothes in the bathroom after your bath!)

◆ A special brush/sweater shaver for removing the 'pilling' from jerseys and cashmeres

◆ A sticky-tape roller

◆ Scotchguard fabric protector

◆ Sewing kit

◆ Button box

◆ Belt hangers

◆ Trouser hangers

◆ Skirt hangers

◆ Dress hangers

◆ A spot remover

◆ A tube of neutral leather cream

◆ A suede brush and spray

◆ Spray waterproofer for leather

◆ Moth-proofing spray (NB use all sprays near a wide open window or preferably outdoors, particularly if you are allergic)

◆ Hanging bags, preferably cloth

making summer bare-able...

As we get older, we love winter more – because it gives us the chance to hide less-than-perfect body bits under opaque tights and high-necked pullovers. But rather than sweat miserably through hot weather under too many layers, we thought we'd ask Belinda Seper – owner of ultra-stylish Belinda Boutique in Sydney's Double Bay, and Womenswear Fashion Director of Georges (the Terence Conran-owned Melbourne department store) – for her advice on how to dress when the mercury's rising...

◆ 'You don't have to go bare-legged if you don't think yours are up to it: look for sheer, 9-denier tights which are like gossamer. They feel as if you're wearing hardly anything but disguise uneven skintone – and seem to suck in those little bits that hang over the kneecap!'

◆ 'Floaty silk palazzo pants are a terrific choice for your bottom half. If you want to wear tighter clothes, go for stretch fabrics because they don't feel so restricting. A pair of the most expensive stretch pants that you can afford is a fantastic investment and will shave years – and inches – off. Today's stretch fabrics look just like any other fabric – but feel fabulous on.'

◆ 'Linen is a terrific summer fabric – if you can live with the crumples. Personally I like that layered linen look of a baggy shirt over trousers – but you have to give up being paranoid about not being perfectly ironed.'

◆ 'Check out tailoring in lightweight wools, which really are almost as cool to wear as cotton – but slightly more structured and business-like, and don't crumple.'

◆ 'For summer jackets, try lightweight wool mixes, silk mixes, linen mixes – blended with viscose or acetate. They're light enough to wear over a T-shirt without expiring, if you'd rather not take your jacket off. An alternative to the summer jacket is a soft, knitted silk or viscose cardigan. With pants and a simple T-shirt in cotton or silk, they're the picture of cool summer dressing.'

◆ 'Spend the maximum on swimwear that you can possibly afford. With swimsuits, you want them fabulously constructed on the inside, with tummy panels and uplift if you need it, plus a flattering cut to the leg. Spend time – and money – finding the right bathing suit. Remember: no swimming costumes at the buffet table. Wear a sarong – or buy a couple of yards of chiffon and tie it around your hips. (And don't forget lashings of SPF15 on the chest.)'

◆ 'Steer clear of anything around the neck: scarves or high necklines. They make for instant hot flushes – even if you're not menopausal...'

◆ 'I prefer clean, simple lines: a T-shirt snug to the body is much more flattering than a loose blouse.'

◆ 'Layer a sheer blouse over a T-shirt if you're self-conscious about your arms. You can put on a bodysuit, a camisole or a skinny underpiece and fling an organza, silk chiffon or georgette shirt over the top. Or drape a piece of chiffon over your arms, shawl-style – it's a wonderful fabric for disguising little bumps and curves and blurring the edges a little.'

◆ 'Beware of dresses that are too loose and floaty – the Ghost look. The risk is that you end up looking like a walking fridge and nobody can tell you've got a shape underneath. Try to buy dresses which are slightly more shaped at the waist, without being tight.'

◆ 'If summer dressing is a problem, go to a professional – or buy a book on how to dress stylishly and soak up the advice. People think that getting dressed and made up comes naturally – but it doesn't. You wouldn't mend your own lavatory; you'd get a plumber. If you don't want to go to a personal shopper, find a fashion sales assistant who's your age and whose style you like – not some skinny sixteen-year-old – for advice.'

◆ 'Age is a state of mind, not a number. Clothes can help – but there comes a point where women have to accept themselves for who they are, and the ageing process is part of that. We're all individual, and if we were all perfect, that would be boring. If I want to wear a sleeveless dress and it's a hot day, I wear it, even if I'm not that happy with my arms. I get a little bit funny about the veins in my legs but I'm too busy to get them fixed. There are plenty of people out there who specialise in helping you look and feel fabulous – so if there's something that really bugs you, deal with it. Otherwise, quit worrying and enjoy life.'

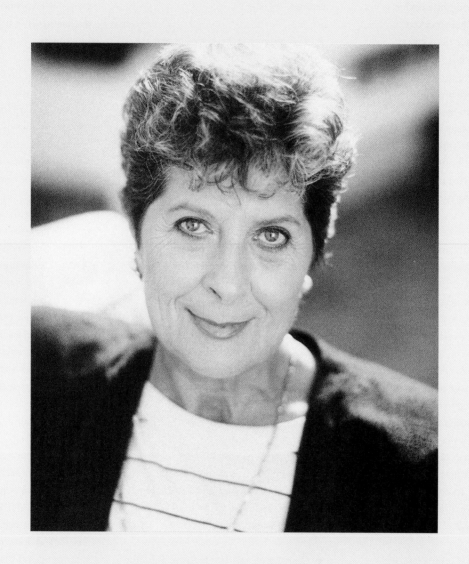

Joan Burstein

Joan Burstein, founder of Browns, the most elegant clothes store in London, is a legend for her style and charm. She has been through tough times – illness, bankruptcy and all the ups and downs of family and business life – but she faces the world with the calm straight gaze of a woman at peace with herself. Now a great grandmother, she glows with the zest and joie de vivre of a teenager.

'I always knew what I liked and how I wanted to look, even as a child. And trends in magazines always influenced me. I was one of the few women to get magazines during the War. I worked in a chemist and wanted the *Ladies Home Journal* and the girl in WH Smith wanted Nivea cream. So we bartered.

'The main thing is your body when it comes to looking stylish and attractive in clothes. You must keep it fit, respect it and become involved in it. You have to be disciplined not to put on weight. I am, because I don't feel comfortable if I get heavier.

'I've always been athletic; I used to run and high jump, and nowadays I swim and walk a lot in the country. I do floor exercises every day for about 20 minutes for a slightly weak back.

'I really believe in reflexology. Sue Reid comes to me at home every week now and if there is a problem she usually manages to pinpoint and unblock it, so the energy flows again.

'My husband taught me the importance of the body's relationship to what you eat, what you do and how you are. He was a vegetarian when I met him. He's a thinking man, very special. Years ago a wonderful naturopath, Gordon Latto, saved my teeth for me. I had very bad gums after my second child was born and my dentist told me I would have to lose my

teeth – at 25. Another specialist agreed. It was put down to poor nourishment during the War which had led to an infection taking hold. But Gordon told me that if I ate only raw vegetables and fruit for nine months, I could save them. No hot food because heat in the mouth encourages the germs. The problem wasn't my teeth, he said, but the gums. To strengthen them the blood had to be regenerated. I did it – and my teeth were fine.

'I'm not a silly eater and some things – like red meat and shellfish – don't suit me so I don't eat them. I love raw vegetables and fruit. All organic if possible – it's the only food one should be eating now.

'I wish I could meditate, but I seem to have too many thoughts in my mind, so I relax by reading. I like all sorts of books for different purposes: holiday books like *Captain Corelli's Mandolin*, aeroplane books like John Grisham's and books for the soul.

'We started Browns in 1970. The inspiration was simply survival. We had had a very large business which unfortunately went into receivership. We lost our home, everything, the children had to come out of school. It was a cruel process but we did learn from it. Browns is wonderful. I have a brilliant, supportive team and I don't come in at the crack of dawn

nowadays except when I'm buying – then it's 12 hour days but I do take time off for R and R!

'I'm on the go all the time so my clothes have got to be comfortable as well as looking good. And I have to feel very at ease in myself. I like simple clothes in beautiful fabrics. You must choose clothes that are your shape – my wardrobe is full of a designer called Zoran because I know that I look good in his clothes and can go anywhere in them. For evenings I wear floppy charmeuse silk pants with a chiffon t-shirt and perhaps a jacket. I used to wear bright colours but my skin tone changes as I get older and I prefer neutrals like navy, black or grey with a touch of colour in a scarf. And I love white: on holiday I wear it all the time, but not in the store because it gets grubby. Shoes are very difficult because I have a large broad foot with a high arch so I wear trousers which disguise them. And I love my pearls – in or out of fashion, I don't care.

'Sometimes when I'm feeling particularly tired I think maybe cosmetic surgery or collagen injections might be nice but then I think 'Well, I'm too old for it'. It satisfies vanity – nothing wrong with that – but it doesn't really change anything. For me the most important thing is health. That's all that truly matters.'

the fabulously simple guide to eating for health, beauty and happiness

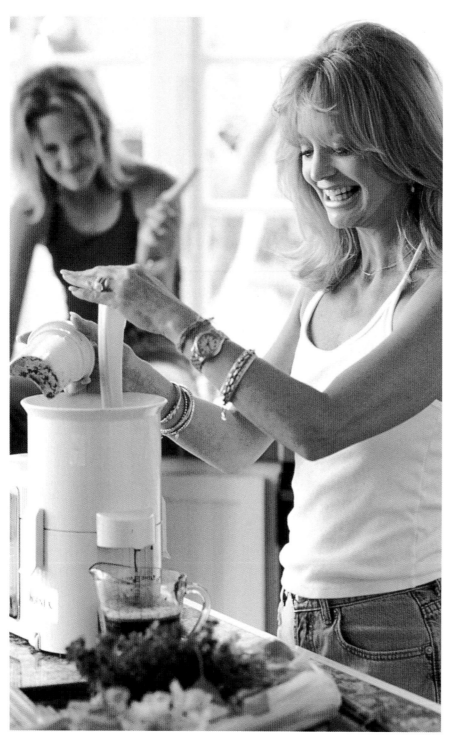

We truly are what we eat. Each one of us is made up of about 63 per cent water, 22 per cent protein, 13 per cent fat and 2 per cent vitamins and minerals. Every bit of that comes from what we eat and drink. But the perfect fuel is not only nutritious – it's totally delicious. So your ultimate feel-good eating plan – to be enjoyed forever – starts here...

What we put in our bodies directly affects the way we look, our health (present and future), energy levels, our moods and even our brain power. So it's vital to get it right. It's politically correct nowadays to say that there is no such thing as good food and bad food. If you don't have enough, then of course *all* food is good. But most of us today actually have too much – and we spend our time trying *not* to eat. So we're going to put our mouths where our money is and say we think there *is* a difference in the quality of food on offer.

Much mass-produced food – vegetables, fruit, meat and particularly cook-chill and processed food – is poor quality. It will keep you going but it may not give you the nourishment you need for gleaming health. The nutrients may have been leeched out by intensive production and by processing. More worryingly, it may well contain added chemicals which could impair our health. For instance, recent research in

Denmark has found that the growing number of sometimes life-threatening antibiotic-resistant 'superbugs', which are sweeping through our hospitals, may be connected with the increasing use of antibiotics in animal feeds.

Good-quality food for us is organic, grown and produced without the addition of unnatural chemicals. Both of us buy, grow and eat organic food. That's not every single mouthful – but as much as possible. (While we try to pick organic dishes on restaurant menus, for instance, we're not about to give up eating out just because there isn't much organic restaurant food around.) We like food the way Nature intended, not put through umpteen chemical processes or genetically engineered. In the main, we eat vegetables, fruit, hardly any meat, a bit of fish and cheese, lots of grains and pulses, and plenty of good olive oil. You could call it eating like an Italian or Greek peasant – which is just fine because they've been proven scientifically to have the healthiest diet of all. We also love Japanese food and eat lots of soya and seaweed *(see p.193)*. And we're very keen on the odd mouthful of organic chocolate too.

Conventionally produced food simply doesn't taste as good as organic, also the battery of chemicals used on non-organic food – pesticides, antibiotics and growth hormones – may harm our health. Could someone please tell us: what's the *point* of intensively produced or genetically engineered food? (Apart from great profit to the food and chemical business of course.)

An eminent member of the industry told us that the reason food is now being genetically engineered is simply because scientists have found out how to do it. And because some international companies have staked literally billions on its success.

Apparently, Bill Clinton is behind GE food because it has been earmarked as one of the big growth industries of the 21st century. But we don't think that's a great reason for using consumers as guinea pigs for a new technology which may harm our health and environment.

The argument against organic is that it's more expensive. That partly depends on what you buy. If, for instance, you cut down on meat, in line with all the medical recommendations, and use it as a garnish instead of the centrepiece of a meal, your bills plummet. Cost also depends on where you shop – supermarket or farm shop. Another way of cutting costs is to grow your own. Increasingly, people are growing at least some of their own vegetables and salads – in back gardens, allotments, window boxes, grow-bags – which not only saves money but is deeply satisfying.

Listening to all the different health lobby groups, you might think that you should eat one way to help protect you against cancer, another for heart disease, and yet another for osteoporosis. And that's before you've got round to thinking about the food that's slimming, and gives you energy, sparkling eyes, glossy hair and clear skin.

The good news is that, actually, the way to fulfil all those food requirements is the same. It's very simple. And it's here in the **feel fabulous forever** food guide. What's more, it's delicious. We know; we eat this way. We never diet – and we're pretty happy with our shapes. We never ever go hungry, we're bursting with energy, and we're always having treats. Try it.

EATING THE NATURAL WAY...

◆ We are designed to graze, not gorge, so eat several – three to five – light meals daily rather than one or two heavy ones.

◆ Breakfast an hour or so after you wake up so your digestion has had a chance to get going; never skip breakfast – you risk weight gain and low energy.

◆ Sit down at lunchtime for at least 45 minutes if possible and try to eat it in good company.

◆ Try not to drink too much with meals – it flushes the food through your body before it can be absorbed.

◆ Eat fruit between meals or at the beginning of a meal: it can get stuck in your digestive tract and ferment if eaten last.

◆ Have your last meal at least two hours before sleep.

IDEAL FIGURES

Experts agree that for optimum health, what we eat should be divided up like this:

carbohydrate	70%
fat	15%
protein	15%

In fact, what most people eat looks like this:

carbohydrate	28%
fat	40%
protein	12%
sugar	20%

what's what in the food you eat

CARBOHYDRATE

Carbohydrate, which consists of sugars and starches, is the body's main fuel. It comes in two forms: 'fast release' and 'slow release'. 'Fast release' foods include sugar, honey, malt, sweets and most refined foods; these give a spurt of energy as your blood sugar levels zoom up and then a slump as they crash down again. 'Slow release' foods include vegetables, fresh fruit and whole grains; these provide more sustained energy because they contain more complex carbohydrates and/or more fibre which help moderate the sugar release into the bloodstream.

Aim to eat 'slow release' carbo-hydrates as the mainstay of your diet; making up 70 per cent of your total daily intake.

PROTEIN

This is absolutely essential, because it contains the 25 amino acids (forms of protein) which are the building blocks of the body. The best quality protein sources are fish, meat, beans, peas, lentils, quinoa, soya and eggs.

Aim to eat 35g (1^1/4oz) of protein daily, with one small serving of meat, fish, cheese or a free-range egg, to make up 15 per cent of your daily diet.

FIBRE

This absorbs water in the digestive tract, making food bulkier and easier to pass through the body; it maintains energy levels, and helps to prevent constipation and putrefaction of food (the underlying cause of many digestive complaints, including diverticulitis, colitis and bowel cancer). Eating a fibre-rich breakfast cereal is a proven way of helping to protect against bowel cancer. Fibre is found in whole grains, vegetables, fruit, nuts, seeds, lentils and beans.

Aim to eat at least 35g (1^1/4oz) of fibre daily, making up 10 per cent of your calorie intake.

FATS

Fats or lipids are essential for the body, but in the right form – (see Eat The Right Fat, p.195).

Bad fats

◆ Saturated fat is hard fat, found mainly in meat and dairy products, and is not essential for the body; it's linked to obesity, heart disease and a wide range of other illnesses.

◆ Hydrogenated (hardened) fats (aka trans fatty acids) are found in processed foods and are thought to cause raised blood cholesterol and contribute to heart disease and some cancers.

Good fats (see also p.195)

◆ Unsaturated fat is found in cold pressed oils, nuts and seeds, and is thought to lower harmful cholesterol.

◆ Omega-3 is an essential fat found in oily fish with teeth (salmon, tuna, mackerel, herrings, sardines), linseeds, walnuts and walnut oil, flax seeds and oil. It is vital for the brain and nervous system, immune system, cardiovascular system and skin.

◆ Omega-6 is another essential fat and is found in sunflower and sesame seeds, and in safflower, soya and linseed.

Aim to eat: good fats only, and reduce fat intake from average 41 per cent of diet to a maximum of 30 per cent, and ideally 15 per cent.

THE BLOOD SUGAR CONNECTION

Stabilising your blood sugar levels is probably the most important factor in maintaining energy and weight levels, according to nutritionist Patrick Holford, as the amount of glucose (sugar) in the blood largely determines your appetite.

Glucose is raw material which your cells convert to energy. When the level drops, you feel hungry. When it's too high, the body converts the excess to glycogen, a short-term fuel stored mainly in the liver and muscle cells, or to fat, our long-term energy reserve. About three in every ten people find difficulty in keeping their blood sugar stable rather than soaring too high and then dropping too low.

Low blood sugar can trigger a whole raft of symptoms including fatigue, poor concentration, irritability, sweating, depression, headaches and digestive problems.

The ideal is to keep our blood sugar levels on an even keel. Eating sugary foods is the biggest offender, with glucose – and foods which contain it – the worst of all. The best foods are pulses – peas, beans and lentils – and whole grains; all are high in complex carbohydrates and release their sugar content slowly. They are also high in fibre, which helps to stabilise blood sugar levels as well as aiding the digestive process. Following the friendly foods in our **feel fabulous forever** food guide should keep you on an even keel. Just remember not to skip meals.

the **big** question

There is a common belief that as women get older, it's inevitable that they get plumper. True or not? Not true, says leading expert Professor Michael Lean, of the Department of Human Nutrition at the University of Glasgow, although we may change *shape*. The shift in hormone levels with the menopause (i.e.falling oestrogen levels and comparatively higher testosterone levels) means that we are more likely to store fat around our middles rather than our hips. But hormone changes don't result in a major shift in appetite – and thus weight. It's more likely that we simply take less exercise and/or eat more, as we get older.

Nevertheless, the big and growing problem of overweight and obesity in the so-called developed world should be taken seriously. Everyone can lose weight, according to Professor Lean, with a 'combined' programme of sensible diet, exercise plus psychological support.

Danger signs for obesity used to be predicted on Body Mass Index. Doctors have now simplified this and say that women of any height whose waist measurement is 80cm (32 inches) or more should try not to get bigger and, if possible, to take off some pounds. This emphatically does not mean crash dieting – it means lifestyle changes along the lines we suggest in **feel fabulous forever**. With a waist of 88cm (35inches) or more, women are in danger of a serious medical problem and should consult their doctors immediately.

Professor Lean cautions most seriously against women consulting slimming clinics without their GP's referral and taking drugs which have not been scientifically validated and may be dangerous. 'Whether these clinics are in a village hall or in Harley Street in London, it's the same thing. They charge huge prices for drugs which cost pennies and patients are unlikely to receive the good multi-disciplinary care they need.'

For truly intractable cases of obesity, two new presription-only slimming pills – Sibutramine and Orlistat – are becoming available and are far preferable to the current choice, says Professor Lean. Surgery is a final option.

food for flatter tums

Washboard stomachs are pretty unrealistic for most older women but almost everyone will be able to reduce a Rubenesque belly. An efficiently working digestion and strong stomach muscles are the way to a flatter tummy. If you bloat easily, try cutting out all foods containing wheat, beans and all carbonated drinks. Explore food combining *(see p.196)* where fruit is eaten as a snack only, never at main meals, and protein foods are not eaten at the same meal as carbohydrates. All exercise will help, while re-bounding on a mini-trampoline has a marvellous effect on constipation. Also check out whether you may have food sensitivities, candida or Irritable Bowel Syndrome (IBS) *(see pp.198–199)*. Then concentrate on the posture exercises on *p.164* to improve your stomach muscles.

THREE GOOD REASONS NEVER TO DIET

◆ It doesn't work: 90 per cent of people who go on diets put the weight back – and more – within two years. (Consider **Liz Taylor**.)

◆ Yo-yo dieting is a body and . mind stressor which contributes to hormonal problems, osteoporosis, cellulite, hair loss and chronic illness – and robs you of energy.

◆ Eating well – and taking exercise – will give you lots of energy and keep your body looking great at its natural weight. If you need to lose weight, try food combining *(see p.196)*. Good food makes you thinner. Fill up on complex carbs rather than quick-fix fatty or sugary snacks. 240 cals of stomach-satisfying potato are almost seven times more filling than the same cals of wouldn't-fill-up-a-bird croissant.

The opposite of fat is healthy – *not* thin.

Eat fruit till noon, salad and berries for lunch and either proteins or carbohydrates for dinner – but don't mix. And water, water everywhere: both sides of your bed, in the kitchen, even in the hallway. Bottled water is easiest – just grab and swig.
LAUREN HUTTON

superfoods for women

Scientists are learning more every day about the role of certain foods as disease-preventers, infection-fighters and potential life-extenders. And a new nutritional concept is emerging: eating more of certain foods so that we feel more vital and healthy and protect ourselves against illness.
We asked three of the world's top nutritionists – Joseph Pizzorno from Bastyr University in Seattle, Patrick Holford from the Institute of Optimum Nutrition in London, and Kathryn Marsden, best-selling author and nutritional consultant – to prescribe the superfoods that every woman needs as she ages...

why we should all eat organic...

In addition to not assaulting our bodies with potentially harmful levels of toxic chemicals, every nutritionist we have ever spoken to is agreed: organic is best – nutritionally too. 'Although so far there's been precious little research comparing the nutrients in organic versus conventionally grown foods, the research that has been done is highly compelling in favour of organics,' explains Dr Joseph Pizzorno. 'One study showed that the selenium content in organic food was four times that of conventional produce. In another study, the zinc content was 50 per cent higher in the organic food. We're talking about huge differences. The message is clear: organically grown foods are safer and much more nutritious.' Adds Patrick Holford, 'Although organic food is often 25 per cent more expensive than non-organic, it usually contains less water and more solid matter – including nutrients. So it really doesn't work out more expensive – yet it's so much better for you...'

SOYA

All three agreed that soy-based products like tofu, tempeh, miso and soya milk – which contain beneficial plant oestrogens called phytoestrogens – have important implications for women's health. During childbearing years, these plant chemicals can help prevent breast cancer; Asian women who eat large amounts of soy have a five-times lower rate of breast cancer than women who eat a typical Western diet. During menopause, when oestrogen levels drop by 60 per cent, phytoestrogens can help make up the difference. The optimum daily intake, according to our experts, is around 100–200mg of soya a day. 'The equivalent of a 350g (12oz) serving of soya milk or a serving of tofu,' explains Patrick Holford. Although many vegetarian foods contain soya in the form of soya protein (burgers, frankfurters, etc.), Dr Pizzorno warns that this may have been highly processed and prefers tofu and soya milk.

CRUCIFEROUS VEGETABLES

'Broccoli, Brussels sprouts, cabbage and cauliflower contain substances which improve the ability of the liver to deal with both the toxins in our environment and those we produce internally,' explains Dr Pizzorno. 'They also contain useful cancer-protecting compounds.' Adds Patrick Holford: 'Research has shown that if you eat cabbage more than once a week, you are reducing your risk of developing colon cancer by two thirds.' Better still, believes Dr Pizzorno, eat between 115–175g (4–6oz) a day – 'in any combination' – preferably raw or juiced, as cooking destroys vital enzymes. (Other cruciferous vegetables are cress, horseradish, kale, kohlrabi, mustard greens, radish and turnip.)

BLUEBERRIES

'Blueberries are rich in anthocyanidins, a type of flavonoid, which help protect the eyes from macular degeneration.' Anthocyanidins are present in all berries with a blue/purple colour, i.e. black grapes, blackcurrants and cranberries,' says Dr Pizzorno. You can also try supplementing with concentrated extracts. (Find berry extracts in natural food stores.) Eat daily, if possible.

BRAZIL NUTS

'An excellent source of selenium,' explains Dr Pizzorno. 'There is amazing data emerging on the link between selenium deficiency and increased rates of cancer. Selenium is a terrific immune-booster. In addition, it helps healthy thyroid function; often, people who have low energy levels may be suffering from selenium deficiency.' A handful of shelled Brazil nuts each day can help.

Patrick Holford adds other nuts – particularly almonds and hazelnuts – to the list of health-boosting nuts, together with seeds like flax, sesame, and sunflower. 'To get a balance, mix together sesame, sunflower and flax seeds and keep them in a sealed jar in the fridge. Eat a heaped tablespoon of these, ground, each day.' (NB Delicious sprinkled on salads.)

GARLIC

Explains Patrick Holford, 'Garlic contains about 200 biologically active compounds, many of which have a role in preventing disease – including cancer and heart disease.' Dr Pizzorno, like Patrick Holford, prescribes a clove a day, cooked or raw.

TOMATOES

Tomatoes help guard the eyes as we age as they are high in substances called lutein and lycopene to protect against macular degeneration. Eat them juiced, raw, in pasta sauce, or in ready made products – around 50g (2oz) a day, to get the protective dose.

BREWER'S YEAST

'I'm a great believer in this old stand-by,' says Dr Pizzorno. 'It's a good source of protein, packed with B vitamins and high in chromium, which helps regulate blood sugar levels.'

SHIITAKE MUSHROOMS

These have immune-system enhancing properties; they contain lentinan, a powerful immunity booster. Shiitake are one of the few vegetable sources of vitamin D, rich in calcium and phosphorus, with high levels of many amino acids. Buy them fresh or dry (soak before cooking); aim for one serving, twice a week.

QUINOA (pronounced keen-wa)

Known as "the mother grain" because of its unique sustaining properties; it contains significantly more protein than any other grain – and the quality of protein is better than meat,' says Patrick Holford. It offers almost four times as much calcium as wheat, plus extra iron, B vitamins and vitamin E. Find it in natural food stores. (It's also

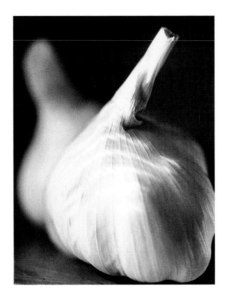

delicious in stir-fries with vegetables and tofu.) Go for one serving, twice a week (more often if you're vegetarian).

FISH (if you're not vegetarian)

In addition to being rich in protein, vitamins and minerals (especially selenium), fish is a good source of brain-enhancing nutrients; oily fish (mackerel, herring, salmon, tuna, shark and swordfish) are rich in Essential Fatty Acids. Aim for three servings a week.

EXTRA VIRGIN OLIVE OIL

This is packed with monounsaturates and is good for the heart. Olive oil seems to help blood sugar levels as well. Use it in cooking or pour it on

salads – 1–2 tablespoons a day.

AVOCADO

'A great skin food,' says Kathryn Marsden. 'Avocado is also rich in monounsaturates. Many women worry that avocado is fattening because of the high oil content, but there are only 190 calories in an average fruit. Avocado is rich in potassium, vitamin E (which is anti hot flush), carotene, folic acid, B5, biotin and vitamin C, plus the thyroid nutrient iodine. Piled high with hummus and a green salad, you've got a perfect, nutritious, filling meal.'

YOGHURT

'Sheep's and goat's yoghurt are best, as they're easier to digest than cow's milk, says Kathryn. A terrific source of calcium, it helps keep the digestive flora healthy, as it contains "friendly" bacteria. The levels of these bacteria diminish the longer you keep it, so buy it fresh in small quantities.'

◆ Our vote for a superfood goes to seaweed: when we're really tired and need to zing the next day, we have a Japanese meal with miso soup, seaweed salad and sizzling tofu steaks in ginger and soy sauce, possibly with a side order of veggie oshinkomaki or California rolls. And we do feel fab the next day. Seaweed is one of the richest sources of calcium. It is full of minerals that help to create and maintain bone mass, lower blood pressure, eliminate varicose veins and haemorrhoids, restore and increase heart efficiency and relieve incontinence, vaginal dryness and persistent hot flushes, according to Virginia M. Soffa, Director of the Breast Cancer Action Group in Burlington, Vermont.

fabulously friendly foods

ALWAYS TRY TO BUY:
Fresh, organic food, locally produced

Vegetables (unlimited)
Raw or lightly cooked. Aim for five portions a day

Beans, peas (fresh or dried)

Lentils

Whole grains (aka cereals)
e.g. brown rice, millet, rye, oats, quinoa, wholemeal bread, corn, wholewheat pasta
Aim for four portions a day

Fruit
Aim for three portions a day as snacks

Soya foods, e.g. tofu, soya milk

Live yoghurt

Seeds (sunflower, sesame, safflower)

Brazil nuts (buy unshelled)

Almonds and hazelnuts

Extra virgin olive oil, cold pressed

Plus, if you're not vegetarian, add in two to three servings weekly of:
Shellfish

Eggs, from organic-fed hens (salmonella and campylobacter are endemic in others)

Organic white meat
e.g. chicken with skin off

DRINK
Choose:
Still pure water – 1.5–2 litres (3–3½ pints) daily
Organic herbal teas
Vegetable juices (try home-made)
Fruit juice diluted with water
A little (under two glasses daily)
Good wine

energy sapping enemy foods

TRY TO AVOID
Processed, refined, ready-prepared, packaged and/or canned foods

Diet foods

Refined white sugar/flour and other quick-fix carbohydrates, e.g. white bread, biscuits, cakes, candy bars

Low-fat cheeses or spreads

Sauces with additives

Cow's milk

Refined wheat or sugar-loaded breakfast cereals

Saturated (hard) fats, e.g. meat and dairy fat

Bran and bran-containing foods: they can interfere with calcium absorption

Artificial flavours, colourings, sweeteners, preservatives

Salt/salty foods

Polyunsaturated spreads

Processed, smoked, coloured fish/cheese/meat

Pork/beef

DRINK
Avoid:
Fizzy drinks which are high in phosphate
Artificially sweetened drinks
Coffee, tea
Beer, lager, spirits

THE FACTS OF FAT

◆ Most of us eat too much of the wrong sort of fat. Over 40 per cent of our calories come from fat, and more than half from saturated fat. Health experts tell us that fat should provide no more than 15–30 per cent of our diet.

◆ Saturated fat is a major 'baddie', particularly in terms of heart disease and strokes: too much meat, eggs and butter can pile up the fatty cholesterol deposits in our arteries and cause weight problems. Saturated fat is present in most animal foods, including meat and dairy products.

◆ Swapping from butter to margarine (which is made from vegetable oil) may not automatically be the answer, if the oil in the margarine has been 'hydrogenated'. Hydrogenation is a process that converts liquid oils into solid oils, but at the same time it produces substances called 'trans-fatty acids', which actually increase blood cholesterol and blood fats and are said to disrupt the vital functions of EFAs. 'Hydrogenated fats act as blockers, stopping the good fats getting through,' says Dr Erasmus. So look for a margarine or spread which says 'non-hydrogenated' on the label – and be aware that many, many processed foods (including biscuits, cakes, ice-cream and many ready-prepared meals) contain hydrogenated vegetable oils. (Margarines are also linked with allergies, according to recent research from Germany.)

◆ Heating oils for cooking – even in stir-frying – destroys EFAs, explains Dr Erasmus, and may actually be harmful. 'Burning oil, where you create smoke, actually makes it carcinogenic,' he says.

eat (the right) fats – and oil your skin from the inside out…

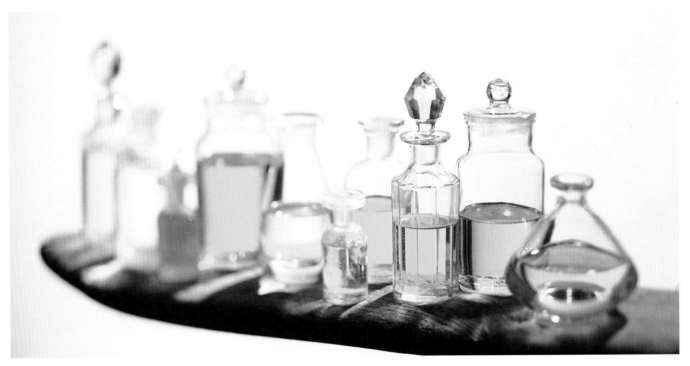

Low-fat mania is sweeping the world. But our bodies – and our complexions – actually need fat. Because without it we may be fast-forwarding ageing…

According to L.A.-based plastic surgeon Richard Ellenbogen, MD, 'Very low-fat diets suck the oils out of the skin. We see people in their thirties on low-fat diets who look like prunes.'

Dr Udo Erasmus, a leading international expert, agrees. 'Our bodies need to be oiled,' he tells us. 'Oils – which contain Essential Fatty Acids (EFAs) – do a wonderful job. If you get the right balance, they form a barrier on the skin against loss of moisture, giving soft, smooth, velvety skin; plus the fine lines and wrinkles that come from dryness will diminish.' Among other vital health-protecting roles, fats transport the vital fat-soluble vitamins A, D, E and K round the body.

EFAs are found in vegetable oils (in particular in flax seed and hemp oils), seeds, nuts and some other foods like oily fish. The EFAs that play such a vital role are omega-6 (gamma-linolenic acid or GLA) and omega-3 (alpha-linolenic acid) fatty acids, and we need a balance: two thirds omega-3, one third omega-6. The good news is that to save us the trouble of working out if we're getting the sums right, balanced mixtures of oil are available in capsules, or as liquid oils*. (These oils can taste quite delicious swallowed from the spoon – or sprinkled on salads; aim for 1–2 tablespoons a day, or the equivalent in capsules.)

Fascinatingly, the fastest way to tell if you're getting enough EFAs is a DIY skin test. 'The skin is the last organ to get the oil; if it gets there, you know it's got everywhere.' Dr Erasmus suggests taking a sauna or a hot bath, towelling skin dry but not applying a body cream or lotion. 'If skin still feels papery and dry, you should up your intake of EFAs. When you're getting enough, you should reach a point where putting a moisturiser on your skin is no longer necessary – because your skin is being lubricated from inside by EFAs.' If taking extra EFAS in the form of seed oils doesn't improve your skin (and therefore all your organs), you may be one of the approximately 20 per cent who can't convert the EFAs from seed oils; instead, try EFAs in the form of 1000mg of evening primrose oil or borage (starflower) oil.

food combining

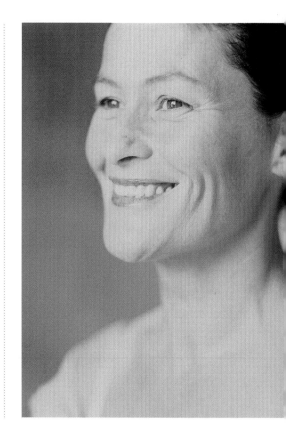

Food combining, also known as the Hay Diet, has been around for some 75 years since Dr William Howard Hay devised it to help patients recover from chronic problems. The basis of it is not mixing foods that Dr Hay and his followers believe fight in your stomach – i.e. proteins and starches – and keeping fruit separate. This way of eating, say its supporters (who include us), eases digestive and other chronic problems including allergies, headaches and skin problems.

Despite the fact that many people have found it of enormous help, most doctors are still adamant that it has no scientific basis and is simply a faddy way of eating, which has no point except that you are bound to lose weight because you are eating less. However, Professor Jonathan Brostoff ** is open-minded: 'It helps about half my patients who suffer from Irritable Bowel Syndrome (IBS) – but the trouble is, I don't know which half. But it certainly can't hurt so I often suggest they get hold of a book on food combining.

Nutritionist Kathryn Marsden, who has written several best-selling books on her own simplified form of food combining, gives us the basics.

◆ Introduce this way of eating into your diet for one or two days a week to start with, to ease yourself into it.
◆ If you find that it suits you, increase that to three, four or five days weekly. But don't put yourself under pressure to follow it slavishly: healthy eating should not be a cult religion or make you feel deprived. Indulgence days are positively to be encouraged.
◆ Increase your intake of fresh fruit but eat it as a snack between meals or as a starter, not with your proteins or starches.
◆ Also try snacking on a handful of dried fruit, nuts or seeds.
◆ Drink plenty of water between meals.
◆ If you want to lose weight, aim each day for: one protein-based meal served with plenty of fresh vegetables or salad, one starch-based meal served with a good-sized portion of fresh veg or salad; plus one meal based on either a vegetable dish, e.g. a big salad, stir-fry or stew, or a selection of any fresh fruits.
◆ If you aren't worried about your weight, try the alternative of one protein-based meal and two starch-based meals per day, with generous portions of fresh salad or vegetables.

HOW TO FOOD COMBINE

Proteins in Column A will mix with anything from Column B. Starches in Column C will mix with anything from Column B. Don't mix Column A with Column C.

A Proteins	B Mix with A or C	C Starches
Fish/shellfish	All veg except potatoes	Potatoes/sweet potatoes
Free-range eggs	and sweet potatoes	All grains including: oats,
Organic poultry	All salads	pasta, brown rice, rye, millet,
Lean lamb	Seeds	couscous, quinoa, bulgar
Cheese	Nuts	Sweetcorn
Yoghurt	Herbs	Flour
All soya products	Fats and oils including:	Bread/crackers
Milk (but keep to	cream, butter,	Pastry
a minimum)	margarine and extra	
	virgin olive oil	

NB Pulses (peas, beans, lentils) combine well with all kinds of veg and salads and with other starches but can cause digestive problems if mixed with protein foods.

prevent dementia with green veg and party games

Alzheimer's disease is the commonest form of dementia in the elderly. But heart disease, stroke and endocrine (hormonal) disorders, as well as rarer conditions such as the human form of BSE, can also bring about the brain deterioration which causes this infinitely distressing condition. Dementia affects about one in ten people over 65, one in five over 75.

Problems include memory loss, personality changes, impaired ability to reason, being disorientated and unable to care for oneself.

Dr Kim Jobst**, previously Clinical Director of the ten-year OPTIMA study (Oxford Project to Investigate Memory and Aging), suggests the following ways of protecting the brain and perhaps preventing dementia.

1 Recent research suggests that B vitamins (mainly folic acid, vitamins B6 and B12) have the same protective effect on the brain as they do against heart disease and stroke, cancer and possibly even multiple sclerosis, by helping lower high blood levels of homocysteine, a damaging amino acid. So eat plenty of foods containing B vitamins, e.g. fresh fruit and vegetables which are also rich in brain-protecting antioxidants. Check your levels of folic acid and vitamin B12 with your GP, a qualified naturopath or nutritionist; if they are low, eat well and consider supplements, preferably under guidance. The current recommended doses are 2.5–5mg folic acid, plus 2mcg daily of B12 for one week, then 400mcg folic acid daily plus a B complex supplement which includes B12. (Folic acid supplements alone may be dangerous if B12 levels are very low.)

2 Keep up oestrogen levels. There is some evidence that HRT may protect the brain against the development of memory problems and Alzheimer's disease, as well as protecting against heart disease and osteoporosis. You can also boost oestrogen levels by eating soya-based products and other phytoestrogens *(see pp.197 and 218)*, which are also very high in folic acid.

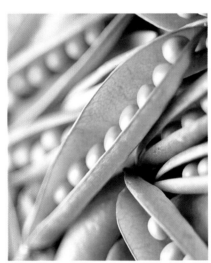

3 Take regular exercise: research suggests that lack of it may be a risk factor for dementia.

4 Avoid prolonged stress and stressful situations, and keep anxiety levels down. Too much stress has a damaging effect on the blood supply to the heart and the brain.

5 Don't vegetate: it's clear that continuous mental exercise helps protect the mind from decay. Try puzzles, crosswords, games, models, three dimensional games, learning routes etc. Kim's game (memorising objects on a tray over a minute or so, then writing them down when the tray is whisked away) is particularly good.

There is evidence that people who set about learning poetry, plays or new skills when they find their memory is beginning to fail, seem able to slow down deterioration or even improve their memory.

6 Keep existing hobbies going and try to learn new skills, especially musical ones. Those who learn to play an instrument seem less likely to get dementia, as do those who educate themselves or study with others. Gardening is particularly good for keeping mind and brain alert.

7 Pray and/or meditate. Time to relax, reflect and be at peace protects against not only dementia, but also heart disease, cancer, depression, general infections and other problems of ageing.

8 Keep in touch with friends and family and organise an active social life. Interact with agreeable people.

9 Consider herbs: there is evidence that ginkgo biloba, the Chinese maidenhair fern tree, improves the blood supply to the brain and may help slow down the progression of Alzheimer's disease. Sage may also help protect the brain. Consult your GP and/or herbalist before taking any supplements. Don't be afraid to ask for more than one opinion!

10 In general: live well, eat well, drink good red wine in moderation, stop smoking, sustain relationships and activities and – above all – be positive and enjoy life, since all these things help keep your immunity up, your blood vessels unclogged, your melatonin and DHEA levels high and your brain active and alive, and so diminish the risk of dementia.

when food is unfriendly

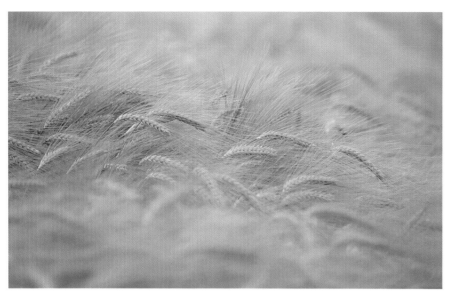

Most of the time food is not only necessary to sustain our bodies, it's also a treat for our minds. But for some people, it seems, things are going wrong...

Some foods (among them tree nuts, shellfish and peanuts) clearly have a harmful effect on people who are allergic to them: they risk going into a potentially life-threatening condition called anaphylactic shock. Equally, migraine sufferers will almost certainly be told by their doctors that cheese, citrus fruit, chocolate and wine are likely to trigger their blinding headaches. Asthma attacks and eczema are also known to be triggered by food allergens. So the link between some foods and ill-health is firmly established. Some doctors, though, have long believed that there may be a wider problem – that in addition to severe food allergy, there may be a more widespread, less severe effect which they term food 'sensitivity' or 'intolerance'.

Until recently this was a cue for most doctors to raise their eyebrows and mutter phrases about quack medicine.

Now all that has changed. The British Government has an on-going research programme into food. It has produced a list of the most common trigger foods which may cause serious reactions in sensitised people: peanuts, tree nuts, fish, shellfish, eggs and seeds, e.g. sesame. Less acute reactions may occur with cow's milk, soya, wheat and other cereals (grains). Further offenders include tomatoes, oranges, chocolate, coffee and tea, plus artificial flavourings, preservatives and additives.

The non-fatal consequences of food intolerance can have a very distressing and debilitating effect on people's lives. According to *The Complete Guide to Food Allergy and Intolerance** by Professor Jonathan Brostoff and Linda Gamlin, the gamut of symptoms, running from top to toe, may include:

◆ Headache, migraine, fatigue, depression/anxiety (and hyperactivity in children); recurrent mouth ulcers

◆ Aching muscles

◆ Vomiting, nausea, stomach ulcers, duodenal ulcers

◆ Diarrhoea, Irritable Bowel Syndrome, constipation, wind, bloating, Crohn's Disease

◆ Joint pain, rheumatoid arthritis

◆ Water retention

Symptoms may not be constant – stress, for instance, may make reactions vary widely. And there may be other symptoms of sensitivity which are not included in this list. Sarah suffers from wheat and other food sensitivities which can provoke extreme brain fuzziness (this is not a joke!), depression, lethargy and skin rashes. Sensitivity may also swing with hormones: it's known that eczema tends to get worse in the pre-menstrual stage and sensitivity to food may be more marked then.

Curiously, some 50 per cent of sufferers find they crave the very food to which they are sensitive. So when they eat – or drink – the offending substance, they may feel better initially, making it doubly hard to trace the culprit and to give it up.

Exactly what causes food intolerance is not yet certain but one thing is crystal clear: it's not all in the mind. So if you have unexplained health problems, explore the food link...

candida — the cinderella illness

Candida, also known as candidiasis, responds both negatively and positively to food. One of the most common female infections, it affects about three in four women at some point in their lives. It's often called the Cinderella illness because doctors have traditionally been reluctant to take it seriously – so many women seek help from natural medicine practitioners and nutritionists.

Candida is caused by over-growth of a yeast-like fungus called *Candida albicans* which can run riot in different parts of the body. It often occurs in the vagina (when it's called thrush), causing a thick white curdy discharge which smells like baking bread, and/or itching in the genital and anal area.

Candida can also collect in the gut and start a fermentation process; this leads to symptoms like those of Irritable Bowel Syndrome. Professor Jonathan Brostoff** suggests that this portmanteau of symptoms, in tandem with tiredness, aching joints and depression, may all belong together as part of a condition he calls 'gut fermentation syndrome'.

Bloating, flatulence and stomach pains are common, as well as irregular bowel habits including constipation and diarrhoea, bad breath and catarrh. You may also have aching joints, always wake up tired, and/or feel generally depressed and below par.

Some sufferers also get cravings, particularly for sugar, bread, alcohol and chocolate; you may put on weight for no apparent reason and not be able to lose it. Periods can become irregular and it may affect your memory, concentration – and even your libido.

If you go to your GP, you may have a swab test to find out whether the fungus is present. The most usual treatments are antifungal creams for thrush and, if those don't work, a course of antifungal pessaries. There is now a single-dose antifungal pessary available called Diflucan, which you can buy at your local chemist.

Conventional antifungal creams or pessaries may work better in combination with a low-yeast, low-sugar diet – because the fungus feeds on yeast and sugar. So try cutting out all forms of sugar (e.g. chocolate, sweets, cakes, biscuits, and puddings), yeast (bread and bread-related food such as pizzas and pasta), dairy products (though you may find goat's or sheep's milk products are easier to digest – or try soya milk instead). Particularly avoid blue cheeses, mushrooms and alcohol.

Many people say that food combining also helps *(see p.196)*. Experiment and see what suits you. Try to eat fresh food rather than ready-prepared or cook-chill; many sufferers prefer organic food. As well as diet, there are some other useful self-help options for thrush. Many women have benefited from the old favourites of using a tampon soaked in organic cider vinegar (one capful of vinegar to four of water) or natural bio yoghurt. Nutritional supplements may be helpful: probiotic supplements with bioacidophilus (to repopulate the gut with good bacteria), and a supplement called Mycopryl which fights the fungus. There is also a new and effective supplement called Candidicin, but this must be taken in the middle of a meal.

how I beat candida

AGE: 41

PROFESSION: FOOD PRODUCER

'As an adult, I've suffered chronically from sinusitis, asthma and lots of symptoms I didn't even realise were candida-linked: sore eyes, aching joints, fatigue, vaginal thrush, wind and diarrhoea.

'But I was starting a business, raising a family and felt too busy to tackle the problem. Then a couple of years ago, I read a magazine article (by Sarah Stacey) which prompted me to track down a nutritional consultant. The diet suggested meant I had to cut out all my favourite foods: fruit, bread, chocolate or other sweet foods – and carrot juice! The upside was that I was in control of my body; in the past, I'd literally felt the candida was saying "feed me", demanding sugary foods.

'The first week, I felt dreadful. Giving up bread was hardest because I had been eating so much of it. I started to base my meals around brown rice, vegetables, salads, unrefined pasta, fish, peanut butter and oatcakes – plus supplements of B6, biotin and immune-boosters. In week four, natural anti-fungal supplements were added in, together with garlic and EFAs. Gradually, the symptoms disappeared – and I lost about a stone, effortlessly.

'It's an amazing feeling to be in control of my health. To anyone who thinks they might have candida, I'd say: try the diet. Don't be a victim. It gives you so much confidence to discover that you can take control again – and live life more fully.'

a fabulous fresh start

We live in a toxic world. Pollutants attack us from every quarter: petrol fumes, power lines, smoking, alcohol, sunlight, pesticides in foods, additives and flavour enhancers, office technology, mercury fillings in teeth, prescription drugs, chemicals used in common household cleaners, paints, glues, plastic containers and furnishings, and the biggest pollutant of today's world – stress – which affects both our minds and our bodies.

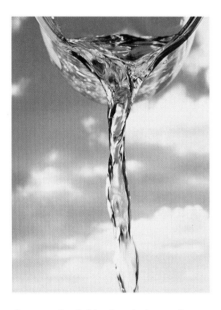

As a result of this chemical assault – and invasion by the toxins produced by inner stress – we are on toxic overload. And the consequences are plain to see. As one friend, a high-powered, busy headmistress, said sadly, 'I can't remember the last time I got out of bed in the morning feeling gleaming.' Lifestyle-related illnesses are booming: at least one in three people suffer from anxiety, one in four from Irritable Bowel Syndrome, and one in five from some form of allergy.

An effective way of combatting this toxic overload is a regular gentle fast and detox which gives both body and mind a chance to regenerate. 'If you keep stuffing food and other toxins into your body, there is no point at which it can rest and sort it all out,'

explains nutritional therapist and psychologist, Dr Marilyn Glenville. 'Fasting and detox can restore balance and give you a renewed feeling of energy and vitality.'

Fasting and detox cleansing are not the same thing. A fast is when you only drink pure water – a minimum of six to eight large (300ml/^{1}/2 pint) glasses a day – and eat nothing. Do this first, for 24 hours in peace: 'Give yourself permission to wind down – put on the answerphone, rest, sleep, have a gentle walk, listen to music,' suggests Dr Susan Horsewood-Lee[**]. 'Or just stare into space.' You can fast at home, at a health hydro or anywhere peaceful.

Follow with a gentle cleansing period lasting from two to ten days or more. During this time the cells of the gut, which in ordinary life are constantly on arduous survival duty and have the fastest turnover of any cells in your body, have a chance to rest. 'You're turning the clock back on your gut so that the cells become youthful and bright,' explains Dr Horsewood-Lee. As you relaunch your system after this clarifying process, remember that everything is more sensitised. 'So go for pure, simple, good food,' she recommends, 'and that applies to colour, texture and taste.'

You may feel worse before you feel better, both emotionally and physically, warn experts (though some side-effects may be allayed by colonic irrigation).

Possible side-effects include insomnia, coated tongue, dizziness and light-headedness at the beginning of the fast, aching limbs and muscles, hunger pains and nasal discharge. They're all good signs, though, that your body is getting to work expelling toxins.

You may also feel upset and tearful. 'So go to a health hydro or set up a lifeline – a friend to call – in case you need it,' says Dr Horsewood-Lee. Deep breathing and meditation (*see pp.162 and 238–239*) are enormously helpful to still disquiet of all sorts.

Naturopath Dr Harald Gaier says it's important to remove as many toxins from your system as possible. As well as chemical-laden foods (buy organic when possible), avoid smoking, alcohol, drugs of all kinds and the stressors that make you feel out of control – whether that's 50 phone calls a day or noisy neighbours.

Also take this time to think about other longer-term detox measures – for instance, having mercury amalgam fillings removed: 'Mercury is a powerful neurotoxin' says Gaier, and research now shows that it lodges in your brain and body (*see p.141*).

At the end of this cleansing process, you can expect clearer skin, better digestion, probably some weight loss and a flatter tummy, heightened senses, and possibly an improvement in problems such as arthritis. Most of all, you have given yourself a fresh start.

cleansing and detox eating plan

Fast first if possible, then follow this two- to ten-day plan – though you can go straight into it if you prefer. This programme, devised by Dr Marilyn Glenville, acts as a cleansing diet to help many inflammatory conditions (including IBS, asthma, eczema and arthritis), and will also reveal whether you are allergic (or sensitive) to certain common foods.

If you feel worse for a few days remember it's a good sign, meaning you were sensitive to something you ate every day. When you stop eating the food, you get withdrawal symptoms. Colds, diarrhoea, headaches or skin break-outs are all signs that your body is discharging toxins.

If you have a digestive problem (e.g. pains, flatulence or bloating), cut down on raw food and poach or steam vegetables instead. Eating blander fruit (apples, bananas and pears) and non-crunchy salads and vegetables helps. If you have migraine or arthritis, avoid citrus and acidic fruits and foods.

BEFORE YOU START
If you are in reasonable health, this is a safe cleansing programme. Don't fast for more than 24 hours to begin with. Consult your doctor first if:
◆ you are taking prescription drugs
◆ you are severely underweight
◆ you are pregnant
◆ you are diabetic
◆ you have TB or cancer

DETOX DAYS 1 and 2:
Eat only raw salads with olive oil and cider vinegar plus fruit; if you have digestive problems or have had a colonic irrigation try steamed or poached and/or puréed vegetables, without fruit. Drink only bottled mineral water.

DETOX DAYS 3–9
If you have been eating only raw salads, add in some lightly steamed vegetables, including potatoes.

DAY 10 ONWARDS
DO EAT: raw salads (or wilted leaves), fruit, vegetables (raw, lightly steamed, puréed, in soups or stews), baked potatoes; fish (steamed, poached, grilled or baked, preferably oily fish such as mackerel, salmon, herrings and sardines); nuts and sunflower seeds; soya milk; rice cakes; sesame paste (tahini); olive and sunflower oil; cider vinegar; pulses (chickpeas, lentils, kidney beans, etc.); brown rice. Flavour food with miso dissolved in hot water, herbs and spices.
DO DRINK: spring water, fruit juice, vegetable juice (make your own or make sure bought versions are additive-free), herbal teas.

NB The liver is the major organ of detoxification so it needs to function 100 per cent during this time. Drinking hot water with a slice of lemon will help, and you may want to take a supplement such as BioCare's Hep 194*, or herbs such as milk thistle or dandelion.
DON'T EAT: dairy products (butter, cheese, milk, etc.), or foods containing dairy; bread or pastry, sauces or gravies made with flour; pasta, cakes or biscuits of any type; anything containing artificial additives (colourings, flavourings, preservatives), flour, wheat or other grains except brown rice; red meat; eggs; sugar; salt; 'instant' or cook-chill foods; sweets or chocolates.
DON'T DRINK:
Tea, coffee, alcohol.

prescription

FOODS TO FIGHT CANCER
Dr Rosy Daniel of the Bristol Cancer Help Centre, England, says scientists insist that what you eat can help you – and your family – fight cancer.

◆ Fresh vegetables and fruit – locally grown and ideally organic – should be at the heart of your diet.
◆ Try to eat a good proportion of vegetables raw. Don't overcook the rest and use cooking liquor in other dishes, e.g. soups or risottos.
◆ Fresh vegetable juices are fantastic because they contain so many nutritious and protective minerals, vitamins and plant chemicals.
◆ To retain the nutrients, store veg in cool humid conditions – the fridge is good – not in a vegetable rack.
◆ Think Oriental and make your diet 40 per cent vegetables, 40 per cent staples such as pulses and grains and 10–20 per cent protein and fat.
◆ An ideal meal contains a grain (brown rice, quinoa, couscous, millet or buckwheat), a pulse (peas, beans or lentils), plus salad or vegetables, and a soya product.
◆ Consider reducing animal fats – i.e. meat and dairy produce – which carry an extra risk factor for breast, colon and prostate cancer.
◆ Replace cow's milk products with soya yoghurts, creams and ice-cream – also try oat milk and rice milk.
◆ 10 per cent extra body fat puts up your risk of hormonal cancers by as much as 50 per cent, possibly because toxins and also hormones are stored in it.
◆ Cut down on excess sugar and alcohol. (Drink grape juice instead.)

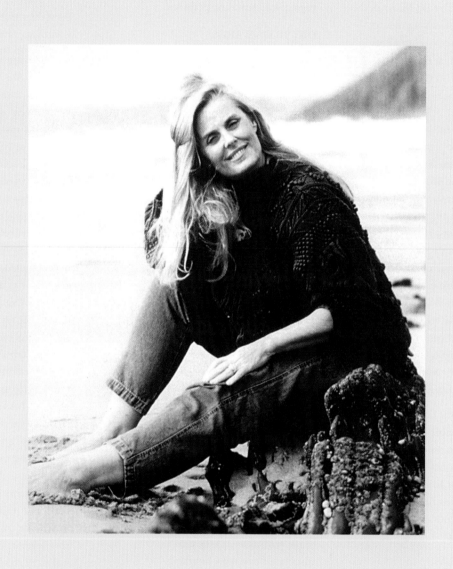

Leslie Kenton

We are inspired by Leslie Kenton because of her pioneering journalism: for almost two decades this international bestselling author has worked to be the first to discover – and explain – the newest discoveries, treatments and foods that may help us feel better, live longer, look lovelier. The ultimate 'natural beauty', she has inspired us with ground-breaking books including *The Joy of Beauty, Raw Energy** and *Passage To Power** – which broke the menopause taboo and talked about alternatives to HRT. When American-born, mother-of-four Leslie isn't globetrotting, she divides her time between London and the wild Welsh coast...

'I am not in the least bit interested in growing old gracefully; I want to grow old disgracefully, with a gleam in my eye. I want to carry my own wood into my cabin on the day that I die. But to be honest, I never think about ageing. There is a real freedom in growing older. We live in a great time because if we're healthy and love what we do, there's nothing to stop us living until we're 120 – and I mean really *living*, not just staying alive or having cosmetic surgery, but vital and vibrant.'

'In my career, I've tried to investigate everything with the potential to make us feel and look better. The one thing that has stuck with me – on a physical and mental level – is detoxification. If you detoxify the body, you rejuvenate and energise it so it heals itself. But it has to be done over and over again because we build up waste that has to be eliminated. So whenever I feel the need I will have nothing but raw food for a few days.

'I try to eat a huge variety of food: fresh vegetables and protein, with a little fruit and different seaweeds. I like to get as many different herbs and vegetables as possible, choosing them because they're beautiful and I love the taste – not because this or that is good

for me. I avoid dairy and eat wheat very rarely; I'm part of the 85 per cent of people that really can't tolerate one or other of them. I don't eat processed food and always buy organic if I can. The soil our food is grown in is so depleted by intensive agriculture that we simply don't get the trace minerals we need for optimum health. What's more, the herbicides and pesticides that are sprayed onto conventionally-grown food are oestrogen mimics, which leads to the hormonal imbalance that causes PMS, menstrual problems and a tricky menopause; I believe eating organic food helps protect you against that. Even if you don't eat organic food you really ought to filter your drinking and cooking water; I purify all mine with a reverse-osmosis water filter and I drink two to three litres a day. The more I drink, the more energy I have.

'The cocooning world of my bed is also very important to me. Ideally I'd sleep seven or eight hours a night. Exercise is also essential: I do a lot of weight-bearing exercise: running along the cliffs where I live and working out with free weights for an hour and a half, three times a week. (I also go mountain biking with my sons!)

'I take supplements, but they vary

from time to time. The one thing I swear by is a product called Pure Synergy, a mix of sixty-two different immune-stimulating herbs, vitamins and minerals, plus algae; I mix it in the blender with spring water, ice cubes and a handful of herbs from the garden. I also take Udo's Choice*, a blend of Essential Fatty Acids: a couple of tablespoons a day, on a salad if I'm feeling lazy. I also put the Udo's Choice oil on my body, which just laps up the EFAs. For my face, I like Clinique Recovery Cream and Estee Lauder Uncircle for dark under-eye circles. I also like The Green People Company's pure, natural, effective cosmetics.

I believe menopause has the potential to be a time of great creativity. If you have hot flushes, look at what it is in your life that needs to be created or brought out in yourself – that could be an outward sign that you're bottling things up inside. If you're waking in the night, then rather than tossing and turning in bed, or even crying, I'd suggest that you get up, go into a room by yourself and start writing, trying to tap into your inner creativity. Above all, start to look ahead at what you want to do with your life – and start to live a life that's authentically yours...'

supplementary benefits

Let's lay our cards on the table. As well as being passionate about eating the best possible diet, we're firm believers in nutritional supplements. Survey after survey in different countries, including Britain and America, shows that, however good their diet, virtually everyone is deficient in key nutrients. This may be due to the way food is produced or to the extra strains of all kinds – from physical pollutants to emotional and mental pressures – that affect us, living at this time in history.

Additionally, there is increasing evidence that some supplements can help in the battle against ageing. The strongest contenders by far are antioxidants which neutralise the harmful free radical molecules that cause cell damage and death (see p.13) affecting our health – and our looks. Says Gladys Block, Professor of Public Health and Nutrition at the University of California: 'We need to prevent cancer and other diseases. There's ample evidence that nutrients can help do this. Policy-makers should back away from the position that you shouldn't take supplements. Antioxidant supplement use in disease prevention is inexpensive insurance.'

Ideally, we suggest you go to a qualified and experienced nutritionist, naturopath or a doctor with detailed knowledge of nutrition. (Not as common as you might think; two eminent British professors – who did not want to be named – guestimated that at most 1 per cent of doctors in Britain had more than the most basic grasp of nutrition.) If this is impossible, start with a good multi-vitamin and mineral supplement and an antioxidant preparation. If your skin is dry, add in Essential Fatty Acids (EFAs see p.195). Always give supplements at least a month to see if they are of benefit. Some may take longer: trials with evening primrose oil (a source of EFAs) showed that it took three to four months to have a significant effect.

We asked nutritionist Stephen Terrass**, the author of many books, and the Technical Director of a leading international supplements company, to give us his tips for supplements to help us feel and look our best.

WHAT TO TAKE WHEN:

Here are supplements that may help you down the decades
REMEMBER: buy as good-quality supplements as you can afford, by a reputable manufacturer. It's important to take supplements as directed. Please *don't* exceed recommended dose levels or you may risk side-effects. More is not better.

TWENTYSOMETHING

+ Multiple vitamin/mineral formula
preferably containing minimum 50mg B complex and 400mcg folic acid. Adequate folic acid is specially important for women of childbearing age because the B vitamin folic acid (folacin) helps prevent neural tube-related birth defects such as spina bifida. The evidence seems to show that even with the best of diets, you can't eat enough folic acid to give optimal protection so a supplement is sensible (see also dementia p.197). Dose: as directed on label.

+ Essential Fatty Acids (e.g. GLA)
In spite of negative publicity, fats are not always bad for you. In fact, certain fats are absolutely essential for your health as well as your skin and hair (see p.195). It's a matter of choosing the right type of fats in the right amount – and in a form that your body can use properly.

The fats you need are known as essential fatty acids (EFAs). Among other things, EFAs are converted in your body to hormone-like substances called prostaglandins, which are responsible for regulating many essential body processes, such as blood clotting, immune function, hormone balance, inflammation, etc. EFAs also form part of the basic structure of your cell membranes.
Dose: 100–150mg per day of GLA (omega-6) (or as directed).

+ Antioxidants
Look for sulphur-rich nutrients plus common antioxidants such as vitamins A, C and E, selenium and carotenoids. Sulphur, especially when found in nutrients such as cysteine, glutathione and lipoic acid, is one of the most powerful detoxifying agents. Sulphur is also a major component of hair, skin and nail tissue.
Dose: to protect against disease/ageing:
◆ vitamin A 800–1000mg
◆ vitamin C 500–2,000mg
◆ vitamin E 100–400iu
◆ selenium 150–200mcg
◆ carotenoids 15–20mg
◆ l-cysteine 100–500mg (contains sulphur)
◆ zinc 15–25mg
◆ copper 1–2mg

- ◆ manganese 10–20mg
- ◆ lipoic acid 50–60mg

+ Dong quai
This versatile phytoestrogenic herb is especially helpful in PMS because it helps balance oestrogen levels.
Dose: as a standardised extract 150–300mg, as a non-standardised extract 500–1000mg

THIRTYSOMETHING
+ Multiple vitamin/mineral formula
with minimum 50mg B complex and 400mcg of folic acid
+ Essential fatty acids (e.g. GLA)
Dose: 100–150mg GLA (omega-6)
+ Antioxidants as before
Although it will not always be detectable, the cumulative damage from free radicals may be significant even at this early stage of life.
+ Siberian ginseng
(*Eleutherococcus senticosus*)
Clinically proven to improve tolerance to several different types of stress, mental, physical and environmental.
Dose: standardised extract 300–500mg, non-standardised 1000–2000mg
+ Calcium and magnesium
Bone density begins to be compromised in this decade, and the best time to start a preventative approach against osteoporosis (*see p.221*) is as early as possible. Magnesium is needed for calcium to be distributed properly in the body.
Dose: calcium 800–1000mg, magnesium 400–500mg

FORTYSOMETHING
+ Multiple vitamin/mineral formula
with minimum 50mg B complex.
+ Essential fatty acids as before
+ Antioxidants
+ Dong quai or black cohosh

These phytoestrogenic herbs are known to exert a positive oestrogenic effect without the risks linked to HRT, and also to regulate hormone balance.
Dose: **Dong quai:** standardised extract 150–300mg, non-standardised 500–1000mg. **Black cohosh:** standardised extract 200–400mg, non-standardised 500–1500mg
+ Calcium and magnesium as before
+ Proanthocyanidins (e.g. grapeseed extract, pine bark extract aka pycnogenol). This plant flavonoid enhances collagen stability in the body, and has a special affinity with the skin and vascular system. Used both internally and externally (e.g. in skin creams) to discourage wrinkling.
Dose: grapeseed extract 100–200mg per day, others as on label.

FIFTYSOMETHING
+ Multiple vitamin/mineral formula
with minimum 50 mg B complex.
+ Essential fatty acids
Omega-3 with omega-6 (GLA) is especially relevant at this stage, due to the former's protective effect against cardiovascular disease.
Dose: 200–600mg omega-3 (EPA) plus 100–150mg omega-6 (GLA)
+ Antioxidants as before
The effects of free-radical damage will normally have been quite established by this stage. Aside from free- radical factors such as skin wrinkling, early stages of osteoarthritis may become apparent during this decade. Sulphur-rich antioxidants may be especially useful during the menopause because sulphur is a major component of joint tissues and lubricating fluid.
+ Black cohosh
This phytoestrogenic herb is clinically proven to relieve hot flushes, depression and vaginal atrophy

associated with menopause, without the risks which may arise with HRT.
Dose: standardised extract 200–400mg, non-standardised 500–1500mg
+ Calcium and magnesium as before
+ Proanthocyanidins as before
Aside from collagen protection and circulatory benefits, proanthocyanidins may also help stabilise joint tissue and may exert an anti-inflammatory effect.

SIXTYSOMETHING
+ Multiple vitamin/mineral formula
with minimum 50mg B complex
+ Essential fatty acids as before
+ Antioxidants as before
+ Black cohosh as before
+ Calcium and magnesium as before
+ Soluble fibre formula (e.g. psyllium seed husks, pectin, flax seed, etc.)
Digestive abilities are typically much weaker in women over 50, often leading to intestinal sluggishness and symptoms such as constipation and/or diarrhoea. Soluble fibre can be used for improving intestinal function and detoxification, as well as relieving constipation and diarrhoea.
Dose: psyllium seed husks 1000–3000mg (with a full glass of water)
+ Proanthocyanidins as before
+ Ginkgo biloba
(*see preventing dementia p.197*)
Dose: standardised extract 60–180mg per day

SEVENTYSOMETHING+
+ Multiple vitamin/mineral formula
with minimum 50mg B complex
+ Essential fatty acids as before
+ Antioxidants as before
+ Calcium and magnesium as before
+ Soluble fibre formula as before
+ Proanthocyanidins as before
+ Ginkgo biloba as before

your **roller-coaster** hormones

According to many men, hormones are the catch-all explanation for whatever ails a woman's mind or body. Whether we like it or not, these chaps may not be far from the truth. Every one of us (that includes men too, of course) is governed by these powerful invisible forces which control every moment of our days: moods, desires, waking and sleeping patterns, the way we age, and, crucially, every woman's reproductive cycle.

From puberty to menopause, women live in a flurry of reproductive hormones – mainly oestrogen and progesterone – going up and down like a pearl diver. In a perfect world, these hormonal carousels wouldn't affect us. But, due probably to the stresses of 20th century life, many women now suffer a raft of problems, from PMS to the discomforts of menopause.

Conventional medicine has made vast strides in treating hormonal upsets from the Pill and Hormone Replacement Therapy to fertility treatment. There is also increasing interest in the so-called miracle hormones: melatonin, DHEA, pregnenolone and growth hormone.

But it's becoming clear that manipulating nature in this way may not be as desirable as doctors hoped. HRT, for instance, once viewed as the elixir of life for menopausal women is now controversial, partly because of unpleasant side-effects, partly because of the increased risk of breast cancer. Many experts also say that while the hormonal system is a delicate precise mechanism, requiring a featherlight touch, HRT is a crude blunderbuss-like treatment.

Today many women want to explore alternative remedies for menopausal symptoms. And many experts believe these can be equally effective, although there is much less scientific evidence – mainly because the pharmaceutical companies do not fund research into alternative therapies.

In this section, we have worked with our experts to put together the bottom-line information that we felt we – and you – really need. The most important thing for any woman to understand is that there are many ways of helping problems. HRT is not the only option. If the treatment you are offered does not feel 'right' for you, do not accept it; ask about other choices.

Remember: it's your life – you should be in charge. So find out about all these different systems and as Professor Howard Jacobs, an international expert in hormones, says: 'Learn to trust your body'.

the main hormones that make us tick

Hormone	Produced by	What it does
Follicle stimulating hormone (FSH)	pituitary gland	stimulates growth of cells surrounding eggs in the ovaries and controls division of sperm in the testes.
Luteinizing hormone (LH)	pituitary gland	triggers ovulation of egg from ovary.
Oestrogen	ovaries	controls menstrual cycle; levels fall after menopause.
Progesterone	ovaries	also controls menstrual cycle; high levels support successful pregnancy.
Testosterone (a male hormone also found in women)	adrenal gland	may cause undesirable male features in women, also greasy hair/skin, acne, excess hair growth.
Thyroxine (and other thyroid hormones)	thyroid gland	controls metabolic rate and levels of activity; too much = restlessness and hyperactivity; too little = weakness and lethargy; essential for normal menstrual cycles and fertility.
Adrenalin and noradrenalin	adrenal gland	increases heartbeat and pressure in response to activity and stress.
Cortisol	adrenal gland	many actions, including increasing the stressful effects of other adrenal hormones.
Insulin	pancreas	controls the rate of sugar absorption.

THE LOW-DOWN ON YOUR ROLLER-COASTER HORMONES

Q What is a hormone?
A Hormones are body chemicals produced by different glands which carry messages from one part of the body to another, via the bloodstream.

Q What do they do?
A They control the chemistry of the trillions of cells in your body, determining, for example, the rate at which some burn up food and release energy, which cells produce milk, hair or other products. They influence your mental and emotional state, your drive to succeed, your sexuality and appearance, as well as your menstrual cycle, immune system and your chances of getting osteoporosis, some cancers and even possibly heart disease. They also have an effect on the way you age.

Q What controls them?
A The headquarters is part of the brain called the hypothalamus which works with the pituitary, also in the brain, to send hormones to other 'endocrine' (hormone) glands in the body including thyroid, adrenals and ovaries.

Q Can I see my hormones?
A No. Hormones are so potent that, in some cases, less than a millionth of an ounce of a hormone is enough to produce an effect. Individual hormone molecules are so small you can't even see them under a microscope.

Q What happens at puberty and menstruation?
A Around the age of 11 or 12, an increase in growth hormone triggers the spurt of growth which happens before the onset of menstruation. Next, the hypothalamus starts producing another hormone called gonadotrophin releasing hormone (GnRH); GnRH stimulates the pituitary to produce follicle stimulating hormone (FSH) and luteinizing hormone (LH). FSH works on the cells which surround the eggs (i.e. the follicles) in both ovaries; all of a woman's eggs are present at birth incidentally, unlike male sperm which are constantly reproduced. Every monthly cycle, FSH ripens an egg ready for release and fertilisation and also tells the ovary to produce the female sex hormone, oestrogen. (There is actually a group of oestrogenic hormones: oestriol, oestradiol and oestrone. They all come under the oestrogen umbrella so, for simplicity's sake, we'll call them all 'oestrogen'.)

Oestrogen levels rise over the first half of the menstrual cycle, causing the lining of the womb to grow ready to receive a fertilised egg. In the middle of the cycle, LH triggers the release of an egg (ovulation). Oestrogen levels then fall off slightly and progesterone, the second female sex hormone, is produced. Progesterone makes the glands in the womb produce a nutritious fluid for the embryo and makes the womb receptive to implantation of the embryo in the lining. If the egg isn't fertilised, progesterone levels fall, causing a period as the womb lining is shed.

Q Okay, so what happens at menopause?
A Menopause comes from the Greek words *'meno'*, meaning month, and *'pausis'*, meaning ending. It happens when the ovaries run out of their supply of eggs. It's a gradual process, between the ages of 44 and 55. The average age of the last period is 50 or 51. Menopause is medically defined as the time when a woman has had no periods for a year. It's considered to have finished one year after the last

period, although some experts advise using contraception for two years. During 'peri-menopause', levels of various hormones change gradually: the ovaries stop releasing eggs and making oestrogens and progesterone. As oestrogen drops, FSH goes up, menstrual flow becomes lighter and often irregular until eventually it stops altogether.

Q Is there a point at which women stop producing oestrogen entirely?
A Oestrogen levels tail off gradually as the ovaries stop working. In the first year after menopause, oestrogen levels are about half to one third of what they were before menopause. By a couple of years later, levels have fallen again. There is always some oestrogen in the body because it's converted from other hormones but progesterone is only made in effective quantities when oestrogen is produced from the ovaries. Women also produce a small quantity of testosterone; during menopause, the ratio of testosterone to oestrogen becomes higher because of the falling levels of oestrogen.

Q How do I know when I'm coming up to menopause?

A Around 44/45, women start to notice changes – often minimal – in their menstrual periods due to erratic hormone production. Periods may be heavier (or lighter), you may get PMS for the first time, cycle length may be shorter, you may miss a period. If you're worried, consult your doctor; diary your symptoms beforehand. You may have a blood test to measure FSH levels and show whether you are in peri-menopause. If there is abnormal bleeding, the doctor may refer you for one or more of the following tests:

Endometrial biopsy: Microscopic examination of sample of womb lining.

Hysteroscopy: The womb is examined through a tiny telescope on a narrow flexible tube inserted into the vagina.

Ultrasound: An imaging probe is inserted through vagina or abdomen.

Professor Jacobs insists that women should not be subjected to Dilatation and Curettage (D&C). 'It's obsolete: if your doctor recommends it, find yourself a new gynaecologist.'

Q What is surgical menopause?

A When periods stop because of a hysterectomy and removal of ovaries. Women whose ovaries are left will continue to produce oestrogen (although they won't menstruate) so will have an FSH test for menopause.

Q Am I bound to get uncomfortable physical symptoms of the menopause?

A About 20 per cent of women have few, if any, symptoms, about half mild ones and the rest severe. If you do have symptoms, you're likely to have them for more than a year; in some women, they can last more than five years, both in peri- and post-menopause.

Q What are the most common ones?

A Hot flushes (or flashes) and night sweats. A survey of 500 women by the Women's Nutritional Advisory Service showed hot flushes affected 87.5 per cent, night sweats 75 per cent.

Q What causes hot flushes?

A Reduced oestrogen affects the body's thermostat. One moment you feel shivery cold, the next like an inferno. About four in five women experience some hot flushes; 70 per cent of these for more than five years. They may go with heart palpitations, dizziness, peculiar crawling and itching sensations under the skin, or momentary losses of awareness.

Q Does the change of life affect sleep?

A Oestrogen deficiency can disrupt sleep patterns, and night sweats make your bed even more of a battleground. Taking oestrogen in some form can help. Reduced oestrogen levels may also cause aches and pains all over the body and may also affect concentration and memory.

Q What about sex?

A Vaginal dryness and lack of libido are common *(see p.208).* More than 50 per cent of women are affected by vaginal dryness, which in turn affects libido. Less blood flow to the vaginal area results in loss of elasticity in skin tissues and cells of vagina and also bladder, which may lead to stress incontinence and/or cystitis.

Q Anything else physical?

A Dry and ageing skin: without oestrogen, the skin becomes thinner and more fragile, more prone to sensitivity, discolorations and broken capillaries, and less able to retain moisture.

Q What about the emotional side?

A Depression and anxiety are the most common complaints. Some women experience rapidly changing moods, irritability, low self-confidence, even panic attacks. Mood swings are exacerbated by any problems including, as one woman growled, 'husbands'!

hormone tests

Hormone levels can go up and down at the drop of a hat so a single test may be a signpost rather than a firm measurement. However, it may help determine the stage of menopause and any marked hormonal deficiency.

Conventional: From doctor/specialist.
Blood tests:

◆ Testing for progesterone on day 21 of cycle to show if you are ovulating.

◆ Ratio of LH to FSH may suggest polycystic ovary disease.

◆ FSH levels indicate approaching menopause; peri-menopause is likely if FSH level is above 25 units per litre (some say above 12); or LH level is above 50 units per litre and oestradiol (oestrogen) level below 150 picomoles per litre (pmol/l).

NB FSH levels vary from month to month so may not be reliable.

◆ Low oestradiol, oestrone and oestriol levels may indicate peri-menopause.

Urine tests:

◆ LH tests show if you are ovulating.

◆ The presence of chorionic gonadotrophin (CG) suggests pregnancy.

Unconventional: From some practitioners specialising in hormones who allege saliva tests in particular are more accurate than one-off blood tests.

◆ Saliva tests measure oestrogen, progesterone and testosterone levels throughout cycle to show changes linked with problem periods, PMS, infertility and menopause.

◆ Hair analysis may suggest nutrient deficiencies.

◆ Tests for food sensitivity may help pinpoint trigger foods affecting PMS and other hormonal problems.

low-down: hormone replacement therapy

HRT aims to prevent the symptoms of menopause by restoring the levels of oestrogen and progesterone. Replacing the oestrogen lost at menopause by HRT is believed to reduce the risk of spine, hip and wrist fractures, possibly by up to 70 per cent. For women at risk of osteoporosis, HRT is usually prescribed for the five to ten years immediately following menopause, or if the ovaries are removed during hysterectomy (surgical menopause). Women may also be prescribed it much later in life.

Oestrogen-only preparations were soon linked to an increased risk of cancer of the womb (four to eight times higher than non-hormone users), and are not recommended for women with wombs. To offset the risk, progesterone was added in the form of synthetic progestogen (also called progestins). Some researchers claim the combined drug still carries the womb cancer risk (three times as great as for women who are not on HRT at all) and that it may raise blood pressure. The synthetic progestogen triggers a monthly withdrawal bleed and several unpleasant side-effects but, despite these problems, it is now the standard therapy for women with wombs.

Although the oestrogen used in HRT is called 'natural', it is in fact synthesised in a laboratory. 'Natural' simply means an exact chemical replica of the oestrogen in your ovaries; it's more properly called 'nature identical'. One popular oestrogen used is Premarin, extracted from the urine of pregnant mares. This contains a specific equine oestrogen and also a natural human-like oestrogen called oestrone sulphate. The HRT trials which suggested a heart-protective effect have predominantly been carried out on Premarin and some doctors believe the equine hormone is the 'magic' ingredient in lowering heart disease.

The use of this product is now declining mainly because of animal welfare concerns. Despite reassurances from the drug companies, animal rights activists have drawn attention to the fact that the mares must spend months tethered in stalls so that their urine can be collected in catheters and that their foals are fattened up and sold for slaughter.

questions to ask your doctor about HRT

◆ What do you think are my long-term health risks, based on my own and my family's medical histories?
◆ Why should I start HRT now, rather than waiting until I'm older?
◆ Do you advise oestrogen on its own, or with synthetic progestogen?
◆ What type of HRT do you advise?
◆ What side-effects are there? May I see the manufacturer's information?
◆ Do any of the side-effects listed need immediate medical attention?
◆ How long would I need HRT?
◆ If I do decide to take HRT, what tests would I have first and what kind of follow-up would I receive?
◆ What alternatives are there to HRT for me?

other drug treatments

Raloxifene
One of a number of alternative 'designer oestrogen' drugs now licensed in America for women at risk of osteoporosis. In a large study, this Selective Estrogen Receptor Modulator (SERM) increased bone density by 1–2 per cent; researchers believe it avoids any increased risk of breast or womb cancer. Potential side-effects include a mild increase in hot flushes at the start, plus a small increased risk of blood clots. Still being trialled in the UK so not currently available.

Alendronate (Fosamax)
This bisphosphonate, approved for treating osteoporosis but not preventing it, appears to build up a woman's spine by 3 per cent per year for three years. Since the drug, which is usually prescribed for women who cannot take oestrogen, is bound into the bone, there are safety concerns and difficulty in taking it has led to nasty side-effects in the oesophagus.

Etidronate (Didronel)
A cousin of alendronate, approved only in Canada and UK to date.

Slow-release sodium fluoride
A bone-building mineral, taken in tablet form; still under research.

Calcitonin
Naturally occurring hormone, sniffed or injected, that increases bone density in the spine by 1.5 per cent per year for two years but gives no benefit to hip or forearm after that time. Does not build as much bone as alendronate but has few side-effects.

On the horizon
Calcitriol, a very active form of vitamin D, stimulates the osteoblast bone-building cells; but in high doses may cause kidney stones.

forms of HRT

1 **Pill** The commonest delivery method in the USA and UK.
Downside: The oestrogen passes through the liver and is converted so loses some of its potency (but passing through the liver could be an advantage because it offsets cholesterol, according to Professor Jacobs); pill must be taken daily; more likely to induce nausea.

2 **Vaginal cream** This delivers oestrogen direct to the vagina and vulva, so good for vaginal lubrication.
Downside: Absorption can be erratic so not suitable long term, or for preventing osteoporosis.

3 **Skin patch or gel** The patch comes in different strengths and is applied once or twice a week to the skin of the lower abdomen, bottom or hips. Patches release a steady supply of oestrogen which bypasses the liver, so avoiding nausea. Gels also administer oestrogen through the skin.
Downside: Progestogen must be given separately, if needed (i.e. for women with wombs) in the form of tablets, pessaries or a separate patch; the patch can become dislodged; oestrogen levels can rise dramatically if skin becomes heated; skin irritation has been reported in 5 per cent of cases.

4 **Implant** Supplies oestrogen for up to six months; placed under skin of abdomen under local anaesthetic.
Downside: Implant can deliver very high levels of oestrogen and when these fall, symptoms may return as a result of oestrogen withdrawal rather than deficiency. Professor Jacobs warns against having this form of HRT.

possible side-effects of HRT include:

- Gastrointestinal upsets
- Nausea and vomiting
- Weight gain
- Breast tenderness and enlargement
- Breakthrough bleeding
- Heavy menstrual bleeding
- Raised blood pressure
- Thrombophlebitis (inflammation of the wall of a vein)
- Headaches or migraine
- Dizziness
- Leg cramps
- Fluid retention
- Depression, irritability, mood change
- Vaginal candidiasis (thrush)
- Bloating
- Abdominal cramps
- Jaundice
- Increase in the size of fibroids in the womb
- Intolerance to contact lenses
- Skin irritation/rashes
- Hair loss *(see p.106)*
- Reduced glucose and carbohydrate tolerance (this could lead to blood sugar imbalances, especially after eating simple 'quick-fix' carbohydrates, e.g. refined foods such as candy bars and also fruit. These fluctuations may also contribute to weight gain)

WARNING

HRT affects blood circulation and also the reproductive parts of your body – breasts, ovaries and womb. These effects may be undesirable and/or dangerous, e.g. increased breast cancer risk (*see below*).

Do not take HRT if you have:
- family or personal history of breast or womb cancer
- thrombosis
- severe cardiac, kidney or liver disease

Think twice about taking HRT if you have:
- high blood pressure (this shouldn't preclude you taking HRT if you have oestrogen deficiency syndrome but get blood pressure treated first)
- vaginal bleeding of uncertain cause
- endometriosis (the lining of the womb growing in other places than the womb); if you have symptoms of oestrogen deficiency syndrome, ask your doctor about a progesterone dominated HRT or a product such as Livial, a non-bleed oestrogen which does not affect the womb. In the future, a SERM (*see p.209*) may be helpful.
- benign (non-cancerous) breast disease, e.g. breast cysts
- fibroids (benign womb growths)
- migraine

HRT AND THE INCREASED RISK OF BREAST CANCER

An analysis of 51 studies worldwide by the Imperial Cancer Research Fund showed an increased risk of breast cancer in women on HRT. Risk is related to the length of time it's taken, and falls within five years of stopping to the same as for non-HRT users. There seemed no added risk for women with a family history of breast cancer. Although breast cancer is rare in women under 40, a recent overview of 54 studies reported that there is a small increased risk of breast cancer in women currently using the Pill.

Time on HRT	Breast cancers diagnosed over the 20 years from age 50 to 70	Extra breast cancers in HRT users
never	45 per 1000	–
5 years	47 per 1000	2 per 1000
10 years	51 per 1000	6 per 1000
15 years	57 per 1000	12 per 1000

what women say about HRT

Angela Barker, 47, nurse

'Three years ago, I started to get hot flushes – I would go red as a beetroot, and feel sick and ghastly. I also got terrible sweats at night and had frightful insomnia. My hair was very dry and my skin creasing like an old lady. I had a little bit of vaginal dryness. Also my character was starting to change: I was very bad tempered and I couldn't control it. The main practical problem was lack of energy – I just couldn't cope.

'My family doctor sent me to see a specialist in HRT. He asked if I would take part in a research programme using Evoril oestrogen patches with a Mirena intra-uterine coil which gave a very small amount of progesterone. I had extensive tests first under anaesthetic: full hormonal blood profile, an endometrial biopsy, hysteroscopy and D&C which showed I was peri-menopausal; the coil was put in at the same time.

'One of the reasons I was so keen on HRT was because there is very severe osteoporosis in my family. I began with 100mg patches, two per week on my bottom, but my breasts got tender so I cut down to one 50mg patch and one 100mg patch weekly. The patches are very adhesive and some women experienced skin irritation. My symptoms all disappeared in six months and it suited me very well. A lot of women gave up, however, because of side-effects, including bleeding and pain from the coil. Because of the increased risk of breast cancer, I had regular mammograms (breast X-rays), and breast ultrasound and full manual breast examination.

'I became much more intolerant of alcohol, which is apparently something to do with having higher levels of oestrogen. But I didn't put on weight.

'I am nervous occasionally about the cancer risks but, all in all, I'm now in pretty good order.'

Caroline Neville, 55, MD of her own public relations company

'My gynaecologist said that we would stage-manage the menopause to suit my lifestyle because I was very busy and had to have a lot of energy. I was 51 when I had a couple of hot flushes and didn't have a period for about three months. I also developed aching hips and knees. My gynae thought it was the lack of oestrogen affecting my joints so he prescribed HRT in tablet form; it cured my aches and stopped the flushes but I felt bloated and put on weight. I went on to a smaller dose patch but my knees and hips started hurting again so I added a small patch beside the big patch. That was getting complicated so I tried this new OestroGel with a pump dispenser which you use like a body cream. I use one pump full for each arm. If I develop aches and pains, I put on a third later in the day. It's very good. Because of the risks of HRT, I have a breast mammography and ultrasound yearly and an internal scan of my ovaries and womb. Some menopausal women are electing to have their ovaries taken out by vacuum. The theory is that, with no ovaries, you miss out on having ovarian cancer. I'm not for unnecessary surgery, but my doctors have made me aware this is a possibility. However, every three months I do take a progesterone pill, which gives me a bleed for a few days, to clear out my system.'

Judie Sandeman-Allen, 50, mother

'I had a late baby at 40 and my periods never returned to normal. Over the next six years they got heavier and heavier and my PMT got dramatically out of hand. I felt like murdering someone. My family doctor never mentioned menopause, just put me on HRT (Nouvelle). I didn't know that periods and PMT can get worse before menopause, and I had no idea of any side-effects of HRT. Nouvelle worked: my PMT disappeared, my periods lasted five days and were considerably lighter. But six months later I was on holiday when I noticed my fingers were puffy. I thought it was just the heat, but over the next year it got worse and worse very gradually, until I would wake up unable to bend them. Then my muscles began to be so painful I could hardly walk and I felt ill and exhausted. The doctor said I had all the symptoms of underactive thyroid. The tests were negative but she put me on thyroxine. It had no effect but the GP just went on changing the dose. Not once did she mention HRT, or suggest I come off it. Finally I went to an endocrinologist who admitted he too was baffled. I was truly frightened, I was becoming a cripple and no-one knew what was wrong with me. I had to give up work because I felt so ill. And I was still swallowing the HRT pills. The third time I saw him, the endocrinologist said: "Perhaps you should stop taking the HRT". Geronimo! My symptoms began to go. I still had hot flushes and it took about six months for the swelling in my fingers to disappear completely, but I'm fine now – though incredibly angry that neither the GP nor the endocrinologist had a clue that HRT could be the cause of my problem.'

HRT: an expert view

The diseases which claim most women's lives increase dramatically after the menopause. The 'lady killers' are coronary heart disease (also called cardiovascular disease), breast cancer followed by some other cancers (lung, colon, ovarian, womb and cervical) and osteoporosis (hip fractures due to thinner bones result in the deaths of more women than cancers of the ovaries, cervix and womb combined). However, this does not mean that you are about to die after menopause – most deaths happen much later in life. The average age of death for British women now is 79, giving women in the 20th century close to 30 years after the menopause. Pro-HRT doctors claim that not only can HRT banish the unpleasant side-effects of the menopause but it can significantly protect against the lady killers. Others deny this emphatically. What should we believe? We asked international expert Professor Howard Jacobs, Professor of Reproductive Endocrinology at the Middlesex Hospital in London, to give us an inside view on the pros and cons of HRT.

'My position is that of an oestrogen sceptic – as opposed to the oestrogen evangelists. I believe replacement therapy can be useful but that it is mis-prescribed for many women – and in the worst case scenario that may lead to cancer. I hold this view because of what I read and because of the patients who are referred to me by those self-same evangelists. They take it as read that all women should be prescribed oestrogen replacement therapy, often with progesterone too. They're good people, but they see women as no more than hormones circulating in the blood. Often, I fear, these are doctor gurus – doctors who "know the answer" – and if women patients complain, then the women don't really understand what "the answer" is.

'Although some women feel wonderful on HRT, the duration of hormone treatment in this country is usually measured in months. *(Only 10 per cent of women in the UK who start HRT continue for more than one year.)* It's not because these women have been told to come off it – it's because they feel terrible. Many feel very congested, their

breasts get too big and their legs swell. Then, if you have a womb, the current wisdom dictates that you have to take progesterone as well, and most women tell me it makes them feel dreadful.

'We're told HRT may prevent heart disease. But there has never been a single study randomly allocating a large number of women to HRT and a control group not taking HRT, then counting the number who have heart disease. The studies have looked at some women who chose to take HRT and some who did not. Sure enough, women who choose to take HRT fall down from a heart attack less frequently than women who choose not to. However, it may be that the type of woman who takes HRT is, in fact, healthier than the woman who doesn't. In the USA, where the studies were done, it's the given wisdom that taking HRT is part of a healthy lifestyle. People who've examined the lifestyles of HRT and non-HRT users have discovered that HRT users have more medical check-ups, smoke fewer cigarettes, eat more fibre, are more physically active and less likely to have

diabetes – all major contributory factors to avoiding heart disease. *(Tellingly, no form of oestrogen therapy is licensed for the prevention of heart disease because no study to date has convinced the American regulatory authority these drugs are effective, according to the peer-reviewed journal of **Alternative Therapies**.)* So the first thing you can say is that there is currently no trial which shows that HRT protects against heart disease. We may suspect that oestrogens are good for the heart but there is no proof and, more importantly, we can't tell how much more helpful HRT would be than, for instance, giving up smoking – the single most important thing you can do to save your life. *(New research from Denmark on 25,000 women shows that smokers have twice the risk of heart disease.)*

'Osteoporosis is more complicated. Firstly, we are not sure the tests on bone density and mineral content actually tell us about bone strength – which is what we want to know. But let's accept for a moment that bone mineral content is a good index of bone strength. If you give oestrogen, there's no doubt you will improve bone mineral content, but as soon as you stop taking the oestrogen then the calcium will leave the bones, and the bone mineral content will go back to its previous level.

'Secondly, there are two kinds of fractures which concern us: fractures of the vertebral spine and fractures of the hip. It's very important to understand that these conditions occur years apart, not together. Hip fractures, for reasons we don't know, occur to women in their seventies and eighties, vertebral spine fractures to women in their sixties. I think HRT probably does increase vertebral bone density and thus reduces the risk of vertebral bone fracture, but again there is no definitive evidence.

'However the position with hip fracture and HRT is pretty problematic. Remember we're talking about giving HRT to a woman of 50 and saying it may have an effect on her body when she is in her eighties. And that effect will only be to delay the onset of symptoms of osteoporosis. So she would need to take HRT for ten years in her fifties – if she can stand it – to potentially delay her hip fracture until she is 90 rather than 80.

'To avoid the risk of osteoporosis, all women should take weight-bearing exercise and eat much more vitamin D and calcium in their diet.

'HRT is clearly advisable, however, when a woman has the distressing symptoms of oestrogen deficiency syndrome – hot flushes, sweating, vaginal dryness and rawness plus, sometimes, bladder problems (see Q&A) and lack of concentration. But just one of these symptoms does not mean oestrogen deficiency. And being miserable, unhappy or tired all the time are not symptoms either. Oestrogen is not the answer for depressive illness.

'The other situations when HRT may be an option are when women are in a high-risk group for heart disease, osteoporosis, and possibly Alzheimer's and colon cancer. The doctor needs to establish whether a woman comes from a family with a history of these conditions and whether they smoke, have high cholesterol, high blood pressure and what their lifestyle is like – whether they take exercise and have a good diet or not. With possible osteoporosis sufferers, the doctor also needs to ask whether she had anorexia nervosa as a teenager (so she never achieved normal bone mass) or her periods stopped at any point; and of course do a bone density test.

'If women have major risk factors and will not improve their lifestyle then, in my opinion, they should probably take oestrogen. But before prescribing HRT, the doctor must also weigh up the risks of taking it if the woman has a family history of breast cancer.

'Fat women tend to produce more oestrogen than thin ones. So oestrogen-related diseases tend to occur more commonly in fat women but oestrogen deprival syndromes, such as osteoporosis, occur much more commonly in thin women. Smoking alters the way that oestrogen is used by the body so smokers with oestrogen deficiency syndrome need twice as much oestrogen as non-smoking women.

'Women who are taking oestrogen for the control of menopausal symptoms (as opposed to preventing osteoporosis) should only take HRT for as long as the symptoms persist without the treatment. I advise my patients to test themselves periodically or so and see if the symptoms recur without the HRT. If they don't, then I suggest they stop the treatment. And it's vital for women to trust their bodies – if they feel bad on HRT then it's probably not doing them much good. I don't believe women should have implants because you can't take them out, you have to wait until the implant is used up.

'If you don't have the symptoms of oestrogen deficiency syndrome, if you have a healthy lifestyle and if you are not at high risk of conditions which are probably related to oestrogen deficiency, I can't see the point of taking oestrogen.'

Summary of Professor Jacobs' views on HRT:

◆ HRT can be a useful therapy for women who suffer from oestrogen deficiency syndrome. The symptoms are: hot flushes (flashes), sweating, vaginal dryness/rawness, possibly bladder problems and loss of concentration.

◆ HRT may also be useful for women at high risk of heart disease, osteoporosis and Alzheimer's with a poor lifestyle in terms of diet and exercise.

◆ HRT is not a suitable treatment for anxiety, depression or fatigue.

◆ Although HRT has not yet been shown definitively to reduce the risk of heart disease and osteoporosis it almost certainly helps – the problem is we just don't know by how much. What is certain, however, is that simple lifestyle changes *will* reduce the risk.

◆ HRT increases the risk of breast and possibly womb cancer.

do you believe in miracles?

The idea of a magic elixir to fight off age is the fulfilment of all our dreams, the Holy Grail of age researchers – and a billion-dollar prospect for pharmaceutical companies. But, despite a slew of much vaunted contenders including the so-called 'miracle' hormones, international experts at a meeting in London in 1997 were sceptical. And so are we...

Antioxidants are the only anti-ageing compounds really worth the hype, according to researchers worldwide, who contributed to a meeting organised by the British Medical Journal. *(For more on antioxidants, see p.13.)* However, there is increasing talk of the so-called 'miracle' hormones – **melatonin, DHEA** (dehydroepiandrosterone), **pregnenolone** and **growth hormone** – which, according to some researchers, can keep us healthy and beautiful, bursting with vim and vigour, with our minds and memories alert. Like all hormones, they decline with age and the pro-lobby believes that giving us back the levels we had at our peak (about 25 to 30 years old), can rejuvenate both body and brain. But the National Institute on Ageing (NIA) in America warns potential consumers: 'The NIA does not recommend taking supplements of DHEA, growth hormone or melatonin because not enough is known about them. People who have a genuine deficiency of human growth hormone should take it only under a doctor's supervision.'

Despite these warnings, melatonin, DHEA and pregnenolone are classed as food supplements and are freely available in America, and by mail order in other countries. The UK Department of Health comments about its ban on melatonin: 'Melatonin is a very powerful hormone which has a marked physiological effect. Therefore it's a medicine, not a substance which compensates for a deficiency in your diet.'

As the NIA also points out, hormone supplements may not have exactly the same effects on us as our own naturally produced hormones because the body may process them differently. Also, high doses of supplements, whatever form they come in, may result in higher amounts of the hormones than are healthy. For instance, the usual dose of 2–5mg of melatonin is thought to be safe by researchers but can result in blood levels of up to 40 times higher than normal.

When that happens, any negative effects may increase. And even tiny amounts of these powerful substances can have widespread effects on the body chemistry.

The bottom line is that there is currently not enough research to substantiate their use. Bear in mind the fatal consequences in body-builders who have taken cocktails of similar hormones. However, large-scale studies are ongoing worldwide and there may come a time when after further research these hormones are shown to be useful and safe. Meanwhile we do caution you to be sceptical about anti-ageing clinics who prescribe these and other powerful drugs. Although some doctors may be extremely knowledgeable, we were worried when we interviewed the owner of one such clinic in London. He routinely prescribed DHEA and also pharmaceutical drugs more or less on demand. Our concern was the lack of information given to patients about proven lifestyle factors, such as nutrition and exercise, and the emphasis on these so-called 'miracle' drugs.

the so-called 'miracle' hormones

Hormone	Produced by	What it does
Melatonin	pineal gland	regulates sleep/wake pattern and influences other hormones, affecting mood, libido, digestion and immune system.
DHEA	adrenal glands	may be converted to hormones, principally oestrogen and testosterone.
Pregnenolone	adrenal glands, ovaries (testes in men)	may be converted to hormones, including oestrogen, testosterone and cortisol.
Growth hormone	pituitary gland in brain	regulates growth and maintenance of skin, connective tissue and organs.

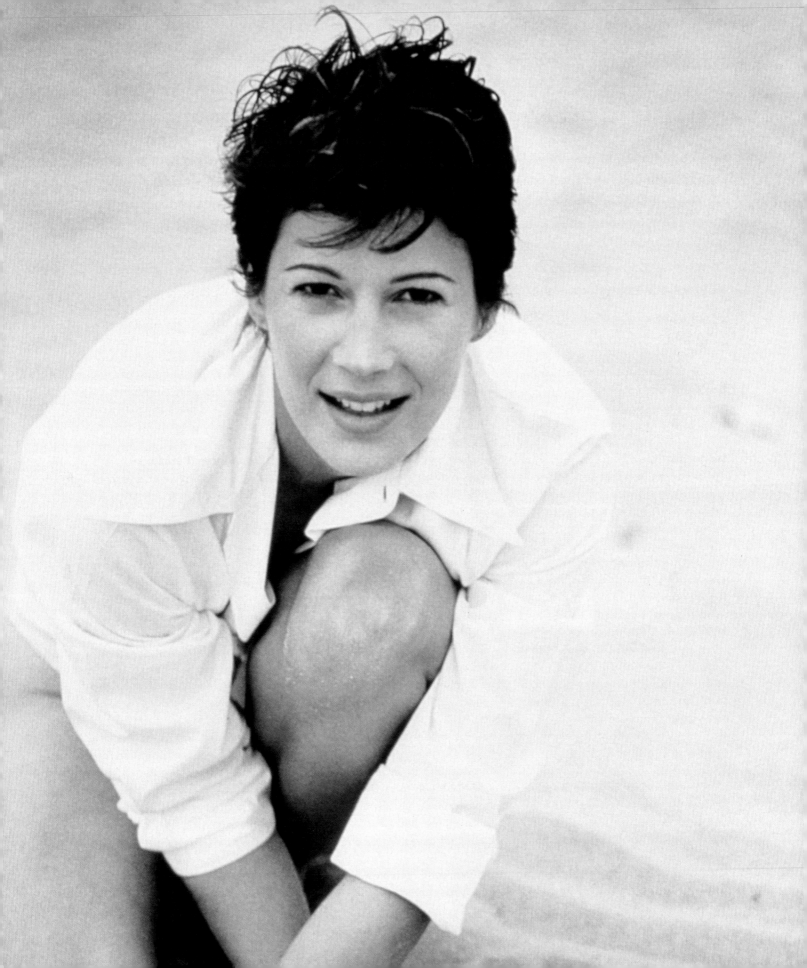

alternative hormone helpers

Many experts feel that an integrated combination of gentle alternative/complementary therapies, aimed at treating both body and mind, can ease the menopause (and of course many other conditions). As well as the stress therapies detailed on *pp.238–239*, there is a range of traditional herbal, homoeopathic and nutritional approaches such as the ones detailed below. It is always wise to consult a doctor with an interest in these remedies, or another appropriate expert – homoeopath, nutritionist, naturopath, herbalist or Chinese medicine expert are the most relevant – before starting out on a new regime. We recommend keeping your family doctor informed about what you are doing.

ALTERNATIVE MEDICAL SYSTEMS

The following systems have given help to women we know. In practice, they may overlap, and practitioners invariably also give general advice about lifestyle measures.

Homoeopathy

The homoeopathic approach involves exploring the woman's feelings about the menopause and what it represents to her, then supporting her with homoeopathic tinctures. Devotees include Queen Elizabeth II who, together with other members of the Royal Family, regularly consults London-based medical doctor and homoeopath, Dr Ronald Davey.

Dr Tessa Katz of the Women's Clinic at the Royal London Homoeopathic Hospital reported in 1997 that about 70 per cent of patients feel a definite improvement in menopausal symptoms while using homoeopathic medicines, about 25 per cent get some benefit and the remaining 5 per cent notice no change. Most of the patients have tried HRT and are either unhappy with taking possibly harmful medication daily, or have suffered 'intolerable' side-effects. Some patients use homoeopathic treatments alongside HRT.

Chinese Medicine

Menopausal symptoms are believed to be linked to kidney, blood and kidney/liver imbalances. Herbs such as *dong quai* (Chinese angelica) and ginseng are commonly prescribed. Acupuncture is used to balance hormones and ease pain. Chi Gung, a system of mind/body meditation and gentle exercise, is also practised as part of Chinese medicine.

Western Herbal Medicine

The emphasis is on stimulating the hormonal changes to progress as easily as possible. Herbs which work like oestrogen are often prescribed for hot flushes, night sweats and flooding, e.g. black cohosh, blue cohosh, agnus castus, hops and wild yam. Infusions of sage or motherwort, which also have an oestrogen-like action, are prescribed for vaginal dryness, and pot marigold cream may be suggested for the vagina. For stress, soothing herbs (e.g. skullcap and vervain) with St John's Wort (one of the best researched herbal antidepressants) for depression. Lavender, rose and ylang ylang oils may be recommended for the bath.

Bio-energetic Medicine

This is based on the principles of homoeopathy and acupuncture, well known in Germany. Practitioners believe that behind every condition is a weakness in the system or a prolonged energy disturbance. The aim is to balance the body so that it functions optimally.

Nutritional Therapy

Higher levels of various vitamins and minerals may help as women get older, particularly the B vitamins 6, 12 and folic acid, vitamins D and E, plus magnesium, chromium and zinc. Vitamin E has been shown to improve vaginal dryness (*see also Seaweed, p.193*), hot flushes, sweating, dizziness and fatigue, as well as protecting against heart disease.

Hydrochloric acid (HCl), which helps digestion and the absorption of minerals including calcium, seems to decline with age. Zinc and/or B12 deficiency, food sensitivities, rheumatoid arthritis, stress, coffee consumption, pollutants, and an over- or underactive thyroid may all affect it; by menopause, some women appear to have virtually no HCl. Eating papaya (pawpaw), which is rich in the digestive enzyme papain, or taking supplements such as HCl and/or pepsin with meals, may help.

alternative 'drugs'

Pharmaceutical drugs are not the only preparations which can have an effect on menopause. Many women – and increasingly medical practitioners – are impressed with the potential of more natural medicines, which include foods.

Natural Progesterone

Progesterone creams for menopausal symptoms are riding on a wave of popularity with some women, including Lesley Kenton *(see p.203)*, Gloria Hope Price *(p.225)* and Gayle Hunnicutt *(p.91)*. However there are others who have either had no benefit or have indeed experienced side-effects.

There is also some controversy about their often touted claim to be a natural plant remedy, which tends to imply that they are actually 'squeezed' out of a bunch of leaves. A more accurate description of these preparations is 'nature-identical'; in fact they contain synthesised progesterone made in a laboratory from raw plant material, originally wild yam, today usually soya beans. *(See Dr Linda Fellows, right.)* Dr John Lee, one of the leading advocates of this therapy, makes it clear that natural progesterone should really be called 'plant-derived' and emphasises that no wild yam or other plant contains actual progesterone. However, he claimed in a letter published by *The Lancet* in 1990 that it can indeed reverse bone loss.

Dr Susan Horsewood-Lee, an independent GP practising in London, finds the research so far encouraging and has no hesitation in recommending it. 'It is a perfectly legitimate and useful option for some women.' The patients she has found it benefits are those who would never agree to take conventional HRT but are at some risk of osteoporosis. 'These are patients who basically look after themselves already; they're eating and taking exercise. They have a bone density scan and it's low; they spend the next 12 months doing some more load-bearing exercise, adding in a supplement with, say, calcium, magnesium and boron, but the next bone density scan is even lower.' At that point, Dr Horsewood-Lee says, her patients are frightened and unsure what more they can do. She then explains that natural progesterone may be able to help and that – although yet again the jury is still out – one of the big London hospitals, the Chelsea & Westminster, is taking this form of progesterone seriously enough to have a large-scale research programme. In her experience, about 90 per cent of her patients have the same or improved bone density after a year on ProGest cream (by Higher Nature).

Additionally, patients (some of whom have not done well on oestrogen) do report feeling better. She has observed anecdotally that they tend to have less hot flushes, possibly because the drop in oestrogen levels happens more gently and may, she suspects, plateau at a higher level.

However, Dr Horsewood-Lee emphasises that natural progesterone is only one of a 'constellation of lifestyle influences' that can help women through the menopause.

what women say…

Dr Linda Fellows, 55, biochemist

'The doctor prescribed Prempak HRT (oestrogen and progestogen pills) when I had hot flushes at 48. I used to get drenched in meetings and it was very embarrassing. I stayed on HRT for about three or four years to try to avoid the hot flushes but I just never felt right. Prempak made me put on weight and feel very congested. It also gave me really bad PMS, not just bloating but irritability and misery to the nth degree.

'Then I discovered what's called natural progesterone cream – though it's not natural in fact, it's made in a lab. It's nature-identical (the same as the oestrogen in HRT), which means that the synthetic molecule is exactly the same structure as your body's. The advantage of nature-identical molecules is that your body is used to dealing with them, whereas it probably views the "unnatural" progestins as foreign substances. I think some cautious tinkering with your body chemistry – under medical supervision, of course – is very helpful. But the other problem about taking any kind of hormone replacement is that your body doesn't go through the menopause properly so you may have to go through another potentially uncomfortable adjustment phase if you stop taking the hormones.

'I now take oestrogen in a very small dose, either orally or via a patch, and I rub on the natural progesterone cream every day before bed and sometimes in the morning too. I also take herbs – a cocktail of black cohosh, sage, hops and wild yam tinctures.

'On a good day, I feel fine now and I am confident that I can find a combination which is absolutely right.'

Gamma-oryzanol
For a gentle way of dealing with severe clusters of hot flushes, Dr Horsewood-Lee suggests taking three capsules daily of this rice extract, which has been extensively researched in Japan.

Plant Oestrogens
Many studies show that soya-based products (e.g. tofu) which are rich in plant (phyto-) oestrogens and calcium have a moderate effect in reducing menopausal symptoms and may help protect against osteoporosis. Some experts have concluded that Japanese women escape hot flushes (there is no Japanese translation) and other menopausal symptoms because their diet is rich in soya and also ginseng. Also the rate of breast and other hormonally dependent cancers and osteoporosis is much lower in Japan.

Phytoestrogen-rich foods include wholegrains (oats, corn, barley, millet, buckwheat, wild rice, brown rice and whole wheat) plus soya flour and flax seed oil; also vegetables (fennel, celery, parsley, sprouts and the legume family – peas, beans and lentils).

Concentrated soya protein is also available in tablet form. Brands include Blackmores Phyto-Life Plus and Solgar's Iso Soy. (See Anne Spencer, right.) A new plant-based product, Promensil, from Australian pharmaceutical company Novogen, is on sale over the counter in Australia, and should be available in America and Britain shortly.

Rhubarb, Rhubarb
A preparation of rhubarb root called Phytoestrol* gives a medium daily dose of plant oestrogens. Although not as fast acting as conventional HRT, it's said to create a lasting improvement in menopausal symptoms.

what women say...

Anne Spencer, 53, health writer
'I had a hysterectomy in 1989 when I was 45, due mainly to fibroids and a prolapsed womb. My ovaries were left intact so I was still producing oestrogen although my periods had stopped. Doctors say that if you have that type of hysterectomy you are likely to bring forward the menopause. Everything went along uneventfully for a while – I used to get a bit hot in the middle of the night and throw off the bedclothes, and over a period of about five years in all, I became slightly more ratty and obsessional, but I was coping and I actively did not want HRT. I don't like the idea of taking hormonal drugs unnecessarily and I didn't feel my symptoms were sufficiently disabling – I could manage quite well.

'Then I went to see Dr Lily Hua Yu, a doctor of Traditional Chinese Medicine at the Acu-Medic Clinic in North London, as part of an article I was writing. She told me I had a frilly tongue – a sign of "yin" deficiency and the root of my long-term lack of energy.

'So I went along as a patient once a week for two months. I had acupuncture and herbal medicine (in tablet form), including herbs such as dong quai, rehmannia and sometimes ginseng, adjusted weekly.

'I felt much much better. My pelvic floor felt toned and literally lifted up. I also slept more soundly. Rather stupidly, I stopped going, partly because it was quite expensive.

'My next great discovery was in Australia at Christmas 1997. By then, I was over the menopause but worried about osteoporosis. I had a heel ultrasound test and a DEXA-scan for bone density, and both were at the lower end of normal. I still didn't want to take HRT and a friend suggested soy protein concentrate – it had changed her life.

'So I bought a bottle of Blackmores Phyto-Life Plus, which also contains calcium, started taking the four tablet dose a day and I feel fantastic. I have more energy, my brain is clearer and people say I look very well.

'Soy is chockful of natural plant (phyto) oestrogens. The key compounds are two isoflavones – genistein and daidzein. They occur naturally in soy products but you need to eat a lot of soy regularly, as Asian women do, to benefit. And the problem about the soy products you eat is that, apparently, the isoflavones may be processed out of them. So it's easier and more reliable to take concentrated soy protein. And you probably can't take too much – you're just taking as a supplement what you would eat in an Asian diet. The calcium content gives you 80 per cent of the Recommended Daily Allowance in the UK; I take Magnesium OK as well, because calcium is better absorbed with magnesium, plus vitamin E and fish oils.

'I've talked to various nutritional experts who believe that these phyto-oestrogens are going to be the big thing. The Imperial Cancer Research Fund in London, who supported the survey of HRT which showed an increased risk of breast cancer, is launching a study of phytoestrogens in treating menopausal symptoms.

'I also swim three mornings a week, and walk for 30–45 minutes on the other days – it makes me feel brilliant. I go to an acupuncturist once a fortnight just to get tweaked. The best advice I ever had for a good night's sleep – from a feng shui expert – is to keep work out of the bedroom.'

what women say…

Sarah Stacey, 49, co-author of feel fabulous forever.

'I went to my doctor in June of 1996 when I was 47 because I was desperate. I was working very hard and couldn't sleep. I would wake up at two every morning and no matter how late – or early – I went to bed or how tired I was, I would thrash around unable to get a wink more sleep. I was terribly depressed and tearful and felt completely unable to cope. I was also having very heavy periods, very often.

'My doctor was very sympathetic, took lots of blood tests, and said he would like me to go on Prozac. I told him I was going to Tom Marshall-Manifold at the Wimbledon Clinic in South London, who practises bio-energetic medicine (see p.219), and would make up my mind after that. Tom gave me a battery of tests and talk. He didn't take blood since my doctor's tests had confirmed I was peri-menopausal, but he did a complicated electro-acupuncture diagnosis. (No, it didn't hurt.) He explained that energy lines – called meridians – run throughout our body, each associated with a different organ. On each line are acupuncture points which hold an electrical – or "energetic" – charge that can be measured with an electronic machine. When you're well, the measurements should all be about the same. Mine were wildly different. The circulation was really overfiring, while the hormone activity was incredibly low. Many other of my body systems were sluggish. In a nutshell, I was unbalanced.

'Tom prescribed complex homoeopathic drops including oestrogen, progesterone, plus other synergistic homoeopathic remedies to regulate the hormones and ingredients to help my pancreas and digestion.

'Additionally, I had herbal tablets, containing agnus castus, damiana, and dong quai plus mimosa bark (a Chinese herb which is a natural antidepressant) and two types of ginseng.

'Nutritional supplements too: evening primrose oil for the essential fatty acids to lubricate my dry eczema-prone skin and to help balance my hormones; and a mineral composition with magnesium to feed nerve tissue, aid the absorption of calcium and also help the hormones, plus chromium to work on my sugar problems.

'Tom explained that this was all aimed at directing my body back into balance. And that, quite simply, is what it did. At the end of the first month, I felt better than I had for years; for the first time, I really understood what it meant to feel balanced in body and mind. At the end of two months, I was beginning to get into the habit of feeling well. The "blipping out" hot flushes subsided and I had begun to sleep well again with the addition of melatonin to the drops and some occasional help from Bioforce's Dormeasan tincture or MedicHerb Valerina. Life really was a bowl of roses.

'I told my doctor about my decision, right at the beginning. He said he thought the naturopathic route might not suit me well, and his instinct was that I was a candidate for HRT. He couldn't explain exactly why: just said it was instinct. I'm hardly ever ill but I go back to Tom every two months or so to have my measurements taken again on the weird machine. I don't question any of it any longer: it may seem extraordinary but it works brilliantly.'

prescription

Internationally renowned natural medicine expert and qualified pharmacist, Jan de Vries, who has received a United Nations award for his work, suggests the following:

For reducing menopausal symptoms
◆ Reduce your intake of animal protein.
◆ Take gamma-oryzanol as directed.
◆ Take evening primrose oil, 1500mg at night.
◆ Take vitamin E (from 200–400 international units daily, rising to 400iu twice daily).
◆ Take a Remifemin (made from the oestrogenic herb black cohosh) tablet twice daily (you can obtain this on a 'named patient' basis from herbal practitioners).
◆ Try homoeopathic Formula MNP415 by Bioforce, 20 drops, three times daily.

For night sweats and hot flushes
◆ Take Menosan (sage extract) by Bioforce, 10–15 drops, three times daily.

For osteoporosis
◆ Take Urticalcin (homoeopathic calcium with stinging nettle) by Bioforce, three tablets, twice daily.
◆ Osteoprime (nutrients for bone health) by Enzymatic Therapy, two tablets twice daily.

For disrupted sleep
◆ Don't eat too much after six p.m.
◆ Take Dormeasan tincture (extract of valerian and hops) by Bioforce, 25 drops, half an hour before going to bed.
◆ Drink herbal teas with melissa and lemon.

osteoporosis

Osteoporosis, or thinning of the bones, affects about one in three post-menopausal women in Britain to some extent, according to the National Osteoporosis Society.

Bones consist of connective tissue (mainly collagen) packed around with solid crystals of minerals, rather like a honeycomb. Despite their inert appearance, bones are as much alive as the rest of our bodies, constantly building (due to the bone-making cells, osteoblasts, which mature into osteocytes) and shedding (due to the third type of bone cell, osteoclasts). They grow with us from birth, stop lengthening at about 16 to 18 but go on increasing in density to reach peak bone mass at about 35. After that, problems may begin because we tend to start losing bone faster than we replace it.

Osteoporosis leads to a reduction in both the connective tissue and mineral content of the bone. This makes bones brittle and easily fractured and also results in curvature of the spine. Although osteoporosis runs in families, it can be prevented by plenty of weight-bearing exercise and good nutrition in early life when bones are forming. Current tests measure bone density, although this may prove not to be the most accurate measurement of bone loss. However, it is useful to have a check, after consultation with your doctor. If your bone density is low, you may be recommended to have follow-ups.

Tests:

1. DEXA: Dual Energy X-ray Absorptiometry, the most widely used scanning technique for measuring bone mineral density; earliest bone loss usually starts in the spine and hip so these are usually scanned. Although believed to be the most accurate current method, the level of precision is such that you can only rely on detecting a change of 2 per cent or more.

2. Photon Absorptiometry: Largely superseded by the more accurate DEXA, this technology is similar, but uses ionising radiation.

3. Quantitive computed tomography (QCT): An expensive system which exposes patients to high radiation doses.

4. Ultrasound scanning: High-speed sound waves are passed through the heel bone which is on the same axis as the hip and is assumed to be representative of the fracture-prone parts of the skeleton. Although this technology may have the potential for widespread use, it is still under investigation.

5. Urine Analysis: Identifies current levels of bone loss (resorption) plus future risk; useful for measuring nutrient levels and dietary profile; the only test to give a broad picture of bone turnover and loss, rather than a one-off measurement.

6. DIY: Height equals roughly the same as the distance from fingertips to fingertips when the arms are spread wide; bone loss means height will decrease in relation to arm span. If you have very lined, aged, facial skin that may be reflected in your bones and you might wish to have a bone density test.

risk factors

You are more likely to develop osteoporosis if:

- it runs in your family
- you are inactive and take little exercise
- you don't get out in the sunlight
- you exercise to extremes
- you go into premature menopause, i.e. before 40
- you smoke
- you eat a diet high in animal protein
- you drink a lot of alcohol and/or coffee
- you add a lot of salt to your meals
- you take certain drugs and medicines including: corticosteroids (e.g. prednisolone), laxatives, diuretics, thyroxine
- you have irregular periods
- you once stopped having periods for more than six months
- you are thin
- you have suffered from an eating disorder such as anorexia or bulimia
- you have a digestive problem e.g. Irritable Bowel Syndrome or a lack of stomach acid (hydrochloric acid)

questions to ask your doctor about osteoporosis

- What do you think is my risk of osteoporosis, based on my own and my family's medical histories?
- What tests do you suggest I have?
- If I am at risk, what treatment do you recommend – and why?
- What will this therapy do – halt bone loss or build bone?
- When would I begin treatment – before or after menopause?
- How long would I have to take it?
- What are the possible side-effects of this treatment?
- Are there any alternatives to conventional therapy?

simple helpers

There is no dispute at all that preventing bone loss through simple lifestyle measures is the best thing you can do at any age – these measures will also help build peak bone mass in the under thirties.

◆ **Take regular weight-bearing exercise.** *(See p.166.)* In one study, 30 post-menopausal women increased their spinal mass by a significant 0.5 per cent in 12 months simply by walking 50 minutes four times a week; in stark comparison, the control group of non-exercisers lost 7 per cent of their bone mass over the year.

◆ **Get out in the fresh air.** Vitamin D from the sun helps calcium absorption.

◆ **Reduce protein foods.** Some nutritionists now believe that a diet high in animal proteins – the typical bacon and eggs, meat at every meal type of diet – may be a primary cause of osteoporosis as well as contributing to bone loss when you have osteoporosis. Protein leads to bone loss because protein-rich foods are acid-forming. The body neutralises this through sodium and calcium. When your reserves of sodium are used up, calcium is taken from the bones. So the more protein you eat, the more calcium you need. Salt also leeches calcium from bones. So cut down on protein and salt, and eat alkaline foods – vegetables and fruits (known to protect bone density), sprouted seeds, yogurt, almonds, Brazil nuts and buckwheat.

One study compared the incidence of osteoporosis in meat-eating women with that in vegetarians. The difference in bone density after age 60 was dramatic, according to Susan Lark, a former faculty member of the Stanford University Medical School. Vegetarian women lost 18 per cent of their bone mass, while meat-eating women lost 35 per cent.

◆ **Don't rely on dairy foods.** The benefits of dairy foods – much touted as the answer for preventing bone loss because of their calcium content – are now disputed. There is, in the words of one expert, 'a dogfight going on out there'. Although some doctors still insist that drinking a pint of skimmed fortified milk daily would solve the bone loss problem, many others disagree, saying there is no evidence that the calcium from dairy products goes onto our bones. They point to Asian women, who don't drink milk or eat cheese, and yet have little problem with osteoporosis.

◆ **Have frequent regular meals** to avoid internal stress which causes an acid body environment

◆ **Cut down on caffeine.**

◆ **Avoid bran and bran-containing foods**. Many nutritionists now believe they may interfere with calcium absorption. Get all-important fibre in your diet by eating lots of fruit and veg.

◆ Drink 1 tablespoonful of **cider vinegar and honey** in a cupful of warm water up to three times daily; naturopaths say this helps digestion and also absorption of calcium.

◆ **Chuck out aluminium pans:** aluminium can leech from cooking pans, foil and containers, and stop the body metabolising calcium. Switch to glass, enamel, stainless steel or cast iron.

◆ **Relax:** stress, strain and feeling under pressure triggers adrenaline production which damages bone.

◆ **Look after your digestion.** As we get older, the levels of beneficial stomach acid (hydrochloric acid) drop, often giving rise to symptoms such as flatulence, bloating and indigestion and interfering with nutrient absorption. Try a food-combining diet *(see p.196)*, which helps many, and a digestive supplement; if the condition continues, consult a nutritionist, naturopath or doctor with expertise in nutrition.

◆ **Don't smoke.** Smoking cigarettes lowers blood oestrogen levels and also has a dampening effect on the cells that make new bone. It can trigger premature menopause by up to five years. By stopping smoking and eating well, women can probably prevent an accelerated menopause – and help to reduce the risk of osteoporosis and the other lady killers.

Supplementary help:
As well as the lifestyle measures above, Dr Marilyn Glenville suggests these daily supplements for menopausal women:

◆ A good multi-vitamin and mineral supplement for the menopause with boron, e.g. Lambert Gynovite, Biocare Femforte, Solgar Earth Source.

◆ 15mg zinc citrate.

◆ Combined magnesium and calcium supplement with a maximum of 500mg calcium citrate (look for a supplement with a 2:1 ratio magnesium to calcium).

◆ 50mg vitamin B complex.

◆ 1000mg linseed oil.

NB If you have a bone loss problem, we suggest you consult a qualified and experienced nutritionist or naturopath for an individual programme.

what to do if you find a breast lump

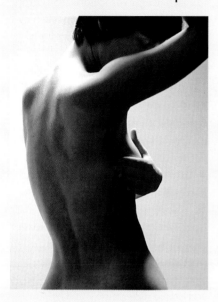

First of all, try to stay calm: 90 per cent of the time it's not serious. If you do need treatment, you have rights and choices.

One in 12 women develops breast cancer in Britain, one in eight or nine in America. Although doctors admit they do not yet have a cure, guidelines have now been agreed by UK medical experts (the British Association of Surgical Oncologists' Breast Group), who say that women should be treated in specialist cancer units by expert multi-disciplinary teams who can give the best possible advice and treatment.

If you find a lump in your breast, make an immediate appointment with your family doctor to discuss it.

WITH YOUR DOCTOR
Detailed notes will be taken of your own and your family's medical history and then you will have a physical examination.

Don't leap to the worst conclusion – nine out of ten breast lumps are benign. What you are feeling may not even be a lump but an area of nodularity; your GP will then suggest examining you again after your next period.

If your GP believes it is a true lump, he or she should refer you immediately to a specialist breast cancer unit. These units are now much quicker at organising appointments and will usually see you within a week although you may have to travel. If your GP is really concerned, appointments and referral letters are now routinely organised by fax.

If your GP does not refer you immediately and you are concerned, you must be persistent, however vulnerable you feel. It is your body.

THE EXPERTS
If you are referred to a specialist unit, you will find the team has several key personnel: one or more consultant surgeons who specialise in breast work, a clinical oncologist (cancer expert), a breast-care nurse, a pathologist (who interprets the results of biopsies), plus a radiographer and radiologist who work on breast x-rays (mammography). Your first appointment will be with the consultant surgeon or a senior member of his or her team. Specialist breast nurses should always be available if you want to see one.

DIAGNOSTIC TECHNIQUES
Firstly, the consultant will examine your breast to confirm that there is a lump. Secondly, needle aspiration will be carried out to draw off some of the cells. (This may be uncomfortable but shouldn't be painful.) If it's a cyst – one of the commonest causes of breast lumps – the fluid can be drawn

off there and then and the problem solved. If it's not a cyst – further investigations will take place. Thirdly, imaging techniques will be used to investigate the situation. If you are under 40, sophisticated ultrasound imaging with sound waves will be used to build up a picture of the breast. For the over-forties, mammography (x-ray of the breast) will be used. (Many surgeons believe that two views should be taken of each breast.) Frequently both ultrasound and mammography are used in both age groups.

From this triangle of information, the consultant surgeon and team decide whether they believe the lump to be benign or malignant. In the most efficient clinics, you will have the result the same day, or within a few days. You should not wait more than one week.

If the results are inconclusive, the consultant may suggest a biopsy under general anaesthetic to remove the lump, for testing. The results should be available within a week to ten days.

If the tests suggest a malignant tumour – in other words, cancer – your next appointment will be with the consultant surgeon, the breast nurse and possibly the oncologist. Although the diagnosis should always be given to you in a warm and caring way, it's a good idea to take a companion with you. Some consultants will give you a tape of the meeting, others are happy if you or your companion take notes. You may want to go in with a list of questions. Now and throughout your treatment, you should be given information and choices and as much support as you feel you need.

CHOOSING A TREATMENT
Treatment options for breast cancer

are surgery, radiotherapy (where x-rays are targeted to destroy the cancer cells), hormone therapy and chemotherapy (by drugs). Treatments may be used alone or in combination. Each case is different and treatment should be individually tailored. The consultant should discuss all the possibilities, and you have every right to ask as many questions as you like about the proposed treatment and any possible alternatives, side-effects – both short and long term, including possible fertility problems – success rate, breast reconstruction (immediate or delayed) or prosthesis fitting service, and arrangements for follow-up after-treatment. The breast nurse will be there to give support and information throughout. Though you may feel pressured to make a decision, you should take as long as you feel is necessary to consider the options. You may find a second opinion reassuring – and most experts will refer you to another specialist without any fuss. If there is a problem, go back to your GP.

Surgery should be offered within two weeks. There are three possible operations: a lumpectomy, or wide excision, where the lump and some surrounding (healthy) tissue are removed; segmentectomy, where a larger area (but less than a quarter of the breast) is removed, leaving a natural shape and cleavage – usually performed when the woman has a lump under 2cm (3/4 inches) round; and a mastectomy, where the breast is removed entirely.

The lymph nodes will also be tested and may be removed to prevent the cancer spreading. Reconstruction of the breast can be performed at the time by a specialist breast surgeon, although some consultants suggest patients wait for six

months before deciding. In this case, the reconstruction may be done by a plastic or specialist breast surgeon.

Radiotherapy is commonly given with a lumpectomy and segmentectomy to stop the disease recurring in the breast. There have been revelations recently about cases where patients have been damaged by massively misjudged doses of radiation, but meticulous checking systems are now in place to prevent mistakes. The number of sessions varies but usually falls between 15 and 30, given over several weeks.

Chemotherapy can be given in tablet form or intravenously and may be prescribed over several months, possibly starting before surgery in order to shrink a large tumour. Side-effects may include sickness, fatigue, depression and hair loss.

Hormone therapy in the shape of the drug tamoxifen, a synthetic hormone, is the most popular back-up treatment today. Tamoxifen, which should be taken for five years, seems to work by blocking the effect of oestrogen (the hormone implicated in most breast cancers) on breast cells. There may be unpleasant side-effects, but tamoxifen appears to prolong the disease-free period and survival (often by several years), and to prevent cancer occurring in the other breast. It's also used in cases of recurrence.

TECHNIQUES TO HELP YOU

Part of the modern overall holistic approach of specialist units is to ensure that new patients meet others who have already undergone similar therapy and to put them in touch with a local or national support group.

Cancer specialists increasingly work alongside complementary therapists to help patients cope with treatment. All

relaxation techniques are helpful. Patients also recommend massage, reflexology, aromatherapy or homoeopathy to help combat nausea and tiredness; chiropractic to help after surgery; a good, balanced diet; nutritional supplements to help build up the immune system; and gentle exercise such as yoga and walking.

GET TO KNOW YOUR BREASTS

Being breast aware and knowing what is normal for you will help you to be aware of any changes. Learn how your breasts look and feel at different times. Examine them whenever is best for you (e.g. in the bath or shower or when dressing).

THE NORMAL BREAST

Before the menopause, normal breasts feel different at different times of the month. The milk-producing tissue becomes active in the days before a period. In some women the breasts then feel tender and lumpy, especially near the armpits. After a hysterectomy, the breasts usually show the same monthly differences until the time periods would have stopped. After the menopause, activity in milk-producing tissue stops. Normal breasts feel soft, less firm and not lumpy.

CHANGES TO LOOK OUT FOR

Appearance: change in the outline or shape of the breast. Enlarged veins, puckering or dimpling of the skin.
Feelings: discomfort or pain in one breast, particularly if new and persistent.
Lumps: lumps, thickening or bumpy areas in one breast or armpit.
Nipple change: an inverted nipple or, very rarely, discharge from, or rash on, the nipple; bleeding or moist reddish areas which don't heal.

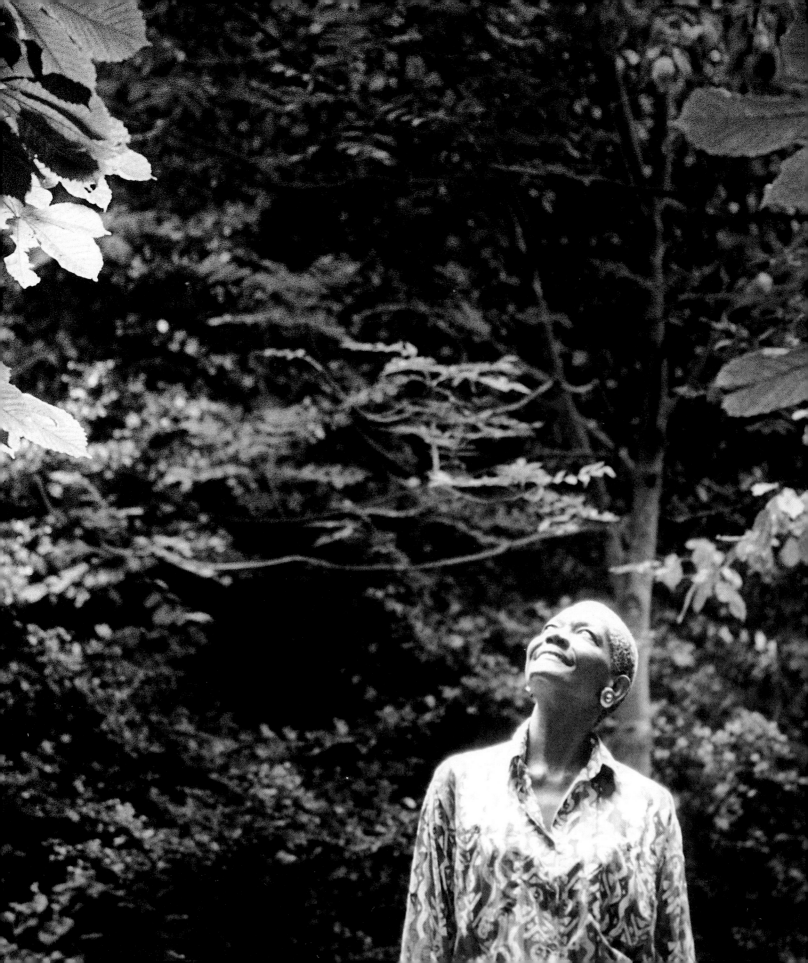

Gloria Hope-Price

We are inspired by Gloria Hope-Price, a psychotherapist and group analyst in her mid-fifties who's passionate about nutrition and mind/body well-being. She and her husband, William, run a tiny health retreat from their home in St James, Barbados*. We love Gloria's Tigger-ish enthusiasm and warmth, her grace – both physical and emotional – and her gloriously down-to-earth approach to life...

'Today I feel more in tune with myself, more alive and alert, freer than ever before. I felt distinctly flat at 40. Everyone had told me "Life begins at 40." So I had a lovely dinner party and waited for the magic moment. Nothing happened and I thought, "I've missed it." You can't get stuck in expectations; you have to be prepared to reinvent yourself and your life. So, at the risk of being called freaky, I started to clear out the garbage in my system with a vegetarian lifestyle.

'The decision to move back to Barbados from London in 1987 was all part of a process of change. I was still going to group therapy twice a week. I began to feel this is all well and good, but my life is about much more than my own – and other people's – neuroses. I decided to become more open with myself: did more socialising, invited my friends to drop in and chat and started dancing which I love.

'It's crucial to give the people around you space for separate lives. Some friends were horrified that we could send Olivia, our only child, to boarding school in England since she was 12 but it was her choice and she has thrived on it.

'I make goat's milk yogurt and cheese here and eat largely raw salads, fruits and vegetables which we grow organically; sometimes I steam vegetables above pure distilled water. We eat raw organic honey, sugar cane, extra virgin olive oil and lemon juice.

'Every 30 days I do a one- to three-day cleanse and detox. I give myself a coffee enema, based on the Gerson cancer therapy, first thing in the morning. After this I add the juice of one freshly squeezed lemon and a pinch of cayenne pepper to a glass of warm water and sip it slowly, followed with some yoga stretches and breathing. I drink plenty of distilled water, freshly juiced fruit and vegetables and salad.

'I started the menopause as we moved here. I was really sweating with the climate change and hot flushes. Do I take hormone replacement therapy? Good God, no. Absolutely not. I really revved up on my nutritional intake with lots of natural oestrogen mimics (*see right*) plus supplements, and an infusion of fennel seeds three times a day. I have weekly aromatherapy massages, with essential oils which contain natural hormones.

'I swim a lot, do yoga and t'ai chi, and I have a rebounder, a mini-trampoline. It's brilliant for cellulite and varicose veins.

'It's so sad to try to hang on to the elusiveness of adolescent beauty. When I was younger, people pursued me to be a model. But I feel much more beautiful now because my soul is alight.'

GLORIA'S SECRETS:
Many foods contain natural plant oestrogens, which may help ease the menopause. Gloria and her nutritionist, Vinson Edghill, are particularly keen on the following, organically grown if possible. They strongly suggest consulting a qualified herbalist, nutritionist or naturopath.
1 Herbal teas: liquorice, aniseed and fennel, caraway, echinacea, black cohosh and dandelion. Three cups daily.
2 Foods: yam, cassava, breadfruit, green bananas, sweet potatoes (not more than once a week), leafy green vegetables, carrots (preferably juiced), sea vegetables. Black strap molasses, unpasteurised raw goat's milk, free range eggs (boiled or poached only). Pineapple, pomegranates, ripe bananas. Oils and seeds: cold pressed oils, e.g. olive; fresh green and black olives; also sunflower and sesame oils and seeds; pumpkin and caraway seeds.
3 Essential oils for balancing hormones: Gloria's aromatherapist, Frederica Bryan, recommends this for the bath: Blend ten drops of lavender and eight drops each of geranium, rosewood, clary sage, rose and jasmine into 100ml grapeseed or sweet almond oils. Add two or three teaspoons of the mixture to a bath two or three times a week and soak for 10–20 minutes. Don't rinse off with soap.

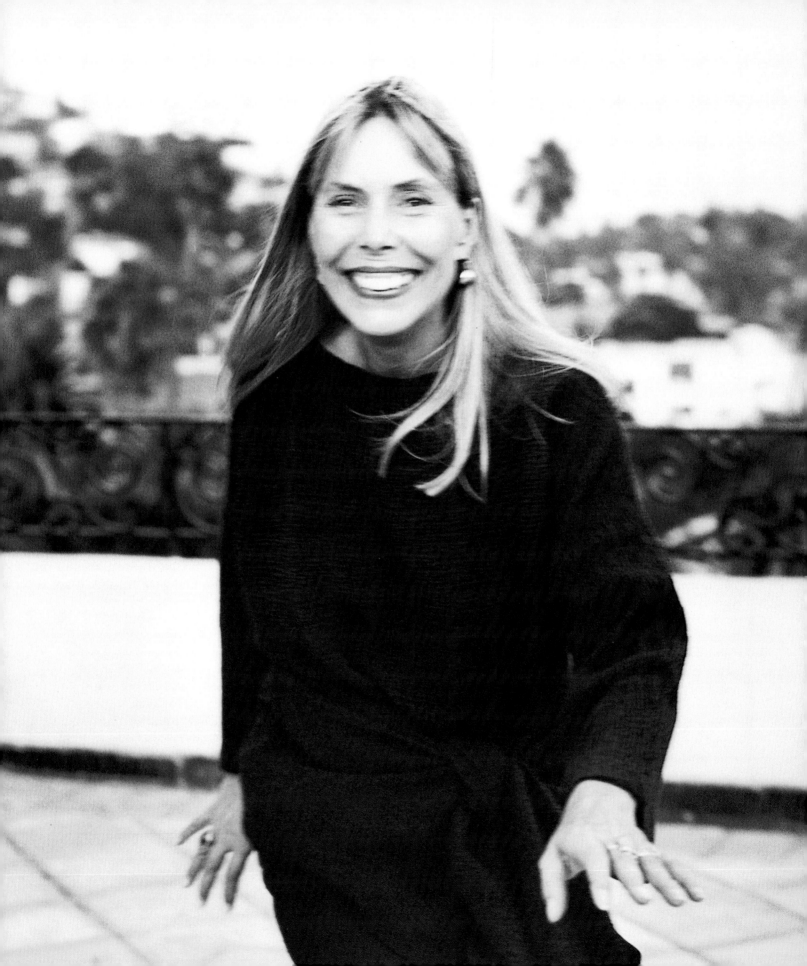

This part of feel fabulous forever **is all about you the human be-ing. (*Not* the human do-ing.)** When all's said and done, friends, lovers, children, employers, even pets won't be with us forever – and the people we're left with are ourselves. Asking our medical experts worldwide for their suggestions on looking after the emotional and

how to **be** fabulous

spiritual side of life inspired the most wonderful input. Looking after yourself is emphatically not selfish, says consultant clinical psychologist Dr Elspeth Stirling: **'You've got to look after yourself first and meet your own needs before you can be fit to look after anybody else's. Stop thinking of others first and you'll do yourself – and them – a favour.'** Neither of us has had a smooth ride (though we're both happy now) and you probably haven't either. This section suggests ways to help your soul sing...

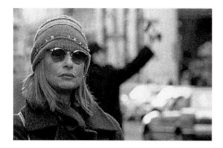

face your demons

Few of us – perhaps none – escape the sort of life experiences that leave us feeling less than blithe and often downright miserable and frightened. They frequently come from childhood as well as the decades of trying to be grown-up. They may be big or small, short- or long-term, but they have a profound influence on the women we are now. Problem is that, however much we suspect they affect our lives, they're often the things we least want to explore. But, as **Lauren Hutton** puts it, 'Every woman has to face her demons.'

Now in her mid-fifties, Lauren is open about the deep-seated problems that led to her consulting a Jungian therapist and resolving the wrinkles in her mind. 'About seven years ago, I was at a very dark time in my life. I broke my leg and for the five months I was recovering, I had to confront myself. I liked nothing about my life. Nothing. I had been in a very long relationship which had broken up. Then I had been with someone else, but I hadn't done what I should have to that. And I didn't like my work.'

'Put out to farm' from modelling at 40, she became 'a cheesy movie queen, making five bad movies a year which I didn't want to see'. But the biggest problems – her 'demons' – were the evils of her childhood: 'That's the thing we put the lid down tight on.'

The factors that really make women look old are psychological, not physical, according to one of the most attractive and interesting women in the world, supermodel Lauren Hutton. Just as we develop wrinkles on our faces so we do in our minds...

She never met her father, who went missing in the Second World War. Her stepfather had a profound effect on her life. 'He was brutal, mad and alcoholic... but he was also a great reader, knew all about the stars and loved nature.' He had a lot to do with her passionate championing of the environment and underprivileged people of all sorts, from women everywhere to the Kalahari tribespeople of Botswana. But at the same time, he made her, she says, into 'Deeply Disturbed of the Ozark Mountains'.

Jungian therapy delves into the subconscious and explores dreams. Lauren Hutton had grown used to regular appalling nightmares of holocaust landscapes, zombie-like men chasing her, and – the worst one – constantly trying to find a place to sleep. Nowadays she dreams of gorgeous houses and beautiful plants.

Hanging on to the wrong man is a bad mistake, she believes. 'If you have a mate and it hasn't worked for ten years, it's not going to change. Bag him, get rid of him! First you'll be much happier alone, second, if you don't it stops you having a shot at real love.'

Hutton is childless but loves children. She deals with that dilemma by being a 'para-parent' to a boy living nearby. 'Para-parenting is happening a lot in Manhattan because over half the people here are single.'

Her ongoing success as a model, and that of others like Dayle Haddon and Carmen dell'Orifice, proves, she believes, that 'womanhood can be celebrated in the bloom, not just in bud'.

Many of us, thank goodness, will not have to face the same demons as Lauren Hutton. Or need the same level of professional therapy. But we believe that everyone benefits from looking at their lives and getting to know themselves better.

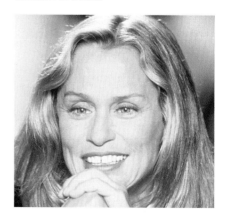

re-start your life

We all want to feel at peace with who we are and how we live our lives. 'I want to really *like* the woman I see in the mirror each morning,' one nearly 50-year-old said to us. And that's what to aim for...

Running away from emotional pain is natural. We may think it's gone but stored-up pain invariably comes back to haunt us. And demons in your cupboard make it pretty well impossible to live in a comfortable state of mind.

Life is about people, and the root of most problems (and much disease) is how we get on with others, according to Dr David Peters, past chair of the British Holistic Medical Association. Sorting out our relationship with ourselves is the first step to getting on well with others.

One of the hallmarks of not valuing ourselves is thinking we have to go through hard times on our own. So face your demons with the help of a confidant(e) – one or more trusted friends, a support group or a professional therapist, doctor or priest.

The key questions are: Do I like myself? and Do I like my life? A good place to start is by sorting out your past, then move on to your present. (Do it vice versa if that's more comfortable.) Write your life story, exploring your feelings about your experiences and about the people who have coloured your life. If you have done things you really dislike yourself for (and who hasn't?), make a list of people to apologise to – you'll feel vastly better.

Be honest and take your time; there's no one to answer to but you.

Now look at the present day. Go through a week or more, being your own emotional shadow. Note your feelings about yourself and your life:

try saying 'I feel...' and see what comes out. Record your dreams. Note what – and who – makes you happy or sad, jolly or snarly, fulfilled or frustrated. Do you, for instance, feel happy at your work? Who do you feel good around? Are you happy with what you do or is there a nagging desire in the back of your mind to do something different? Are you a perfectionist – always trying to achieve the impossible for two women, let alone one? Do you give yourself time to relax and do what you want to do?

Pay attention to your senses: record the music you like, the paintings, books, films, which *enhance* your life.

When you're writing, try not to worry about what *has* happened, or what *may* happen. Live in the present moment: it's the only reality we have. If you find that worries keep popping up, make a list of them, then you can plan how to tackle them – if necessary.

You could write your life story in the third person if you want (using 'she' rather than 'I'); it sometimes helps objectivity. If you find it hard writing things down, say them into a tape-recorder. Or try drawing or painting them.

Discuss what's happening with your confidant(e). If you feel really troubled consider consulting a professional therapist for a short time at least. Brief cognitive behavioural therapy, usually three one-hour sessions with a follow-up three months later, is an increasingly popular option and can be very helpful.

the 'difficult' questions

We found these tough to face up to but also the most constructive:

◆ Do I criticise myself over much? Or am I complacent and/or boastful?

◆ Do I worry what other people think of me? Or do I tend not to consider other people's feelings and wishes?

◆ Do I have enough self-confidence to do what I want as long as it doesn't hurt anyone else? Or do I often give in to what other people want?

◆ Do I usually tell the truth?

◆ Do I say I'm sorry when I've done something wrong?

◆ Am I loyal to family, friends and colleagues? Or do I gossip and/or criticise them behind their backs?

◆ Do I know what I want in most of my life? Or do I feel aimless?

◆ Do I think that I'll get on with most people? Or do I feel I have to be a saint for other people to like me?

◆ Am I contented by and large – and do I say so? Or do I complain a lot?

◆ Do I like what I do? Which bits of my life and which people make me feel up, engaged, passionate? Which make me feel bored, irritable, anxious?

◆ Do I feel in charge of my life? Or have I let someone/something else take control?

When to look for professional 'talking' help:

◆ If you feel your emotions are out of control.

◆ If the inability to make a decision is affecting work and/or relationships.

◆ If you're trapped in a painful situation and can't see a way out.

◆ If you have a pattern of unhappy relationships.

NB Be sure to consult a qualified counsellor or psychotherapist.

the next step

All of this should help you come to terms with the demons from your past. Now, armed with all this information, you are in a good position to see the parts of your life you may want to change. Remember: small changes make a big difference.

One of the big problems about changing our lives is that by the time we see the red light flashing we are usually at such a pitch of desperation that wholesale 100 per cent change seems like the only option. Fast. And all at once. Job, house, man, haircut, clothes, that thread vein on your cheek that's been bothering you for so long. And on, and on. It happens to most of us.

You can't do it, of course, and the only alternative seems to be to do nothing. So you do. Or rather don't. And feel worse. But there is another way. Consider changing 5 per cent. Keep on with what you're doing but change a few small things – the ones you've identified in your life audit. A small change really can make a big difference. Think of it as the art of doing what's possible.

'We're conditioned to thinking in absolutes,' says psychologist Professor Cary Cooper, 'but in fact most people who contemplate major change are unsuccessful in achieving it. A major change work-wise might be something like "I'm going to leave my job entirely and have a good life" or "I'm going to stop being a primary school teacher and become a lawyer." For some people that will be achievable but the vast bulk don't know what that change will bring. So their vision of what will

Live in the present. The only time you have is now.

happen with total change doesn't dovetail with reality and they end up thinking, "My God, I wish I'd known."'

The trick, he says, is to bite off what's chewable. 'Chew that first mouthful and if it feels good, chew another chunk and

Perfection is impossible – admitting to imperfection is human and lovable.

so on.' So when you're considering major change, try smaller ones to begin with. 'Aim at getting the practical information to know what the change might mean to you, get a taste of it without burning your bridges – you might need them as a support system when you're in transition.'

If you're one of the great biters-off-of-more-than-you-can-chew, there's a tendency to feel dejected if you don't achieve 100 per cent. You know from experience you won't manage it – so you procrastinate with everything. The joy of 5 per cent change is that it's almost always achievable. And the rewards tend to be greater than the initial effort. Think of how your life would change if you threw out the tube of toothpaste which has lost its cap and is oozing all over your mascara, in your make-up bag. Or put the door key where you could find it – every time. Or took your alarm clock to the menders. See?

'It sounds good to try for 100 per cent but you'll never achieve it in anything,' says Professor Cooper. 'If you have any sort of big task in front of you, break it down into do-able chunks.'

Einstein's most important question

Scientist Albert Einstein said the most important question for all of us is whether we think the world is a friendly place or not. If you truly believe it is friendly, you will be able to relax and be optimistic about your future – for the next ten minutes and the next ten years. Optimists believe the world is essentially good even if they don't understand why. People who send out positive messages very often get positive responses, so optimism is a self-fulfilling prophecy. But those who think the universe is unfriendly expect the worst and tend to focus on bad things that have happened to them and to other people; so pessimism, like optimism, is largely self-fulfilling.

Gratitude is the key emotion linked to optimism, and so is feeling in control of a situation and not blaming yourself. Revenge is associated with pessimism, also depression and anger plus *not* feeling in control. Pessimism can be transformed into optimism with the help of cognitive therapy and also relaxation techniques.

The neat thing is that you can apply this to pretty well everything in your life. Nothing is too small to be insignificant. For someone who's feeling like a worm,

The only person you can really change is yourself.

simply getting out of bed can seem impossible – let alone getting dressed. So the 5 per cent change could be rolling out on the floor and down to the kitchen. Next day, it could be getting dressed before noon. The next, going out of the house.

Never underestimate what changing a situation slightly can do. 'Shifting a small log at the bottom of the pile causes the whole lot to move,' points out psychologist Dr Keith Stoll. Behaving in a more pleasant way and being good at negotiating, compromising and giving way are recognised as very important factors in improving close personal relationships. 'Pay compliments instead of criticising, smile instead of scowling, take an interest and listen without judging while other people tell you about themselves. Do nice things for other people, such as giving them little presents and looking after them,' suggests Professor Michael Argyle, author of *The Psychology of Happiness*.

Don't live in the problem, live in the solution.

The reason we feel the burden of having to do 100 per cent perfectly – or often 120 per cent – is of course insecurity. It's all very well saying smugly that to be human is to be insecure, but it's not very useful. 'Give yourself permission not to be perfect,' advises Philip Bacon, counsellor and family therapist. 'Many of us are too good at criticising ourselves, which sets up constant conflict in our minds. It's okay to feel selfish, cross, guilty or any other negative emotion. The trick is to acknowledge it, both to yourself and, if it's appropriate, to other people. Then move on.'

A useful 5 per cent tip is to say 'no' occasionally. With adulthood comes the obligation to please people – at home and at work. Most of us feel guilty if we say 'no', resentful when we give in and say 'yes'. Sorting things out every morning in your mind into the things you definitely want to do and those

Happiness is just another way of saying you have your stress load under control.

you don't can help clarify issues. American stress management expert David Sobel says he makes more time for important things – like himself and his family – by assessing invitations and demands, asking himself: 'In five years' time, will I care if I did or didn't do this?' He turns down a lot of things that way. The fear that other people will dislike us for saying no – nicely – is usually unjustified. Invariably they like and respect you more for knowing your own mind.

Following the 5 per cent rule helps put you back in control of your life. And that's the key to dealing with stress, according to experts. It's also a way of being kind to yourself. Which is about the most important thing you can do.

hear yourself

Listening is essential to peace of mind and body. Listen to yourself and to other people without interrupting or riding roughshod over the messages, spoken and unspoken. Bodies usually shout their needs (food, water, loo, sleep, etc.); minds may whisper. Listening to other people's unspoken messages is called using your intuition. Women are very good at it, according to biophysicist Dr Luca Turin. (But not always so good at using it for their own benefit.)

mind and body

Remember that mind and body are never separate. Aches and pains in your body affect your mind and vice versa. Falling in love, for instance, can banish your back pain, and chronic illnesses often disappear on holiday. (But you're twice as likely to get a cold...) Food and drink can make you behave differently: you may feel speedy after coffee, lethargic after wheat. Exercising makes most of us feel (and look) brighter. You can use this mind/body synergy positively to help transform your life. Before you start saying 'I can't possibly change', try this simple example. Sit on a chair facing a window with a view. Ask someone to put their hands on your shoulders. Focus all your attention on a far, high-up point – the top of a building or a tall tree. Both of you will feel the immediate change in your body as your mental and physical energy focuses positively. Our testers found their shoulders went right down and head up.

small changes in difficult times

Physical

● Start by breathing – anxiety is often allied to shallow breathing.

● Untense your body from top to toe, uncrossing arms and legs, straightening spine and neck.

● Take more exercise generally – it's been proved to lift your mood as well as tone your body.

● Ask a friend to give you a hand, foot or shoulder massage for a minimum of 15 minutes once a week, and reciprocate. Allow yourself to relax completely and accept it as a present you deserve.

● Investigate possible food allergies: wheat, for instance, can profoundly depress some people, and simply cutting it out of your diet can lift the depression. Read *Food Allergies and Intolerance** by Professor J. Brostoff.

● Quit smoking, drinking alcohol and caffeinated drinks (coffee, tea, cola, chocolate) which have been linked to depression.

● Drink lots of still pure water.

● Get enough sleep – try to go to bed early, ten p.m. is ideal.

● Improve your diet, making sure you have enough EFAs (oily fish, olive oil and linseed are good sources) and consider taking food supplements. Low levels of B vitamins have been linked to depression; other important mood food supplements are vitamin C, calcium, magnesium, copper, potassium and the omega-6 fatty acids. Consult a qualified nutritionist if small changes don't improve the situation.

● Always take a lunch-break – try for 45 minutes at least.

Mental

◆ Lie or sit comfortably and picture in your mind somewhere you love being, where you have once been happy.

◆ Take a worry break: confront one of your worst fears and really worry about it for the next five minutes. The deal is, however, that the worry is confined to that time only and you don't worry again for the rest of the day.

◆ Unclutter your work and living space.

◆ Count to five, or preferably take five minutes, before yelling at anyone.

◆ Don't watch the news.

◆ Read an enjoyable novel.

◆ Smile at someone; laugh at a joke; see a funny film. Smiling and laughing (even if you fake it) trigger feel-good hormones. Try shouting 'Happy!' and beaming.

◆ Listen to music you enjoy – the rhythm can help your mind.

Emotional

■ Remember you're not the only one – one out of every three women you see every day is likely to have felt the same way.

■ Be your own best friend: imagine the help, love and support you would give a friend in the same situation and know that you deserve the same.

■ Don't write yourself roles in other people's movies when you needn't even have a walk-on part in their lives, or get caught up in their problems.

■ Take a few calming drops of Bach Flower Rescue Remedy or Jan de Vries Emergency Essence in water.

■ Practise feeling joy in small things – a phone call from a friend, a beautiful flower, not getting a parking ticket, a delicious meal.

■ Burn vetiver essential oil, the oil of tranquillity, in a vaporiser – or simply put some on your heel.

■ Allow yourself to wear your favourite clothes, do your hair and put on make-up.

Spiritual

▲ Light a candle in a holy or inspiring place – which could be your own home.

▲ Make a wish to whatever force you believe gave you life.

▲ Believe that there are other people on your side.

instant lifts

✻ Drop 'if only' from your vocabulary.

✻ Turn on some music and dance.

✻ Buy yourself your favourite flowers.

✻ Think of five things you've done well – anything from exquisite ironing, to cooking a delicious meal; adding up your bank statements, to helping a friend; not losing your temper with someone really irritating, to finishing a job of work.

✻ Sit in the sun (with an SPF on, please).

✻ Wrap your arms round yourself and give yourself a hug.

✻ Tune in to your favourite comedy show.

✻ Think about times and places when you are happy; store away the memories to revisit when you feel low.

✻ Think of one thing you can do – big or small – which would make you feel better, and either do it, or take positive steps to make it happen.

✻ Plan a trip or holiday.

✻ Go to sleep with a happy thought in your mind: a compliment someone paid you; a joke; a lovely view; a person you like.

✻ Wake up and decide to enjoy the day as much as you possibly can.

✻ Do something you really want to do, whether it's learning something new (*see Creativity, pp.240–241*) or playing your favourite record.

✻ Consider cognitive therapy – tweaking the way you view the world and your place in it can re-colour your life.

✻ Try a herbal anti-depressant such as St John's Wort, which 23 studies have shown to be as effective as most anti-depressants with far fewer side-effects.

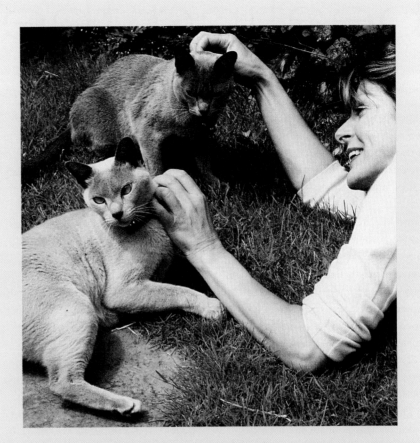

get a life, get a pet

Simply watching a dog bound joyfully round a park or a cat stretch in the sun is cheering. But evidence is now growing that being close to an animal is positively health-enhancing. 'Having a pet can improve your life,' says Professor Donald Broom, who researches into people's physiological responses to animals. By making people calmer, animals can help lower blood pressure and boost the immune system. Plus, of course, some animals prompt owners to take more exercise.

And animals can be powerful antidepressants. Research with elderly women showed that puppies could persuade even the most depressed and reclusive to come out of their shells. 'A warm and wiggly puppy has the power to make an old and tired spirit soar,' said Professor Gloria Francis of Virginia Commonwealth University.

beating the blues

Can't be bothered to get out of bed in the morning? Nothing seems worthwhile? Feel you're trying to turn a mighty river upstream? Millions of others feel the same. But there are positive answers.

Although we are both on a pretty even keel now we have personal experience of depression and stress. According to Government figures, one in five women suffers 'unwelcome stress', and the peak time is between 35 and 54. The World Health Organisation forecasts that depression will be the leading cause of incapacity by 2020. Virtually everyone feels blues-y at times but a staggering one in three women will experience a more severe form of low mood in her life. Twice as many women as men suffer from depression, probably because they have more stress, less support and more hormonal ups and downs.

The anxiety-to-depression spectrum is a complex one. Both are internal states: anxiety is being wound up too tight, and depression is sinking down into a low mood. They are both responses to external stressors. Depending on how we cope with stress, it can be positive – the sort of thing that makes you rise to an occasion – or negative – when we feel things are out of control and too much is expected of us.

'Feeling low' is one of the most common reasons women consult their doctor and, in a hectic world where most doctors have little time to talk, anti-depressant prescriptions are rocketing. Drugs may temporarily mask the pain but they won't tackle the root cause. The encouraging news is that there is a range of non-drug ways to improve it. For women, it's frequently allied to exhaustion – simply doing too much and having too high standards. And, of course, being expected to live a double life as carers and workers. Talk to your doctor if he/she is sympathetic and also consider exploring naturopathy, homeopathy, herbalism as well as counselling or psychotherapy.

Reasons for feeling low

Disentangling the strands in the web of depression may be difficult. Obvious problems are the four big stressful life events: moving house, job worries or unemployment, bereavement, divorce or separation. Stressful life events can all be exacerbated by physical conditions including hormonal changes *(see pp.206–223)*, not eating properly, food allergies, specific vitamin/mineral deficiencies, pollution, not taking exercise or simply being tired out.

Share any worries and also be a good listener for those who may need you.
FRANCES HUNT**

Other physical problems which may result in a low mood include an underactive thyroid, anaemia, candidiasis, hypoglycaemia (the shortage of sugar most often linked to diabetes) and also post-viral symptoms.

Pain – whether it's back, shoulder or neck ache, or the pain of long-term or life-threatening illness – is both a cause and a symptom of depression. Skin problems such as acne rosacea and psoriasis also often depress patients, according to London GP Dr Susan Horsewood-Lee. Post-natal depression may linger for years if not treated.

Alcohol can lower rather than enhance your mood, and too much too often can result in profound depression.

Symptoms of anxiety

- feeling wound up and restless
- thinking and worrying about tomorrow
- feeling panicky
- having trouble getting to sleep
- wanting to avoid people and challenges
- getting indigestion
- setting unrealistic expectations for oneself
- feeling constricted in the throat; hyperventilating

Symptoms of depression

- feeling isolated and misunderstood
- feeling tired or exhausted
- sleeping badly; waking too early
- feeling sad for no apparent reason
- losing your appetite and losing weight or eating much more than usual and gaining weight
- not wanting to do anything or be interested in anything
- having no motivation at work
- feeling worthless and/or hopeless
- having no self-confidence
- having thoughts of suicide

winter depression

Depressed between autumn and spring? So lethargic and sleepy you can hardly function? Comfort-eating like crazy? Any of these can be symptoms of Seasonal Affective Disorder. Now recognised by the medical profession, SAD is sometimes known as 'winter depression' because it tends to strike when the days shorten and the nights draw in, and can endure until the lambs are frolicking in the fields the following spring.

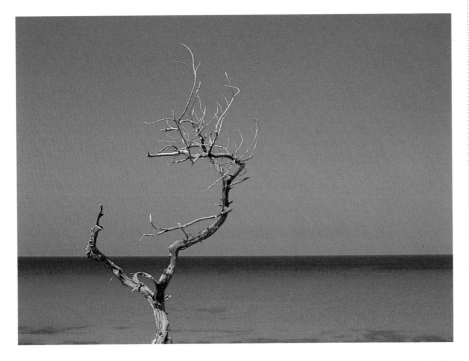

It's thought to affect as many as 10 per cent of us, three times as many women as men, although doctors don't yet know why. But unlike other forms of depression, the cure is simple – good old daylight.

SAD is triggered by lack of daylight. During the night, the pineal gland – our 'third eye' – produces a hormone called melatonin, which makes us drowsy. At daybreak, the bright light of dawn causes the gland to stop producing melatonin. But on dull winter days, especially when we're indoors, not enough light is received to trigger this waking-up process. New research is also starting to link bright light with the increased production of serotonin, a neuro-transmitter; lack of serotonin is known to be a cause of depression. While most people adjust perfectly to the seasonally changing day-length, the body-clock mechanism which tells SAD sufferers when to wake up and when to sleep doesn't function properly.

The solution, for as many as 85 per cent of sufferers, has proved to be light, or photo-, therapy. This means getting out into bright light as much as possible. But since that isn't always practical, consider investing in a full-spectrum light box, which sits on your desk, or some other convenient place where the light can reach your eyes for a minimum of 30–45 minutes daily. The light must be suitably bright; at least 2500 lux (the technical measure of brightness) is needed, about five times brighter than a well-lit office. It must also be full spectrum, which gives you the same light waves as daylight, unlike normal electric light bulbs. (It's not like a sun-bed light, however, and won't either tan you or hurt your eyes.) We both suffer from SAD during winter months and have invested in full-spectrum lights for our desks; we've found them literally life-changing.

SAD symptoms

If you experience these five major symptoms during autumn and winter months you could be suffering from SAD, according to Dr Norman Rosenthal, a US government researcher generally credited with discovering SAD.

1 Noticeable lack of energy to the point of debilitation.
2 A fairly constant feeling of sadness or depression.
3 A desire to sleep as much as possible – or to sleep briefly and become nocturnal.
4 Feeling listless and less creative than usual.
5 Having less control of your appetite – perhaps to the point of weight gain.

NB If you suffer from a skin or eye condition which might be affected by exposure to bright light, check with your doctor before beginning light therapy.

how is it for you?

Probably the biggest myth in the world is that everyone else is having an earthshaking sex life. And it becomes truer as we get older. That's not to say, however, that more – or different – wouldn't be better. We talked to experienced psycho-sexual therapist Frances Emeleus, accredited by the British Association of Sexual and Marital Therapists, about the particular problems of sexual love and ageing.

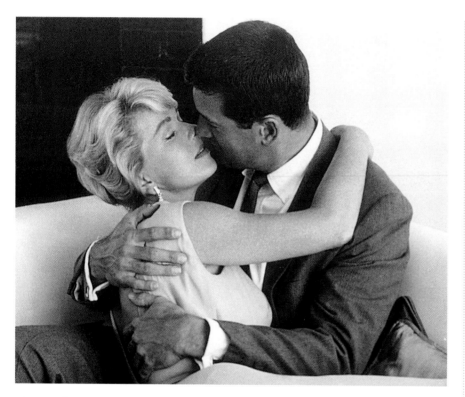

'Our sex lives can lose their sparkle as we get older and, in consequence, become relegated to late at night when both partners are tired. Also, most women struggle to a great or lesser extent with the menopause and that can affect our body image so a lot of middle-aged women no longer feel sexually attractive,' says Frances. The reason for this, she suggests, is largely the media. 'Magazines in particular have constructed a culture which says only one thing is attractive – youth and slimness. It can be difficult for women who don't think they match that idealised photofit to feel sexy. And that's very destructive.'

To help overcome this, she suggests that women look at themselves in the bath, or in front of a mirror naked, and attempt to suspend judgement on their bodies. So, instead of saying 'Oh help!' and rushing for the nearest total tent-like cover-up, she recommends describing your body objectively – 'as if it were a building or a statue; for example "those are nice long curves, that's a striking shape and there's an interesting slope"' – because in doing so you move away from judging your body, and finding it wanting.

Afterwards, she suggests, 'Let yourself think about the woman you saw in the mirror as if she was a close friend – you might be surprised at just how many pluses there are.'

'Being sexy doesn't mean wearing black lace suspenders,' she continues. 'It does mean each of us seeing sexuality as an integral part of our bodies – and souls. Sexual energy is creative energy – part of the life force even when we can't have children any longer.'

Touching and stroking are 'absolutely crucial' to loving your body and discovering its sexuality. And that applies to both partners. 'Remember that men feel exactly the same thing about their bodies – their tummies, their waistlines, their balding heads – but if you can spend time celebrating rather than criticising and condemning, you begin to develop something to help you over your feeling of regret for your youthful body.'

After menopause, women may find that intercourse is uncomfortable as vaginal walls thin and there may be less vaginal lubrication. Frances recommends two lubricating products: Senselle and Sylk *(see Directory)*.

A lot of people have very mixed messages going through their heads about touching themselves and others. Frances recommends sensate focusing exercises (described in the box below) which involve stroking each other's bodies (or your own), in silence, without progressing to intercourse. 'This hurtling towards penetrative sex is like going for a plane or train – it's just how to get from here to there in the shortest possible time. As if we're saying, "This is the only bit that counts and everything else is irrelevant."' A good sex life is also about tenderness and intimacy, she emphasises.

The most important relationship to cherish is the one nearest you. 'Spend time and thought and care on your partner and that will help your sex life.' And communicate! 'Couples have often adapted to "doing it" in a particular way, with very little conversation, very little knowledge of what the other wants and an attitude of he (or she) should know what I like...*by now*. But they never ask what the other one wants or likes, or say what *they* would like. So neither of them knows.'

What's my ultimate health secret? Sex. It keeps you young. Let's face it, after an orgasm you feel better.

ZSA ZSA GABOR

Many women may have a satisfying sex life but feel that there is still something missing. This may be because they are not fully connected with their own bodies and emotions or with their partner's, Frances believes. One of the problems, she says, is that many couples subconsciously base their relationship on getting the other to do what they want. 'All of us want our own way all of the time. A good relationship is where I acknowledge that you have a different point of view from me and I don't need you to hold my view in order for me to feel secure. Sex is not about overwhelming the other, but recognising that you are each different people with different needs.'

Frances also recommends relaxation breathing exercises (*see p.162*; specific techniques are detailed in *The Joy of Sexual Ecstasy* by Margo Anand). And, although the idea of sexual therapy is still a big taboo, Frances believes it could help many people. 'I've seen people turn their sexuality around after 25, 30, even 40 years of mediocre sexual relations.'

Finally, Frances recommends taking your love-making out of the fifteenth division. 'Bodies are magnificent things and sex shouldn't be a third-class activity. It should be a celebration, so spend time and imagination on it.'

sensate focusing exercises

These can be done to another person or to yourself. Remember, do these for yourself, don't get tempted into giving the other person a massage.

TOUCHING: WITH A PARTNER

▲ Take it in turns to silently explore all over your partner's body with different degrees of touch, hard and gentle, circular or long strokes; spend 15 minutes each on the back and 15 minutes on the front, caressing everywhere except breasts and genitals. If you can, talk about it afterwards.

▲ Notice which parts gave you the most pleasure – or not.

▲ Indulge all your senses while you're doing this, with music, warmth, soft lighting and body or massage lotion for your stroking hand.

TOUCHING: ON YOUR OWN

▲ Do the same and remember that being on your own doesn't mean you have to go without sex; solo sex can be a rich and rewarding experience.

questions to ask yourself about your sexuality:

■ What do I really think about sex?

■ Has that view changed over the years?

■ Is this what I really want to think?

■ Am I fulfilling my sexual desires?

■ Has my sex life gone wrong?

■ Where and when did that start?

■ Am I giving in if I give up sex now?

■ Would it be possible for me to change?

■ Do I really want to become a sexual being?

holistic help for stressed-out minds and bodies

Our state of mind is a major factor in our state of health. When you're feeling like screeching – or climbing into a deep, dark, miserable pit – some TLC from an expert pair of hands can soothe your mind and boost your health. There is also a range of complementary therapies to help well-being: some you can do yourself, like meditation, others are done to you, like acupuncture.

We asked three experts, Dr James Hawkins, a member of the British Holistic Medical Association, Dr George Lewith of the Centre for the Study of Complementary Medicine in Southampton, England, and Anne Woodham, author of *Stress at Work* and *The Encyclopedia of Complementary Medicine**, for their top suggestions, see right.

Stress-related and chronic conditions, including high blood pressure, allergies, muscle tension, pain, migraine and headaches, tend to respond particularly well to these types of therapy.

We've tried out many complementary therapies and are great supporters. As well as helping the way we feel, these tension busters can help the way we all look, smoothing out worry lines and putting a sparkle in tired eyes. Our particular favourites are aromatherapy massage, Bach Flowers, reflexology, healing and herbal medicine.

HANDS-ON THERAPIES
Healing
Massage
Reflexology
Tragerwork

ALTERNATIVE THERAPIES
Acupuncture
Bach Flower Remedies
Homeopathy
Herbalism
Music Therapy
Nutritional Therapy
Flotation Therapy

SELF-HELP
Autogenic Training
Tai Chi
Qigong (pronounced chee gong)

DIY...NOW!
Meditation
Meditation helps calm mind and body: circulation improves and muscle tension disappears. As a result, you can deal better with whatever the day hurls at you. Some doctors already recommend meditation to patients to combat stress-related illness. Try the basic principles below, and then decide whether you want to go further.

1 Don't attempt to meditate with a full tummy or when you're hungry.
2 Find a quiet spot where you won't be interrupted; unplug the phone and put up a Do Not Disturb notice.
3 Experiment with dimmed lighting and closed curtains or blinds.
4 Lie or sit comfortably, hands in lap; make certain your body is relaxed, uncross arms and legs, straighten your spine. (Meditation teachers often suggest sitting so you won't drop off!)
5 Breathing gently, imagine your whole body relaxing; start with scalp, hairline, every feature, then move down your body, feeling tension ebb away.
6 The aim of meditation is to stop stimulating thoughts or niggling problems taking up mind space. The easiest way is to concentrate on one calm thought, e.g. the colour blue, mountain tops, a sunset, the sea.
7 Transcendental Meditation gives you a mantra (word) to repeat over and over in your mind. Try choosing a word you find soothing and repeating it.
8 Allow your breathing to settle into a natural rhythm. Focus on your breath: feel the air as it enters your nostrils moving down to fill the lungs; rest a moment then let it go gently, emptying your body. Try to breathe from abdomen rather than chest and feel your tummy swell as you inhale. Count slowly as you breathe: count to four as you inhale, rest for a beat or two, then exhale to a count of four.
9 Whenever a distracting thought breaks in, simply acknowledge it and let it go. American meditation master Ram Dass suggests transforming the thought into a cloud and watching it float away in your mind's eye.
10 Start with a couple of minutes and gradually spend longer. Don't worry if you feel you can't focus at first, just go on practising. Try to establish a regular time to start off with: early morning and last thing at night are very helpful.

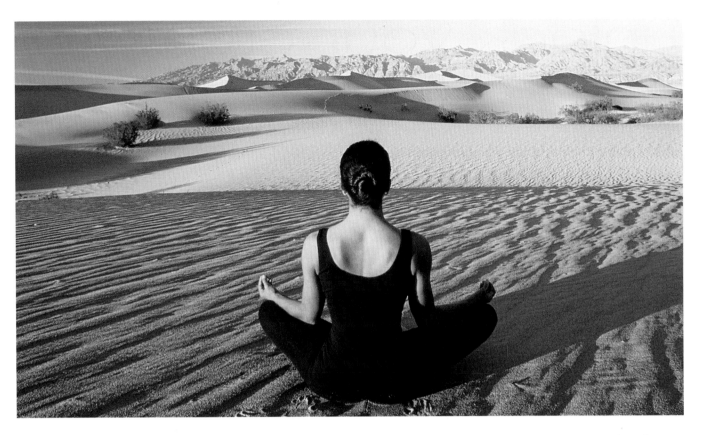

Creative Visualisation

This can be a form of meditation and uses the same general principles detailed above. With visualisation, however, you are going to focus on creating healing pictures in your mind and employ other senses to recreate that memory of wellness. These visualisations or mind pictures can come in thousands of different forms – whatever suits you. Think of it as targeted daydreaming. Once you get used to it, you can do this virtually anywhere, any time, even when there's noise and people around you. Try variations on these themes, then make up your own.

◆ When you feel flustered, think of a place where you have been happy and secure and calm, e.g. a garden in the summer, a beach, a meadow; now feel the sun and the breeze, smell the flowers, hear the mew of seagulls or the buzz of bees; let your mind and body sink into the 'film' in your head.

◆ If you have a problem, or more than one, bedevilling you as you try to go to sleep, try putting it/them into an air balloon, releasing the balloon and watching it drift away, far up into the sky and out of sight.

◆ Alternatively, take your problem and put it into a file, put the file in a folder, and the folder in a lower desk drawer or filing cabinet, shut the drawer, turn the key and put that away. You can do this at any time, but the deal is that you must sort out the problem at the next practical opportunity.

◆ If your left – organising – brain is on overtime and you can't stop your mind whirring, try transferring over to your right – creative – brain like this. Feel yourself in your left brain then turn your back and walk along a path – whatever you like – over to your right brain. Go through a door – turn the handle, open the door, and shut the door again behind you. Notice where you find yourself, in a walled garden, perhaps, or a peaceful room. Make yourself comfortable and either do nothing – smell the roses – or wander round and see who else is there.

◆ If you're frightened or uncomfortable in a situation, visualise winding a lovely lavender-coloured cocoon around yourself, up and down, round and round, until you feel entirely safe.

◆ Or do as actress Amanda Burton does and imagine beautiful golden angels putting their wings around her and shielding her from all harm.

See Directory for contact details for all organisations.

unlock your creativity

We are all creative. But exploring that playful, artistic, creative side often gets put on a back burner in a flurry of family commitments, deadlines and the general, overwhelming feeling that there isn't the time to do the things we have to do – let alone the things we'd like to do. But if you want to experience a real jump in your quality of life, it's time to tap into your creativity.

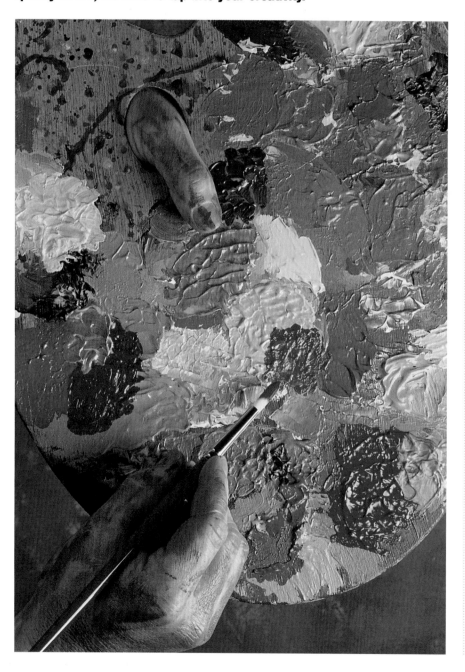

Psychologists believe that we should all make time to indulge and explore our creative potential. 'You never know where that may lead,' says Nick Williams, who runs highly successful seminars to help people unlock their creative potential. 'Sometimes, women discover a whole new path in life – and turn what started as an enjoyable hobby into a career. Others simply find a way of dealing with stress, not just forgetting their problems for a while, but discovering creative solutions – a whole new way of tackling them...'

'As children,' explains Nick, 'we are all naturally creative and have no problems singing/drawing/being natural. But we lose that as we grow up. My recommendation to women is that they get back in touch with creativity in some area of their life – whether through singing or dancing or writing or flower arranging.'

Nick agrees with Leslie Kenton that mid-life can be a time of tremendous creative potential. 'The children have flown the nest – or maybe you're not striving so hard to get to the top of the career ladder, which may allow you more time for creative pursuits.'

BLUEPRINT

So many of us, however, just don't know where to start. So here is Nick Williams' blueprint – to encourage each and every one of us to tap into our creativity...

■ **Start now.** 'We do sometimes forget that life is not a rehearsal. Don't wait for a crisis – an illness, a bereavement – to do the things you really want to do.'

■ **Give up on perfectionism.** 'What often deters people is the idea that if they paint a picture, it won't be "good enough". Paint for yourself, not because you want to put a painting in an exhibition. There is no right or wrong way of being creative – it's about self-expression. You don't have to show anyone: write for your own joy, arrange flowers for your own joy, sing to your heart's content – out of earshot, if you prefer. However you connect with your soul is just fine.'

■ **Never tell yourself 'I'm not creative'.** '*Everyone's* naturally creative – but we often lose touch with that, over the busy years. If you're not sure which area to express your creativity in cast your mind back ten, fifteen, twenty – maybe thirty – years and ask yourself, "What did I love doing then?" I believe that everyone has a vein of gold – their creativity – running through them; sometimes they just have to dig a little deeper to find it.'

■ **Keep a creativity journal.** 'I am a big fan of Julia Cameron's book *The Artist's Way**. This is a 12-step programme for rediscovering creativity, and a key step is to get up every morning and write – about whatever you want to write about; how you feel, whether you're in a lousy or a great mood, what inspires you. Sometimes you feel totally uninspired and hate doing it – and other days you are brimming with ideas and possibilities. Because creativity is like a muscle that needs to be exercised…'

creative inspirations…

It really is never too late – or too early, for that matter – to find out what you love to do, what fires you up and makes you tingle with alive-ness. So: here are some shining examples of adventurous, creative, daring women who've inspired us…

Anna Murdoch – who gave up journalism to marry Rupert Murdoch, but tapped into her creativity again in her forties – and became a bestseller: 'I have a lot of energy and I think women should do things. I don't write to be independent or for the money. I do it for the satisfaction.'

Karin Clements (above right), painter, b. 1944, whose canvases now sell for over £1,000: 'I'd never picked up a pencil in my life till I was 47 and signed up for drawing classes at a local Adult Education institute. I went on to take an A Level in Art, not for the qualification but to learn more. Suddenly, I felt there had been a huge hole in my life that had been filled. My upbringing was: you grow up, get married, have children, it's your job and you should enjoy it. But at the end of the day, I didn't; I would ask myself, 'Why aren't I blissfully happy?' But painting changed my life. And although I now make my living out of painting – I've been commissioned to paint portraits of Gillian Shepard MP and The Duke of Kent, and had sell-out exhibitions – I do it because I want to, not to make money. I can completely lose myself in my painting. If you can just find that fulfilment, it absolutely shines out of you and makes you so much more attractive as a person. My

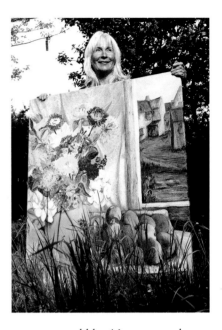

message would be: it's never too late to start something new – and get so much more out of life…'

Maria Platt-Evans (pictured over), photographer, b. 1950, who used to work inspecting sparkplugs in a factory in the North of England and is now an in-demand documentary photographer: 'At 35, I took up photography at night school – and two years later went on to study it full-time at college. My son had grown up; I wasn't anyone's Mum any more, or wife, or daughter, I was just starting to be me, and that was very liberating. The only way I could make a career of documentary photography was to move to London. So I did, and now work for women's magazines. But my passion has never left me; I can be down in the dumps – maybe I haven't been paid and I'm overdrawn at the bank, or I'm shattered and tired – but I can go on a shoot and come away on a high. In a way, I think I get more out of

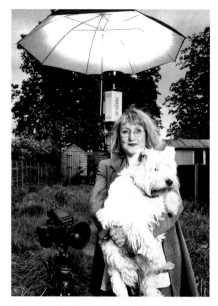

photography because I took it up later; I brought my life's experience to it. My advice is: whatever you long to do, just do it. You have to stop making excuses. The number of women who say, "I'd love to do what you do…" The women at Champion Sparkplugs who used to say that to me are still working there. But I have a whole new life.'

Creativity is good for the soul and work is a process of self-definition, of finding out who you are. But once you find out – you can lie down…

BETTE MIDLER

MORE CREATIVE INSPIRATIONS…

For every one of us, there is a way of expressing our creativity, waiting to be discovered. We could have written a whole book just about the women listed here – and we defy anyone not to be inspired by them… **Lenore Schaeffer**, of Phoenix, Arizona, who's

over 100, took up ballroom dancing after being widowed at 82. Her home's filled with trophies for the foxtrot, the rhumba and the *merengue*. 'I've danced from Santa Monica to Miami. Ballroom dancing gave me a whole new life…' **Mary Wesley**, who had her first novel published at 70 (and has written a bestseller almost every year since). **Betty Boothroyd**, no-nonsense Speaker of the House of Commons – the woman who has many an MP quaking in their boots – is passionate about parascending (in which she's towed by a boat and soars into the skies on a parachute, before drifting slowly back down into the water). **Rosemary Trollope** – mother of bestselling novelist Joanna – took up writing at 79, collating scenes from her childhood in *Starting From Glasgow* (Sutton). **Torun Bülow-Hübe**, Swedish-born former muse who rubbed shoulders with Matisse, Braque, Sartre, Picasso, is seventysomething; she's not only the oldest active silversmith working for Danish company Georg Jensen, but escapes the cruel Scandinavian winters by disappearing to Jakarta – where she passes on her skills to local underprivileged teenagers. Californian **Sally Alexander**, eightysomething, who – when she lost her bid for the House of Representatives in November 1997 – challenged her opponent to a surfing competition. (He didn't show up. But Sally's still surfing – a pastime she's been passionate about since the age of seven.) Brooklyn-born photographic legend **Lillian Bassman**, whose work appeared in virtually every issue of *Harper's Bazaar* from the late forties to the 1960s – and who revived her career at 80, photographing an advertising campaign for Nieman Marcus and working for glossy New York fashion

magazines. Artist **Evelyn Roth**, sixtysomething resident of South Australia's Maslin Beach, who creates giant inflatable installations out of nylon fabric, a career shift inspired when she attended a creative workshop after her marriage broke down 'and I discovered who I was and what I wanted out of life'. (Whereupon she wrote a book on recycling, crocheted a cover for her car out of old videotape – yes, really – and made a short film, showcasing her movement sculptures and choreography.) **Margie Jenkins**, who published her first children's book – *Fun At Bedtime* (The Book Guild) – at an amazing 96… When she turned 60, **Marlies Beschorner** decided 'now or never' – and set off backpacking. 'All my life I had responsibilities, including bringing up two daughters. Now, I could fulfil my old dream of travelling round the world' – so she set off on a 14-month backpacking trip across Iran, Pakistan, South-East Asia and China. Another intrepid traveller: seventysomething **Irene 'Morphy' Richards**, who has notched up thousands of miles since retiring from the Electricity Board over 20 years ago. 'What worries me is all the young people you meet spending their twenties backpacking round the world. What are they going to do when they retire?' Follow the example of **Natalie Hodgson**, perhaps, who's now in her mid-eighties and who took up water-skiing at 69. 'I read that it was for anyone between the ages of seven and 70, so I thought I'd better get a move on.' And when her husband died in 1989 – after 50 years of marriage – Natalie set about creating a bee and lavender farm, in Astley Abbotts, Shropshire. 'I wasn't prepared to sit around and wait to be carried off.'

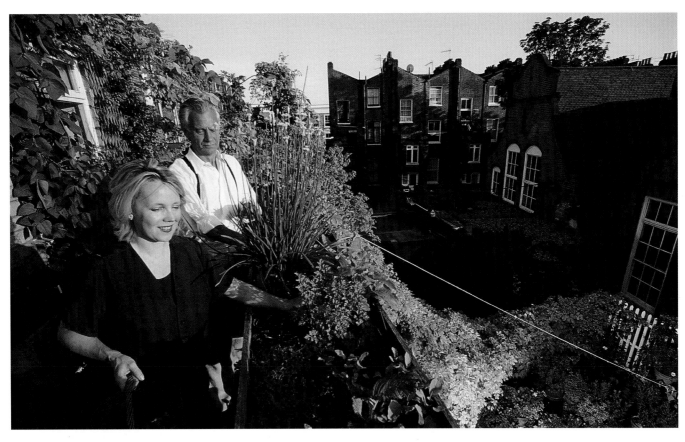

IF IN DOUBT, GARDEN

When the going gets tough, where will you find us? Up to our wrists in dirt, dead-heading the roses, worrying out the stringy roots of bindweed or planting out lettuce seedlings (that's Jo, above, on her Portobello Road roof-deck vegetable garden). It's small wonder, perhaps, that gardening – one of the most accessible forms of creativity for many of us – is soaring in popularity. As May Sarton said in her *Journal of A Solitude*, 'Everything that slows us down and forces patience, everything that sets us back into the slow cycles of nature is a help. Gardening is an instrument of grace.'

Whether of window-ledge proportions or a matter of acres, gardening offers tremendous potential for stress-busting and creativity. We can switch off – or use that time, in touch with nature, to think about how we want to spend the rest of our lives. (We admire fashion entrepreneur **Dianne Benson**, who – having owned four stores in Manhattan – changed tack in her late forties, turning a hobby into a career by writing an utterly inspirational book on gardening – *Dirt* *, a great read for the green-fingered if you can find a copy.)

But more than that, gardening also has the potential to heal our souls. There is actually a new movement – 'horticultural therapy' – creating gardens in unlikely places, such as prisons and inner-city community centres, where stress levels might otherwise soar. Horticultural therapists use gardening to improve people's physical, mental and emotional well-being. Explains Kathleen Fisher, editor of *The American Horticulturalist*, 'Research shows that we don't just imagine that plants make us feel good, but that their presence can hasten physical healing and produce psychological changes similar to those brought about by meditation or other highly relaxed states.'

Nancy Stevenson, Friends' Chairperson of the American Horticultural Therapy Association, believes that gardening is a powerful restorative for the body and spirit. 'In the garden, we witness the natural, cyclic rhythms of birth, life, sickness and death. We see ourselves as part of that process, fit our own lives into the bigger picture of experience. It is a deeply comforting experience.' And at the end of it, we have roses for our house and (organic) vegetables for our table. And as creative pursuits go, beat that.

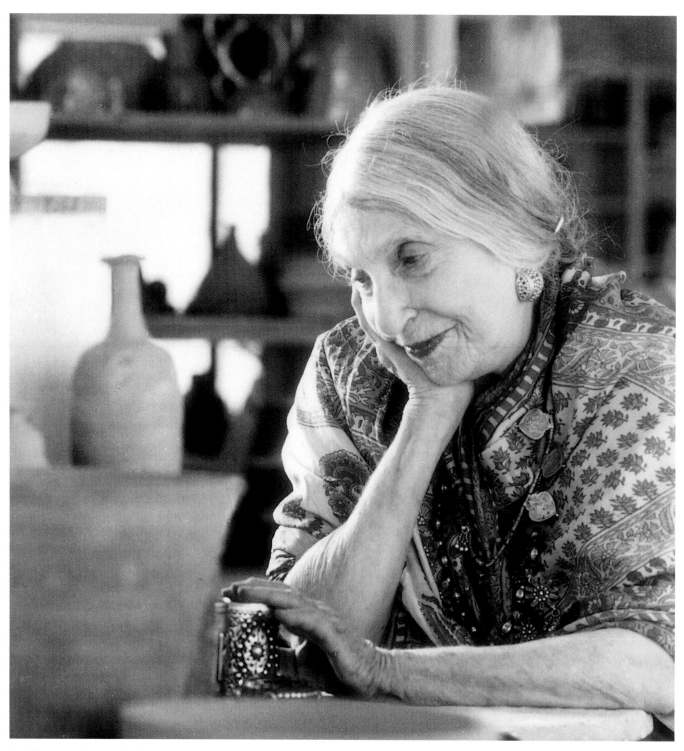

Last but not least – the late Beatrice Wood, known as the 'Mama of Dada', an artist and sculptress who died at the age of 105 just before we were due to interview her for this book. And who was sculpting, drawing and flexing her creative muscle right up to that day...

how to give yourself more time

What wouldn't you give for another hour a day? Not many people know this – as Michael Caine might say – but our bodies think there are 25 hours in each day; the natural body clock runs to a 25-hour not a 24-hour cycle. For reasons known only to evolution, Something Went Wrong and most of us ended up like the White Rabbit in *Alice in Wonderland* – late with life.

But there are tricks to claw back that hour and reduce stress – 'worry hurry sickness' as one psychologist calls it. The simple answer is to get up earlier. Try setting your alarm clock five minutes earlier every day. By the end of a fortnight (lie in on Sundays but not too long or you risk the whole exercise), you will have re-set your waking mechanism by an hour. Great time-saving tips:

1 Do one thing at a time, focus all your attention on that task and finish it before moving on.

2 Make a to do list each day. With each job, ask yourself: Is it really necessary? What would happen if: I junked it? asked someone else to do it? took a short cut? Does it really need to be done today? If not, decide when you should tackle it – and do it then.

3 Plan what you need to prepare today to make tomorrow easier, e.g. collect dry cleaning, plan supper, check route.

4 Keep running short- and long-term lists in your diary: e.g. shopping, birthday and Christmas presents, when to collect shoes and laundry.

5 Practise saying 'no', the greatest time-saver ever invented. It's absolutely legitimate to say 'no' at home or at work when: the request is unreasonable; it's less important than the job you're working on; you don't have the required knowledge, skills or information; you're angry or upset; or it need not be done by you at all.

6 Make a place to put everything – think of the time you spend looking for the car keys, your diary, guarantees.

7 Fill the car with fuel before it's on its last gasp and you spend hours looking for a petrol station.

8 Don't get cross, resentful or give in to road rage: they all waste energy as well as time.

9 Allow other people to do things for you, even if they don't do them quite as well as you would. And always accept offers of help with washing up saucepans: it saves your very valuable time and your equally valuable hands.

10 Make a year plan including time off daily, weekly, monthly and proper holidays. We all know about 'lost' time; now try 'found' time, which means those periods of a few minutes – usually waiting for something or someone – which can either irritate the hell out of you or make your day. Make the most of found time by always carrying a notebook, pen, postcards, address book and a good paperback or magazine plus a personal stereo and tapes if you can.

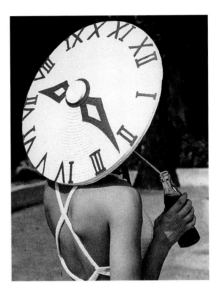

FIND TIME!

1 Sit on a bench in the sun and daydream – it's good for your health.
2 Do your pelvic-floor exercises – pull up your internal muscles and think thin *(see p.178)*.
3 Plan tomorrow.
4 Deep breathe, meditate or do a spot of creative visualisation *(see p.239)*.
5 Read your book or magazine.
6 Plan any big event coming up, e.g. your birthday party.
7 Write 'keep in touch' postcards.
8 Between appointments, stock up on birthday cards, wrapping paper, presents.
9 Give yourself a head massage.
10 Listen to a tape of a book or your favourite music.

directory

When writing to any of the organisations listed in this book, always enclose a large stamped addressed envelope.

NB Virtually all the nutritional supplements listed in this book are available from:
The Nutri-Centre
7 Park Crescent, London W1N 3HE
Tel: 0171 436 5122
who offer worldwide mailorder.

TRIED AND TESTED

Aveda
AVD Cosmetics
7 Munton Road, London SE17 1PR
Tel: 0171 410 1600

Avon
Avon Cosmetics Ltd
Earlstrees Road
Corby
Northants NN17 4AZ
Hotline: 0845 6050400

CACI
For nearest salon contact:
Micromode Medical Ltd
11 Heath Street
London NW3 6TP
Tel: 0171 431 1033

Caudalie
Rhapsody Health Ltd
74 Victoria Road
Ferndown, Dorset BH22 9JA
Tel: 01202 890339

Cellex-C
Cellex-C (UK) Limited
14 High Street, Top Floor
East Grinstead, West Sussex RH19 3AW
Tel: 0345 402214

Crème de la Mer
For international mail order:
Saks Fifth Avenue
611 Fifth Avenue, New York, NY 10022
Tel: 001 212 753 4000

Decleor
Decleor UK Ltd
59a Connaught Street, London W2 2BB
Tel: 0171 262 0403

Dr Hauschka
Haselor, College Road
Bromsgrove, Worcestershire B60 2NF
Tel: 01527 832863

Eyesential
Beauty Direct (International)
17 Park Street
Leamington Spa
CV23 4QN
Tel: 01926 332331

Fenjal
Chemist Brokers
Food Broker House
North Harbour Road
North Harbour
Portsmouth PO6 3TD
Tel: 01705 222500

Gatineau
9-11 Alma Road
Windsor
Berks SL4 3HU
Tel: 0800 731 5805

Glico-Lift
For mail order:
Beauty World Direct Ltd
Freepost SL2009
Maidenhead
Berkshire SL6 1YD
Tel: 0845 600 0039

Guinot
R. Robson Ltd
The Clock House, Ascot
Berkshire SL5 7HU
Tel: 01344 873123

Integra Plus Facecare System
Scanda Sol Professional Ltd
Albion Mews, 12a–14 Legge Lane
Hockley, Birmingham B1 3LD
Tel: 0345 711117

Jan Marini
Jan Marini UK Ltd
P.O Box 9, Barnet, Herts EN4 8BF
Tel: 0181 364 9000

Kanebo
5 Bone Lane
Newbury, Berkshire RG14 5TD
Tel: 01635 46362

Karin Herzog
Floren Marketing Ltd
77 County Park Avenue
The Abbeyfields
Halesowen, West Midlands B62 8SX
Freephone: 0800 0562428
Tel: 0121 602 6882

Jurlique
Naturopathic Health & Beauty Co
Willowtree Marina
West Quay Drive
Yeading, Middx UB4 9TB
Tel: 0181 841 6644

La Prairie
Kenneth Green Associates
3 Thames Mews
Esher, Surrey KT10 9AD
Tel: 01372 469222

L'Occitane
L'Occitane Limited
237 Regent Street
London W1R 7AG
Tel: 0171 290 1421

Medi-Wave
Medi-Wave Research Ltd
5 Buckingham Road, Cheadle Hulme
Cheadle, Cheshire SK8 5EG
Tel: 0161 482 8329

Neostrata
Cosmeceuticals Ltd
The Pavillion, Josselin Road
Basildon, Essex SS13 1QB
Tel: 01268723232

Nina Ricci
Widely available and at Harrods, who
offer a worldwide mail order service
Tel: 0171 730 1234

Neal's Yard Remedies
For stockists, contact:
26-34 Ingate Place
Battersea
London SW8 3NS
Tel: 0171 627 1949
Mail order: 0161 831 7875

Ö-LYS Light Therapy
Ö-Lys Limited, Murlain House
Union Street, Chester CH1 1OP
Tel: 0800 731 3048

Prescriptives
73 Grosvenor Street. London W1X 0BH
Tel: 0800 371 573

Shiseido
Shiseido U.K. Co. Ltd
Gillingham House
Gillingham Street, London SW1V 1HU
Tel: 0171 630 1515

Vichy
Widely available and at Harrods,
See listing for Nina Ricci, left

Vitace Body Lotion
From Cosmeceuticals Ltd., *see left*

Wrinkle Miracle
Available from Boots/Superdrug or by
mail order from:
Dream Nails & Beauty Ltd
44 Ilford Hill
Ilford, Essex IG1 2AT
Tel: 0181 553 3652

Yves Rocher
Yves Rocher (London) Ltd
664 Victoria Road
South Ruislip, Middx HA4 0NY
Tel: 0181 845 1222

INSPIRING WOMEN

Gloria Hope-Price
Windward Natural Health
Green Acre, Sunset Ridge
St. James, Barbados, West Indies
Tel: 001 246 432 6425

Green People's Company
For worldwide mail order:
The Green People's Company
Brighton Road
Handcross, West Sussex RH17 6BZ
Tel: 01444 401444

Logona
Logona UK, Crowe Street
Stowmarket, Suffolk IP14 1DL
Tel: 01449 677773

No Jet-Lag
NZ Health Products Ltd.
34 Raymond Avenue
London E18 2HG
Tel: 0181 530 4593

Sunrider
195 Knightsbridge, London SW7
0171 838 0900

Pure Synergy
Xynergy Health Products
Elsted, Midhurst, West Sussex GU29 0JT
Tel: 01703 813642

Udo's Choice
Savant Distribution Ltd.
15 Iveson Approach, Leeds LS16 6LJ
Tel: 0113 230 1993

Ultra Clear Plus
Available through nutritionists

Urtekram
Whole Earth Foods Ltd
269 Portobello Road
London W11 1LR
Tel: 0171 229 7545

SKINCARE

Aesop
Nicola Wynn Ltd
49 Palace Gardens Terrace
London W8 4SB
Tel: 0171 221 4142

Anne Sémonin
108 Rue du Faubourg Saint-Honoré
75008 Paris
Tel: 00 331 42 66 24 22

Aromatherapy Associates
P.O. Box 14981, London SW6 2WH
Tel: 0171 371 9878

Aveda
See Tried & Tested listing, left

Bach Flower Remedies
A Nelson & Co Ltd, Broadheath House
83 Parkside, London SW19 5LP
Tel: 0181 780 4200

BioCare
From The Nutri-Centre, *see above left*

Blackmores
Naturopathic Health & Beauty Co.
Willowtree Marina, West Quay Drive,
Yeading, Middx. UB4 9TB
Tel: 0181 842 3956

Bliss Spa
568 Broadway
Suite 207, SoHo, New York
Tel: 001 888 243 8825

Caudalie
See Tried & Tested listing, left

Cellex-C
See Tried & Tested listing, left

Crème de la Mer
See Tried & Tested listing, left

Collâge (by Seven Seas)
Available from larger branches of Boots,
Harvey Nichols and Harrods (*see left*)

Decleor
See Tried & Tested listing, left

Dr Hauschka
See Tried & Tested listing, left

Electrolysis
British Association of Electrolysists
2a Tudor Way
Hillingdon, Middlesex UB10 9AB
Tel: 01895 239966

Emu Oil
Pioneer Trading Company
5a High Street, Tattershall
Lincoln LN4 4LE
Tel: 01526 345613

Epil-Pro
Available at The Hale Clinic
7 Park Crescent
London W1
Tel: 0171 631 0156/631 3377

Ruby Laser
Epitouch Ruby laser
Arden Medical International Offices
12 Market Street,
Nottingham NG1 2AD
Tel: 0115 953 9494

E'SPA
Kent Place,
Guildford Road Trading Estate
Farnham, Surrey GU9 9PZ
Tel: 01252 741600

Eva Fraser
Videos, tapes and books available by
mail order from:
The Studio, St Mary Abbots
Vicarage Gate, London W8 4HN
Tel: 0171 937 6616

Eve Lom
2 Spanish Place,
London W1M 5AN
Tel: 0 171 935 9988
Mail order: 3 Westmead Corner,
Carshalton, Surrey
Tel: 0181 661 7991
Also available from Space NK, Barkers
of Kensington, Dickins & Jones and The
Dorchester Spa at The Dorchester Hotel

Frownies
Available by mail order from:
Eva Fraser, *see above*

Georgette Klinger Salon
501 Madison Avenue
NY 10022, New York
Tel: 001 212 838 3200

Imedeen
Widely available in larger Boots,
Holland and Barrett and Harrods

Jan Marini
See Tried & Tested listing, opposite

Janet Sartin
500 Park Avenue
New York NY 10022,
Tel: 001 212 751.5858

Joy Salem
At The Hale Clinic, *see listing above*

Jurlique
See Tried & Tested listing, opposite

Kanebo
See Tried & Tested listing, opposite

Karin Herzog
See Tried & Tested listing, opposite

Kiehl's
Available from Space NK, *see right*

La Prairie
See Tried & Tested listing, opposite

Manual Lymphatic Drainage (MLD)
MLD UK, PO Box 149
Wallingford, Oxfordshire

Nuxe
Available at Space NK, *see right*

Origins
At Harrods, John Lewis or for further
stockists (who all offer mail order)
Tel: 0800 731 4039

Osmotics
Available at (or by mail order from):
Dickins & Jones
244 Regent Street, London W1A 1DB
Tel: 0171 734 7070

Pharma Nord
From The Nutri-Centre, *see p. 246*

Philosophy
Available from Liberty, Harrods and by
mail order from Space NK, *see below*

Remède
Available at Space NK, *see below*

Repêchage
Repêchage Europe Ltd
5 Hugh Business Park
Bacup Road, Waterfoot
Rossendale BB4 7BX
Hotline: 0800 731 7546

Retinova
Retinova Advisory Service
Freephone: 0500 080 040
Or write to:
The Photo-Ageing Information Service
c/o 150 Falcon Road
London SW11 2LW

Shisiedo
See Tried & Tested listing, left

SoftLight Laser
ThermoLase Ltd, 45–47 Cheval Place,
London SW7 1EW
Tel: 0171 581 4499

Solgar
Solgar Vitamins Ltd
Aldbury, Tring, Herts HP23 5PT
Tel: 01442 890355

Space NK
Space NK Apothecary
P.O Box 18025, London EC2A 3RJ
Tel: 0171 636 2523

Verde
75 Northcote Road, London SW11 6PJ
Tel: 0171 924 4379
Mail order: 0870 603 9186

MAKE-UP

Action for Blind People
14-16 Verney Road, London SE16 3DZ
Tel: 0171 732 8771

Barbara Daly
Make-up brushes available at Tesco –
for customer enquiries:
Tel: 0800 505555

BeneFit Cosmetics
At Selfridges, Space NK and Harrods
Tel: 0171 7301234

Bobbi Brown Essentials
Available at Harrods, who will mail
order (*see above*) and selected House of
Fraser stores

**British Association of Skin
Camouflage (BASC)**
PO Box 202
Macclesfield, Cheshire SK11 6FP
Tel: 01625 267880

Cosmetics à la Carte
19b Motcomb Street,
London SW1X 8LB
Tel: 0171 622 2318

Disfigurement Guidance Centre
P.O. Box 7. Cupar, Fife KY15 4PF
Helpline 7.30am-12.00pm:
01337 870281

D.R. Harris's Eye Drops:
29 St James Street
London SW1A 1HB
Tel: 0171 930 3915

Eylure
Original Additions Ltd
Ventura House, Bullsbrook Road,
Hayes, Middlesex UB4 0UJ
Tel: 0181 573 9907

Fashion Fair
Collier House, 163-169 Brompton Road
London SW3 1PY
Tel: 0171 591 4456

Kanebo
See Tried & Tested listing, left

Laura Mercier
Available from Space NK, *see left*

Look Good...Feel Better
To find a workshop in your area, and/or
to obtain a copy of their free leaflet:
Look Good...Feel Better
Josaron House, 5-7 John Princes Street
London W1M 9HD

M.A.C (Make-up Arts Cosmetics)
109 Kings Road, London SW3 4PA
Tel: 0171 349 0601

Make Up For Ever
40 Clarendon Street
Dublin 2, County Dublin, Ireland
Tel: 00 353 1679 9043

Nars
Available from Space NK, *see left*

Origins
See Skincare listing, left

Poppy
Available from Space NK, *see left*

Rubis
Available from Space NK, *see left*

Stephen Glass
Face Facts
73 Wigmore Street, London W1H 9LH
Tel: 0171 486 8287

Stila
Available from Space NK, *see left*

Trish McEvoy
Harvey Nichols
67 Brompton Road, London SW3 1EF
Tel: 0171 235 5000

Tweezerman
AVD Cosmetics
7 Munton Road, London SE17 1PR
Tel: 0171 410 1600

Shu Uemura
Unit 19, 49 Atalanta Street
London SW6 6TU
Tel: 0171 379 6627

Vincent Longo
At Selfridges, or for mail order/stockists:
E'SPA, Kent Place
Guildford Road Trading Estate
Farnham, Surrey GU9 9PZ
Tel: 01252 741601

FRAGRANCE

**Annick Goutal, Chanel, Christian
Dior** and **Guerlain** are widely available.

Coudray, Creed, Diptyque and
Maitre Parfumeur et Gantier are all
available at Les Senteurs, who offer a
mail order service:
227 Ebury Street, London SW1W 8UT
Tel: 0171 730 2322

Demeter
Harvey Nichols
67 Brompton Road, London SW3 1EF
Tel: 0171 235 5000

L'Artisan Parfumeur
L'Artisan Parfumeur
17 Cale Street
London SW3 3QR
Tel: 0171 352 4196

HAIR

Aesop
See Skincare listing, opposite

Aveda
See Tried & Tested listing, opposite

Bioforce
Bioforce UK Ltd, 2 Brewster Place
Irvine, Ayrshire, KA11 5DD
Tel: 01294 277344

Botanical Hair Care Company
Unit 6
Fromside Industrial Estate
Wallbridge, Stroud, GL5 3JX
Tel: 01453 763 670

Bumble and Bumble
Available from Space NK, *see left*

Charles Worthington
Products available at Boots, Selfridges
and John Lewis

Daniel Field
8-12 Broadwick Street
London W1V 1FH
Tel: 0171 439 8223
Mail order: 01844 212300

Dr Hugh Rushton
Harmont House, Harley Street
London W1
Tel: 0171 637 0491

E'SPA
See Skincare listing, p.247

Hairline International
(for advice about hair loss)
Lyons Court
1668 High Street, Knowle
West Midlands B93 0LY
Tel: 01564 775281

Jo Hansford
19 Mount Street, London W1Y 5RA
Tel: 0171 495 7774

John Freida
4 Aldford Street, London W1Y 5PU
Tel: 0171 491 0840
Products available from Boots
and Superdrug

Laurent D. Volumateur
From Privé Salon in Los Angeles
8458 Melrose Place, CA 90069
Tel: 001 213 651 5045

J-F Lazartigue
20 James Street,
London W1M 5HN
Tel: 0171 629 2250

Léonor Greyl
15 Rue Tronchet, 75008 Paris
Tel: 00 331 42 65 32 26
Available at Space NK, *see p.247*

Look Good Feel Better
See Make-up listing, p.247

Michael diCesare
Available from House of Fraser, Harrods
and QVC Shopping Channel

Nature's Best
1 Lamberts Road, Tunbridge Wells,
Kent TN2 3BE
Tel: 01892 552118

Paul Mitchell
Paul Mitchell UK Ltd
Unit1-2 Millenium Point
Broadfields, Aylesbury
Bucks HP19 3ZU
For nearest stockist tel: 01296 696677

Phytologie
69a Eccleston Square,
London SW1V 1PJ
For mail order and stockists tel: 0171
592 9800

Philip Kingsley
54 Green Street, London W1Y 3RH
Tel: 0171 629 4004

René Furterer
For information, call 001-800 522 8285

Romanda Healthcare
Romanda House, Ashley Walk
London NW7 1DU
Tel/Fax/Advice line: 0181 346 0784

Sebastian
California Lines Ltd
Bessemer Road, Basingstoke
Hampshire RG22 4AF.
Tel: 0345 125545

Tween-Time Crayon
From Beauty World Direct, *see p.246*

Urtekram
See Inspiring Women listing, p.245

FEET

Chelsea Nail Studio
5 Pond Place, London SW3 6QR
Tel: 0171 225 3889

Diamancel (foot files)
Available from Space NK, *see p.247*

Reflexology
The British Reflexology Association
Monks Orchard
Whitbourne, Worcester WR6 5RB
Tel: 01886 821207

Scholl
Scholl Consumer Products Ltd
475 Capability Green
Luton, Bedfordshire, LU1 3LU
Customer enquiries: 0800 074 2040

Super Nail of Los Angeles
101 Crawford Street
London W1H 1AN
Tel: 0171 723 1163

The Foot Health Council
53 Welbeck Street
London W1M 7HE
Tel: 0171 486 3381

HANDS

BioCare
From The Nutri-Centre, *see p. 246*

**Chelsea Nail Bar International
Fingercare**
See Chelsea Nail Studio listing, above

Chelsea Nail Studio
See Feet listing, above

Efamol
Efamol Ltd, Weyvern House
Weyvern Park, Portsmouth Road
Guildford, Surrey GU3 1NA
Information service: 0870 6060128

Hale Clinic
7 Park Crescent
London W1N 3HE
Tel: 0171 631 0156

Jessica
For nearest salon and advice:
The Natural Nail Company Ltd
47 Theobald Street, Borehamwood
Herts WD6 4RT
Tel: 0181 381 7793

Jessica Nail Clinic
8627 Sunset Boulevard
West Hollyood, Los Angeles
California 90069
Tel: 001 310 659 9292

Jurlique
See Tried & Tested listing, p.246

O.P.I
37 Pinner Green
Pinner, Middlesex HA5 2AF
Hotline: 0181 868 3400

Paint Job
Available at Space NK, *see p.247*

Privé
8458 Melrose Place
Los Angeles
CA 90069
Tel: 001 213 651 5045

EYES

Bates Method
For information send £1 with an s.a.e to:
The Bates Association of Great Britain
PO Box 25, Shoreham-by-Sea
West Sussex, BN43 6ZF
Tel: 01273 422090

Cutler & Gross
16 Knightsbridge Green
London SW1 XQL
Tel: 0171 823 8445

Dollond & Aitchison
For details of your nearest branch:
1323 Coventry Road
Yardley
Birmingham B25 8LP
Tel: 0121 706 6133

Q Switch Ruby Laser
Used by Professor Nicholas Lowe at
The Cranley Clinic, *see right*

**Specialist Herbal Supplies' Eye
Wash Mixture**
From The Nutri-Centre, *see p.246*

Trayner Pinhole Glasses
The Old Brewery
Newtown
Bradford-on-Avon, Wiltshire BA15 1NF
Tel: 01749 850822

TEETH

David Klaff
1st Floor Suite, 57a Wimpole Street
London W1M 7DF
Tel: 0171 636 9933

Dr Mervyn Druian
The Fresh Breath Centre
93 Haverstock Hill, London NW3 4RL
Tel: 0171 586 7237

**Janina International Oral
Cosmetique**
At Boots, Selfridges and independent
pharmacies or, for information:
Tel: 0181 699 6222

REJUEVENATING SURGERY

Mr John Scurr
Lister Hospital
Chelsea Bridge Road
London SW1W 8RH
Tel: 0171 730 3417

**British Association of Plastic
Surgeons**
The Royal College of Surgeons
34-35 Lincoln's Inn Fields
London WC2A 3PN
Tel: 0171 831 5161

**British Association of Aesthetic
Plastic Surgeons**
Send large 1st class sae for list of fully
accredited cosmetic plastic surgeons to:
35 Lincoln's Inn Fields
London WC2A 3PN
Tel: 0171 405 2234.

British Dental Association
64 Wimpole Street, London W1M 8AL
Tel: 0171 935 3963

**British Association of
Dermatologists**
19 Fitzroy Square, London W1P 5HQ
Tel: 0171 383 0266

**British Academy of Aesthetic
Dentistry**
Suite 152, 84 Marylebone High Street
London W1M 3DE

Dr Andrew Markey
At The Lister Hospital, *see above*

Dr Barry Jones
14a Upper Wimpole Street
London W1M 1AB

Professor Nicholas Lowe
The Cranley Clinic, 3 Harcourt House
19a Cavendish Square,
London W1M 9AD
0171 499 3223

SLEEP

Acupressure
See Acupuncture

Acupuncture
British Acupuncture Council
Park House, 206-208 Latimer Road
London W10 6RE
Tel: 0181 964 0222

Autogenics
The British Association for Autogenic
Training and Therapy
Royal London Homoeopathic Hospital
NHS Trust
Great Ormond Street,
London WC1N 3HR
Tel: 0171 837 8833

Bioforce
See Hair listing, p. 247

Bach Flower Remedies
See Skincare listing, p. 246

Hypnotherapy
Central Register of Advanced
Hypnotherapists
28 Finsbury Park Road
London N4 2JX
Tel: 0171 359 6991

or The National Register of
Hypnotherapists & Psychotherapists
12 Cross Street, Nelson, Lancs BB9 7EN
Tel: 01282 699378

Neal's Yard
See Tried & Tested listing, p.246

EXERCISE/BODY

Amanda Platt (wardrobe doctor)
Tel: 0171-229 8109

Anne Marie Petash (Pilates instructor)
Tel: 0171 229 5243

Aromatherapy Associates
See Skincare listing, p.246

Czech & Speake
39c Jermyn Street
London SW1Y 6DN
Tel: 0800 919 728

Ecco Footwear
Shoon Ltd, Dinder House
Dinder, Somerset BA5 3PB
Tel: 0800 387368

Full Spectrum Lighting
See Winter Depression listing, p.250

Ionothermie (for cellulite)
Ionithermie Ltd
9-11 Alma Road, Windsor
Berkshire SL3 8TS
Tel: 01753 833900

Mesotherapy (for cellulite)
Dr Elisabeth Dancey
55 Wimpole Street
London W1M 7DF
Tel: 0171 224 1330

Manual Lymphatic Drainage
See Skincare listing, p.247

Pilates
The Pilates Foundation
80 Camden Road, London E17 7NF
Tel: 07071 781859

Or: Association of Pilates Teachers
17 Queensbury Mews West
London SW7 2DY
Tel: 0171 581 7041

SAD Association
See Winter Depression listing, p.250

Thalgo
Thalgo UK Ltd, Elgin House
51 Mill Harbour, London E14 9TD
Tel: 0171 512 0872

Walkfit
Walkfit Ltd, 98-102 Station Road
Oxted, Surrey RH8 OQA
Tel: 01883 730666

Estilo Salon
7402 Beverly Boulevard
Los Angeles, CA 90036
Tel: 001 213 936 6775

FOOD

Colon Cleansing Capsules
From The Nutri-Centre, *see p.246*

For a list of qualified colonic irrigation
practitioners in the UK:
The Colonic International Association
16 England's Lane, London NW3 4TG

Organic Food
For information about where to obtain
organic food or to help locate a local
organic box scheme, contact:
The Soil Association
Bristol House, 40-56 Victoria Street
Bristol BS1 6BY
Tel: 0117-929 0661

Pharma Nord
From The Nutri-Centre, *see p. 246*

Phytolife Plus
From Blackmores, *see p.246*

Magnesium OK
Widely available

Western Herbal Medicine
*See National Institue of Medical
Herbalists, right*

Losemore Herbs
From the Nutri-Centre, *see p.246*

Udo's Choice
See Inspiring Women listing p.246

Solgar
See Skincare listing, p.247

Spectrum Oils (EFAs)
Whole Earth Foods
269 Portobello Road, London W11 1LR
Tel: 0171-229 7545

HORMONES

The Back Shop
14 New Cavendish Street
London W1M 7LJ
Tel: 0171 935 9120

Blackmores
See Skincare listing, p.246

Bioenergetic Medicine
Institute of Bioenergetic Medicine
103 North Road
Parkstone, Poole, Dorset BH14 OLU
Tel: 01202 733762

Bristol Cancer Help Centre
Grove House, Cornwallis Grove,
Clifton, Bristol BS8 4PG
Tel: 0117 980 9505

Chinese Herbal Medicine
Register of Chinese Herbal Medicine
PO Box 400, Wembley,
Middx HA9 9NZ
Tel: 0171 224 0803

**Dormeasan, Femforte, Formula
MNP415, Gamma-Oryzanol,
Gynovite, Menosan, Osteoprime,
Phytoestrol, Remifemin, Urticalcin**
Like virtually all the supplements
mentioned in this book, they are
available from The Nutri-Centre, *see
listing at the top of p.246*

Imperial Cancer Research Fund
P.O Box 123, Lincoln's Inn Fields
London WC2A 3PX
Tel: 0171 242 0200

Jan de Vries
Auchenkyle, Southwoods Road
Troon, Ayrshire KA10 7EL
Tel: 01292 317670

National Institute On Ageing (USA)
National Institute of Health
31 Center Drive, Building 31
Room 5C27 Bethesda
MD 20892-2292
Tel: 001 301 496 1751

National Osteoporosis Society
P.O Box 10, Radstock,
Bath BA3 3YB
Tel: 01761 471771

Natural Medicine Directory
Natural Medicine Directory
c/o SPNT, P.O Box 47, Heathfield
East Sussex TN21 8ZX

**Natural Progesterone Information
Service**
PO Box 131, Etchingham TN19 7ZN
Tel: 01435 883189

Nutritional Therapy
See Stress Therapies, p. 250

ProGest Cream by Higher Nature
The Nutrition Centre, Burwash
Common
East Sussex TN19 7LX
Tel: 01435 882880

Solgar
See Skincare listing, p. 247

FACE YOUR DEMONS

**British Holistic Medical
Association**
See Stress Therapiest listing, below

Jungian Therapy
UK Council for Psychotherapy
167-169 Great Portland Street
London W1N 5FB
Tel: 0171 436 3002

STRESS THERAPIES

Absent Healing
See Healing, right

Acupressure
See Acupuncture listing in Sleep, p. 248

Acupuncture
See Sleep listing, p. 248

Aromatherapy
Umbrella Organisation with 4,500
practitioners:
Aromatherapy Organisations Council
P.O Box 355
Croydon, Surrey CR9 2QP
Tel/fax: 0181 251 7912

For stockists/mail order of blended oils:
Aromatherapy Associates, *see p. 246*

Aura Healing
See Healing, below

Autogenic Training
See Sleep listing, p. 248

Ayurvedic Massage
Ayurvedic Medical Association UK
Hale Clinic, 7 Park Crescent
London W1N 3HE
Tel: 0171 631 0156

Bach Flower Remedies
See Skincare listing, p. 246

**Biodynamic Psychotherapy (and
Massage)**
Gerda Boyesen Centre
For info on practitioners,:
Acacia House, Centre Avenue
London W3 7JX
Tel: 0181 743 2437

British Holistic Medical Asociation
59 Lansdowne Place, Hove
East Sussex BN3 1FL
Tel: 01273 725951

**Centre for the Study of
Complementary Medicine**
51 Bedford Place
Southampton, Hampshire SO15 2DT
Tel: 01703 334752

Chinese Massage
See Massage, p. 250

Faith Healing
See Healing, below

Flotation Therapy
Float Tank Association
P.O. Box 11024, London SW4 7ZF
Tel: 0171 627 4962

Healing
Confederation of Healing Organizations
(Government recognised body)
Suite J, 2nd Floor
113 High Street
Berkhamsted, Hertfordshire HP4 2DJ
01442 870660

Herbalists
National Institute of Medical Herbalists
56 Longbrook Street
Exeter Devon EX4 6AH
Tel: 01392 426022

Homoeopathy
Society of Homoeopaths
2 Artizan Road
Northampton NN1 4HU
Tel: 01604 621400

Or: The UK Homoeopathy
Medical Association
6 Livingston Road, Gravesend
Kent DA12 5DZ
Tel: 01474 560336

Or, to find a doctor who is also a
homoeopath:
Faculty of Homoeopathy
2 Powis Place, Great Ormond Street
London WC1N 3HT
Tel: 0171 837 9469

Massage
For a list of local practitioners of Eastern and Western massage:
British Massage Therapy Council
Greenbank House, 65a Adelphi Street
Preston PR1 7BH
Tel: 01772 881063

Meditation
School of Meditation
158 Holland Park Avenue
London W11 4UH
Tel: 0171 603 6116

Transcendental Meditation
Beacon House, Willow Walk
Woodley Park, Skelmersdale
Lanc WN8 6UR
Tel: 0800 269303

Music Therapy
Association of Music Professional Therapists
38 Pierce Lane, Fulbourn
Cambridge CB1 5DL

Nutritional Therapy
Society for the Promotion of Nutritional Therapy
P.O Box 47, Heathfield
East Sussex TN21 8ZX
Send large sae and £1 cheque/PO

Institute for Optimum Nutrition
Blades Court, Deodar Road
London SW15 2NU
Tel: 0181 877 9993
for in-depth health checks including hair analysis

Reflexology
See Feet listing, p. 248

Reiki
The Reiki Association
2 Manor Cottages, Stockley Hill
Peterchurch, Hereford HR2 0SS

Shiatsu
The Shiatsu Society
Barber House, Storeys Bar Road
Sengate, Peterborough PE1 5YN
Tel: 01858 465731

or for a list of graduates:
British School of Shiatsu
6 Erskine Road, London NW3 3AJ
Tel: 0171 483 3776

Spiritual Healing
See Healing, previous page

Sports Massage
See Massage, previous page

Swedish Massage
See Massage, previous page

T'ai Chi
The UK T'ai Chi Association
PO Box 159, Bromley, Kent BR1 3XX

Thai Massage
See Massage, previous page

Therapeutic Touch
The Didsbury Trust
Redmirs, Mungrisdale, Penrith
Cumbria CA11 0TB

Tibetan Buddhism
Samye Ling, Eskdalemuir
Dumfrieshire, DG13 0QR
Tel: 013873 73232

Tragerwork
The Trager Association UK
64 Wilbury Rd, Hove, Sussex BN3 3PY

Transcendental Meditation
See Meditation

Yoga
The British Wheel of Yoga
1 Hamilton Place, Boston Road
Sleaford, Lincolnshire NG34 7ES
Tel: 01529 306851

HOW IS IT FOR YOU?

British Association of Sexual and Marital Therapists
P.O Box 13686, London SW20 9ZH
Tel: 0181 543 2707

Relate National Marriage Guidance
Herbert Gray College
Little Church Street, Rugby CV21 3AP
Tel: 01788 573241

Senselle by Durex
London Rubber Company
Enquiry line: 0800 338 739

SYLK
Freepost, PO Box 340
Rickmansworth, Herts WD3 5WD
Tel: 01923 285544

WINTER DEPRESSION

Full Spectrum Lighting
S.A.D. Lightbox Co. Ltd
19 Lincoln Road
Cressex Business Park, High Wycombe
Buckinghamshire HP12 3FX
Tel: 01494 448727/526051

SAD Association
PO Box 989, Steyning
West Sussex BN44 3HG
Tel: 01903 814942

CREATIVITY

Nick Williams
For information on workshops:
Alternatives Workshops
197 Piccadilly, London W1V 0LL
Tel: 0171 287 6711

HEALTH AND BEAUTY BOOKSHELF

Anam Cara: Spiritual Wisdom from The Celtic World
by John O'Donohue
(Bantam Press 1997)

The Art of Hair Colouring
by David Adams and Jacki Wadeson
(Macmillan Press 1988)

The Art of Sexual Ecstasy: The Path of Sacred Sexuality for Western Lovers
by Margo Anand (Aquarian Press 1990)

The Artist's Way
by Julia Cameron (Pan 1995)

The Beauty Bible
by Sarah Stacey and Josephine Fairley
(Kyle Cathie 1996)

Better Sight Without Glasses
by Harry Benjamin (Thorsons 1992)

Bobbi Brown Beauty: The Ultimate Beauty Resource
by Bobbi Brown & Annemarie Iverson
(Ebury Press 1997)

The Complete Guide to Food Allergy and Intolerance
by Prof Jonathan Brostoff and Linda Gamlin (Bloomsbury 1998)

Dirt – The Lowdown on Growing a Garden With Style
by Dianne Benson
(Dell Publishing 1984 – out of print)

Eco-Friendly Houseplants
Bill Wolverton (Pheonix 1997)

Encyclopaedia of Complementary Medicine
by Anne Woodham and Dr David Peters
(Dorling Kindersley 1997)

The Encyclopaedia of Flower Remedies
by Clare G. Harvey and Amanda Cochrane
(Thorsons 1995)

The Encyclopaedia of Natural Medicine
by Michael Murray and Joseph Pizzorno
(Optima 1990)

Fats That Heal, Fats That Kill
by Dr. Udo Erasmus
(Alive Books 1993)

Healing Environments: Your Guide to Indoor Well-being
by Carol Venolia
(Celestial Arts 1988)

Hotline to Health
by Kathryn Marsden
(Pan 1998)

How to Keep Your Feet & Legs Healthy for a Lifetime
by Gary Null and Dr Howard Robins
(Seven Stories Press 1990)

Journal of A Solitude
by May Sarton
(Women's Press 1995)

Juice High
by Leslie Kenton and Russell Cronin
(Ebury Press 1996)

The Meditator's Handbook: A Comprehensive Guide to Eastern & Western Meditation Techniques
by Dr David Fontana
(Element Books 1994)

Menopause
by Jan de Vries
(Mainstream Publishing 1993)

Mind-Body Medicine – A Clinician's Guide to Psychoneuroimmunology
edited by Dr. Alan Watkins
(Churchill Livingstone 1997)

Natural Alternatives to HRT
by Marilyn Glenville
(Kyle Cathie 1997)

Passage To Power
by Leslie Kenton
(Century Vermillion 1998)

Raw Energy
by Leslie Kenton
(Century Vermillion 1994)

The Optimum Nutrition Bible
by Patrick Holford
(Piatkus 1997)

The Psychology of Happiness
by Prof Michael Argyle
(Routledge 1986)

The Reflexology Partnership
by Suzanne Adamson and Eilish Harris
(Kyle Cathie 1995)

Secrets of a Fashion Therapist
by Betty Halbreich
(Aurum 1998)

Sleep Thieves
by Stanley Coren
(Simon & Schuster 1996)

The Spiritual Tourist
by Mick Brown
(Bloomsbury 1998)

Stress at Work: Causes, Effects and Prevention
by Michael Kompies
(European Communities 1995)

SuperYou
by Anne Naylor
(Thorsons 1996)

The Wellness Book – The Comprehensive Guide to Maintaining Health and Treating Stress-Related Illness
by Herbert Benson and Eileen M Stuart
(Birch Lane Press 1992)

Total Wellness
by Joseph Pizzorno
(Prima 1998)

You Can Look Younger At Any Age
by Nelson Lee Novick, MD
(Henry Holt & Company 1996)

Your Skin: An Owner's Guide
by Joseph Bark
(Prentice Hall USA 1995)

American books can be ordered direct from the US from Reader's Catalog
Tel: 001 212 262 7198
Or over the Internet, via:
www.amazon.com

acknowledgements

This mammoth project wouldn't have been possible without a great deal of help and co-operation. Firstly, we would like to thank the 1,002 women who volunteered to join our testing panel, and who diligently reported back on their experiences with the lotions and potions they were sent to try; we would love to have named them all individually. We continue to be inspired by our **Inspiring Women**, and would like to thank Bernadette Rendall, Gayle Hunnicutt, Gloria Hope-Price, Jennifer Guerrini-Maraldi, Joan Burstein, Leslie Kenton, Lisbeth Damsgaard and Suzanne Adamson. In addition we would like to thank the following, who were all interviewed specifically for this book:

The make-up artists: Barbara Daly, Bobbi Brown, Darac, Jenny Jordan, Kevyn Aucoin, Laura Mercier, Liz Collinge, Mary Greenwell, Noriko Okubo, Olivier Echaudemaison, Ruby Hammer, Stephen Glass, Tricia Sawyer, Trish McEvoy, Vincent Longo. **The fashion experts:** Amanda Platt, Betty Halbreich, Belinda Seper. **The hairdressers:** Andrew Collinge, Charles Worthington, Christophe Robin, Daniel Field, George at John Barrett, John Barrett, John Frieda, Jo Hansford, Léonor Greyl, Louis Licari, Nicky Clarke, Susan Baldwin. **The foot and nail experts:** Clare Wolford (Educational Director of Supernail of LA), Mara Caskin at John Barrett, Robyn Opie, Katharine Royston-Airey **The skincare professionals:** Barbara Simpson-Birks, Christina Carlino, Edith Poyer (Assistant Director of Product development for Fashion Fair), Eve Lom, Eva Fraser, Dr Daniel Maes (Vice-President of Research and development for Estée Lauder Worldwide), Dr John McCook (Elizabeth Arden), Dr Karen Burke, Lydia Sarfati, Marcia Kilgore, Germaine Rich of Aromatherapy Associates, Dr Jurgen Klein (founder of Jurlique cosmetics), Dr Patricia Wexler (New York), Susan Harmsworth (founder of E'SPA, UK).

The doctors, scientists, fitness, nutritional and personal development experts: Philip Bacon (Galsworthy House Hospital, London), Prof Joan Bassey (Nottingham Medical School), Glenda Baum (London), Prof Etienne-Emile Baulieu (Paris), Dr Mary Ellen Brademas (New York City), Dr Carol Brayne (University of Cambridge Medical School), Prof Jonathan Brostoff (Middlesex Hospital and University College London), Dr S R Burzynski (Burzynski Research Inst, Texas), Dr Robert Butler (Chairman Dept of Geriatrics, Mt Sinai School of Medicine, New York City), Dr Rosy Daniels (Bristol Cancer Help Centre, UK), Dr Stephen Davies (Dept of Psychology, Princess Alexandra Hospital, Harlow, Essex), Jan de Vries (Glasgow,) Dr Ciaran F Donegan (Queens Medical Centre, Nottingham), Dr Mervyn Druian (London Breath Centre), Torje Eike (chartered physiotherapist, London), Frances Emeleus (British Association of Sexual and Marital Therapists, UK), Dr Udo Erasmus, Dr Linda Fellows (Meridian Associates, UK), Prof Michael Fossel (Dept of Clinical Medicine, Michigan State), Prof Mary Gilhooly (Centre of Gerontology and Community Health, Studies, University of Paisley), Harald Gaier (Hale Clinic, London), Dr H.B. Gibson (University of the Third Age, Cambridge), Dr Chris Gilleard (Springfield University Hospital, London), Dr Marilyn Glenville (Hale Clinic, London), Prof Jean-Alexis Grimaud (University of Paris), Dr James Hawkins (British Holistic Medical Association), Dr Leonard Hayflick (University of California), Patrick Holford (Institute of Optimum Nutrition, London), Dr Susan Horsewood-Lee (London), Frances Hunt (UK Manager 'Ageing Well Programme'), Prof Howard Jacobs (Dept of Reproductive Endocrinology, Middlesex Hospital, London), Prof Vivian James (England), Dorothy Jerrome (Age Concern, Brighton), Dr Kim Jobst (Glasgow Homoeopathic Hospital and Glasgow University, Department of Medicine and Therapeutics), Mr Barry Jones (London), Dr Kevin Kelleher (Consultant Physician, Queen Mary's Sidcup NHS Trust), Prof Kay-Tee Khaw (Clinical Gerontology Unit, University of Cambridge), Dr Tom Kitwood, (Senior Lecturer in Psychology, University of Bradford), David Klaff (President British Academy of Aesthetic Dentists, London), Dr Peter Laslett (Trinity College, Cambridge), Prof Michael Lean (Dept of Human Nutrition, University of Glasgow), Dr George Lewith (Centre for the Study of Complementary Medicine, Southampton), Prof David A Lipschitz (Director, Center on Ageing, University of Arkansas for Medical Sciences), Dr Geraldine Littler (Department of Sociology, University of Liverpool), Prof Nicholas Lowe (Cranley Clinic, London), Dr Tony Maltby (Depart of Social Policy and Social Work, University of Birmingham), Dr Andrew Markey (Director of Dermatological Surgery and Laser Unit at the St. John's Institute of Dermatology), Kathryn Marsden (Wiltshire, UK), Warrick McNeill (Physioworks, London), Prof Lorraine Faxon Meisner (University of Wisconsin, Madison, US), Prof Peter Millard (St Georges Hospital Medical School, Division of Geriatric Medicine, London), Prof Graham Mulley (St James University Hospital, Leeds), Anne Naylor (France), Kate Neil (Institute of Optimum Nutrition, London), Chrissie Painell, Prof Ian Philp (Northern General Hospital, Sheffield), Joseph Pizzorno (Bastyr University, Seattle, Washington), Prof David Purdie (Centre for Metabolic Bone Disease, Hull Royal Infirmary), Anne O'Dowd RSA, Dr Anthony Quinn (St. Bartholomew's and the Royal London Hospital of Medicine), Prof Elaine Rankin (Chair of Cancer Medicine at the University of Dundee), Ms Linnea Renton (Active Age Manager, Age Concern, Liverpool), Dr Deborah Rozman (Institute of HeartMath, Boulder, Colorado), Dr Hugh Rushton (London), Mr John Scurr (Lister Hospital, London), Dr Elspeth Stirling (consultant clinical psychologist, Royal Dundee Liff Hospital) Dr Ian Stuart-Hamilton (Prinicpal Lecturer in Psychology, Worcester College of High Education), Stephen Terrass (Technical Director, Solgar), Gloria Thomas (London), Mary Thomas (Dark Horse Venture, UK), Prof Anthea Tinker (Institute of Gerontology), Joanna Walker, (Pre-Retirement Association. Guildford), Dr Alan Watkins (Lecturer in Medicine at Southampton University), Dr Ian White (consultant dermatologist, British Dermatological Association), Nick Williams (Alternatives, London), Dr Alex Withnal (Dept of Applied Social Studies, Keele University), Anne Woodham (Hon Chair, Guild of Health Writers), Cynthia Wyld (British Association for Service to the Elderly, UK).

Thanks also the following organisations: Action Research, Age Concern, Society for Endocrinology, British Geriatric Society, British Heart Foundation, British Psychological Society, British Society for Research into Ageing, Institute of Gerontology, Institute of Human Ageing, Public Health Forum, Research Into Ageing. **And to:** Roja Dove of Guerlain for letting us raid the archives in Paris, Mary-Ellen Lapsansky (The Fragrance Foundation, NYC), Jilly Fraysse, Joy Salem, Lizzie Vann (Baby Organix).

We would also like to say thank you, thank you, thank you to the colleagues, family and friends who have given unstinting time and effort including our doughty researchers, Cluny Brown, Hilly Boyd and Catherine Slocock. Thanks to the design team at Button: Anne, Gill, Reg, Rick, Ian and 'supremo' Sue, to David Downton for another set of fabulous illustrations, and to Kirsten Abbott and Julia Scott at Kyle Cathie. Thanks to Dee Nolan, for her patience, and to Rosie Boycott. Craig Sams and Clive Syddall are mentioned glowingly in dispatches. And finally, a big thank you to our agent, Kay McCauley, for being there…

index

photographic acknowledgements

The publishers wish to thank the photographers and organisations for their kind permission to reproduce the following photographs in this book

2 The Image Bank/Meola Studio; 8 Stay Still/Evan Arnstein; 10 Tony Stone Images/Laurence Monneret; 11 Robert Harding Picture Library/Wesley Hitt; 13 The Image Bank/Bokelberg; 14 Francesca Yorke; 19 Francesca Yorke; 23 Robert Harding Picture Library/ Caroline Hughes/© IPC Magazines Ltd/Options; 24 Tony Stone Images/Bill Heinsohn; 25 John Swannell for Yardley; 26 Tony Stone Images/Mark Lewis; 27 Guerlain; 28 Francesca Yorke; 30 Images/Jay Freis; 33 Science Photo Library/Alfred Pasieka; 34 Francesca Yorke; 36–37 Tony Stone Images/Matt Lambert; 39 Marie France/Barbro Anderson/Dominique Eveque; 42 Tony Stone Images/James Darell; 44 Corbis; 47 Andrew Lawson; 49 Angela Hampton Family Life Pictures; 52 Anders Bach; 54–55 Jekka McVikar; 59 Superstock; 61 Tony Stone Images/Jerome Tisné; 63 Hulton Getty; 65 Robert Harding Picture Library/Jake Chessum/© IPC Magazines Ltd; 66 Telegraph Picture Library/Bavaria/Bildagentur; 71 Robert Harding Picture Library/Rene Dupont/© IPC Magazines Ltd/Options; 72 Francesca Yorke; 75 Francesca Yorke; 77 TonyStone Images/Jerome Tisné; 78 The Kobal Collection; 80 Tony Stone Images/Steven Peters; 81 London Features International/Jacqui Brown; 82 Telegraph Colour Library/JP Frouhet; 84 Francesca Yorke; 88 Attard; 89 London Features International; 90 Francesca Yorke; 92 Guerlain; 93 Tony Stone Images/Dennis O'Clair; 94 Action for Blind People; 95 Tony Stone Images/Claudia Kunin; 98 Associated Press; 100 Retna Pictures/Phil Loftus; 104 Francesca Yorke; 107 The Stock Market; 109 Marie France/Barbro Anderson/Catherine de Chabaneix; 111 Alpha/Patrick Sicolli/Angeli; 114 Tony Stone Images/Christopher Bissell; 116 Retna/Bruno Gaget; 117 London Features International/Ken Weingart; 118 Retna/Patrick Swire/MPA; 119 Francesca Yorke; 120 John Swannell; 122 Retna /Jenny Acheson; 123 Retna /Jenny Acheson;124 *above* Tony Stone Images/Donna Day; *below* Retna/Jenny Acheson; 125 Retna/Jenny Acheson; 126 Tony Stone Images/Antonia Deutsch; 129 Robert Harding Picture Library/© IPC Magazines Ltd/Woman's Journal; 132 Superstock; 135 Tony Stone Images/Laurence Monneret; 137 Hulton Getty; 138 Tony Stone Images/Jerome Tisné; 143 Tony Stone Images/Christopher Bissell; 154 Tony Stone Images/Laurence Monneret; 156 Attard; 158 Francesca Yorke; 160 Garden Picture Library/Lynne Brotchie; 162 The Image Bank/M Regine; 168 The Image Bank/John P Kelley; 171 Francesca Yorke; 176 Francesca Yorke; 180 Francesca Yorke; 181 The Image Bank/Tracy Frankel; 182 The Image Bank/Gio Barto; 184 *Belle*; 188 Katz/Outline/Art Streiber; 193 Tony Stone Images/Robert Holmgren; 195 Robert Harding Picture Library/© IPC Magazines Ltd/Options; 196 Tony Stone Images/Catherine Panchout; 197 Tony Stone Images/Chris Everard; 198 The Image Bank/Dingo; 200 The Image Bank/Tcherevkoff Ltd; 202 Huw Evans; 215 The Stock Market/Sanai Shahram; 222 Tony Stone Images/Stephanie Rushton; 224 Francesca Yorke; 226 Katz/Outline/Jeffrey Thurnher; 228 *above* Colorific; *below* Rex Features/Sipa Press; 233 Francesca Yorke; 235 Explorer/Bordes; 236 The Kobal Collection; 239 The Stock Market/ML Sinibaldi; 240 The Image Bank/Weinberg/Clark; 241 George Brooks; 242 George Brooks; 243 Francesca Yorke; 244 Marlene Wallace; 245 Hulton Getty